SO-BAM-567

ADVANCES IN LIBRARY ADMINISTRATION AND ORGANIZATION

ADVANCES IN LIBRARY ADMINISTRATION AND ORGANIZATION

Series Editors: Edward D. Garten,
Delmus E. Williams and
James M. Nyce

ADVANCES IN LIBRARY ADMINISTRATION AND
ORGANIZATION   VOLUME 23

ADVANCES IN LIBRARY ADMINISTRATION AND ORGANIZATION

EDITED BY

EDWARD D. GARTEN

University of Dayton Libraries, Ohio, USA

DELMUS E. WILLIAMS

University of Akron Libraries, Ohio, USA

JAMES M. NYCE

*School of Library and Information Management,
Emporia State University, Kansas, USA*

ELSEVIER
JAI

Amsterdam – Boston – Heidelberg – London – New York – Oxford
Paris – San Diego – San Francisco – Singapore – Sydney – Tokyo

JAI Press is an imprint of Elsevier

JAI Press is an imprint of Elsevier
The Boulevard, Langford Lane, Kidlington, Oxford OX5 1GB, UK
Radarweg 29, PO Box 211, 1000 AE Amsterdam, The Netherlands
525 B Street, Suite 1900, San Diego, CA 92101-4495, USA

First edition 2006

Notice
No responsibility is assumed by the publisher for any injury and/or damage to persons
or property as a matter of products liability, negligence or otherwise, or from any use
or operation of any methods, products, instructions or ideas contained in the material
herein. Because of rapid advances in the medical sciences, in particular, independent
verification of diagnoses and drug dosages should be made

British Library Cataloguing in Publication Data
A catalogue record for this book is available from the British Library

ISBN-13: 978-0-7623-1297-9
ISBN-10: 0-7623-1297-1
ISSN: 0732-0671 (Series)

For information on all JAI Press publications
visit our website at books.elsevier.com

Printed and bound in the Netherlands

06 07 08 09 10 10 9 8 7 6 5 4 3 2 1

Working together to grow
libraries in developing countries
www.elsevier.com | www.bookaid.org | www.sabre.org

ELSEVIER   BOOK AID International   Sabre Foundation

CONTENTS

LIST OF CONTRIBUTORS

Michael Carpenter	Louisiana State University, LA, USA
Linda K. Colding	University of Central Florida, FL, USA
Janine Golden	State Library and Archives of Florida, FL, USA
Jeff Luzius	Gadsden State Community College, AL, USA
Betsy Van der Veer Martens	University of Oklahoma, Tulsa, OK, USA
Jean Mulhern	S. Arthur Watson Library, Wilmington College, OH, USA
James M. Nyce	School of Library and Information Management, Emporia State University, KS, USA
Joan Stenson	Loughborough University, Leicestershire, UK
James H. Walther	Greenberg, Traurig, LLP, NY, USA
Robert C. Ward	Louisiana State University, LA, USA
Larry Nash White	East Carolina University, NC, USA

INTRODUCTION

The introduction to Volume 22 of this series is situated with reference to science, commonsense and the role each has or should have in the work we do as Library and Information Science (LIS) professionals. What we have this year is a series of papers that reports research results from work done mostly in public and academic libraries. It seems that the research done in one domain can have much to say about the other. This is not to say that there are no differences between these two types of libraries, nor is it to say that these differences cannot at times be significant. However, it seems clear that many of the institutional aspects and the challenges that they both face today transcend the boundaries that we usually think mark these two type of institutions off from one another.

Marten's paper uses the work that bibliometric researchers have published to raise questions about what in the LIS community is considered to be truthful and useful when it comes to organizational theory. She uses innovation theory and a communications model to track how LIS practitioners (and others) acquire the organizational theories that informs the work they do. From her data, Marten then raises questions about theory, practice and the relationships they have to each other in the LIS community.

Mulhern's paper is a counterpoint to Marten's. While Mulhern's paper covers some of the same ground as Marten's, she uses autobiography to discuss the issues of knowledge and practice and the appropriate relationship between them. Mulhern, the director of a small academic library for 20 years, uses her return to graduate school as an occasion to reflect on how various readings of what theory and practice emerges from (and informs) every day professional life.

The papers we publish here on academic libraries have much to say to those working in the public library community. The reverse, we believe, is also true. For example, what White has to say in this volume about performance assessment in public libraries has salience for those who work in academic institutions. White looks at how performance has been measured in Florida's public libraries. He is particularly interested in the impact performance measurement efforts have had on these institutions, a topic which so far has not received a great deal of attention. However, performance was assessed, White's data suggest that the use of performance measurement has had little perceived positive impact on this state's public libraries and the services they provide. This may in part be because of how performance in these public libraries is defined, assessed and measured (one library administrative unit used 11 different types of performance indicators). However, White's findings suggest that we may need to rethink what we mean by performance and to revisit how we assess performance in public as well as academic libraries.

Ward and Carpenter take an issue up in their paper that again has relevance to both academic and public libraries. This is outsourcing, a policy that the authors trace back to the 1970/1980s New Public Management (NPM) movement. In eight US cases (only seven are discussed here) where the management of a public library has been outsourced, Ward and Carpenter look to see whether outsourcing has increased services or decreased public accountability. What they found depended very much on how one defines service, accountability and success – terms like performance are contested and not readily susceptible to cost/benefit analysis however refined. In the seven cases studied, accountability – at least legal accountability – seems to have increased. Having said that, the authors also found that stakeholder satisfaction and resource use declined in all the cases. Ward and Carpenter point out that this raises questions for those who advocate outsourcing of any kind – questions to which the LIS community has received few authoritative answers.

Golden looks at middle management and career development strategies in public libraries. She identifies a variety of strategies middle managers could employ given a number of external and internal (within the organization) factors. Golden discusses how these various strategies and factors contribute to middle management career success. She surveyed a sample of public library directors – those in cities and towns of more than 100,000. Of these 390, 215 (55%) responded. Golden reports on the strategies directors themselves used. She also ranked the importance these strategies had in the directors' own career development. Of various strategies, mentoring was reported by 61.1% respondents. But only 8.5% of the directors rated this strategy positively, and just a few respondents (4.6) recommended it. This raises a question about whether we are equipping middle managers with the "right" resources to advance. This question takes on additional importance today when flattening hierarchy (i.e. the disposal and dispersal of middle managers) has become a legitimate, if not the only legitimate, means to reorganize libraries, whether they be public or academic.

Luzius also looks at careers and career choices but this time in academic libraries. Luzius used an internet-based instrument to survey a sample ($n = 1,054$) of librarians who were employed at Association of Research Libraries (ARL) institutions or belonged to the Association of College & Research Libraries. Luzius found that his respondents chose the career they had because it was perceived as one where you help people, can do research, use new technologies and enjoy the benefits of working at a university. From the data he collected, Luzius gives us some recommendations re: recruitment of the next generation of academic librarians.

Colding also discusses recruitment and retention in academic libraries. The paper looks at the issue of turnover in particular. Building on previous work, Colding surveyed online 300 librarians who work at public universities. Multiple regression analysis led to the following conclusions. There are a number of factors, concerning job leaving among academic librarians that appear to be unique. These have been masked in previous research on turnover in professional careers. Colding adds that knowing what indicators "predict" turnover can help library and university administrators retain staff. To keep staff, Colding advises administrators to promote job and work (task) satisfaction.

Golden, Luzius and Colding have all reported on personnel issues that are important to the profession. While the three papers differ from each other in problem domain, scale, methodology and theory, all three address issues that should interest anyone who works or manages a library, whether it be a public or academic library. Walther adds to the mixture by bringing together clients and consumers of library services. The strength of Walther's paper is that he investigates how collection policy, especially cancellation policy, is perceived by both staff and consumers. While the population, collection development librarians and science faculty at one university, is small ($n = 38$), Walther uses multiple data collection techniques to validate his results. This gives Walther's finding more salience than what his sample size might otherwise suggest. From his data, Walther provides a model for joint decision making regarding library resources that should interest those who manage public and academic library collections.

Stenson takes us away from the library community. She interviewed and surveyed 45 senior managers at four public/private organizations in the United Kingdom. Senior management identified which information assets were critical to their businesses, the role information assets played in various divisions of their firms and how information technology supported or did not support information delivery and use. These managers believe that intangible assets (knowledge/information) are critical if their firms are to be efficient, competitive and to deliver value to their customers. Having said that, Stenson's research did not find a direct push-pull relation between the good management of information asset and an organization's marketplace performance. This raises several questions, long of interest to the LIS community, regarding information "quality" and how it can be assessed, measured and delivered.

One of the enlightenment's central tenant is that reason, not belief, is a superior guide to action. To put it another way, when we have a choice between what science tells us and "common sense," science should prevail. Golden found that informants often relied on strategies to advance their careers that her research suggests had little positive benefit. In short, Golden's research and its assessment of various career strategies may be more useful to job candidates than their own and others' commonsense, knowledge and beliefs. It would be harder to find a better example where "science" is not only "stronger" analytically but also more useful in a pragmatic sense.

The ends of "science" and the "profession": would be well served if we looked more closely at what in both the academic and public libraries communities is regarded as common sense. The skepticism the LIS community has regarding science and research, it could be argued, might be assuaged if more work of this kind was carried out and if the findings of that research were more broadly disseminated.

If I may speak for all three editors, I would like to thank the authors for the contributions they have made to this volume and, to E for its support of ALAO. I would also like to thank the readers of ALAO for the comments and suggestions they have sent us and ALAO authors.

James M. Nyce
Co-editor

THEORIES IN PRACTICE: THEORY FUNCTIONS AND DIFFUSION OF INNOVATION

Betsy Van der Veer Martens

INTRODUCTION

The study of the diffusion of innovations into libraries has become a cottage industry of sorts, as libraries have always provided a fascinating test-bed of nonprofit institutions attempting improvement through the use of new policies, practices, and assorted apparatus (Malinconico, 1997). For example, Paul Sturges (1996) has focused on the evolution of public library services over the course of 70 years across England, while Verna Pungitore (1995) presented the development of standardization of library planning policies in contemporary America. For the past several decades, however, the study of diffusion in libraries has tended to focus on the implementation of information technologies (e.g., Clayton, 1997; Tran, 2005; White, 2001) and their associated competencies (e.g., Marshall, 1990; Wildemuth, 1992), the improvements in performance associated with their use (e.g., Damanpour, 1985, 1988; Damanpour & Evan, 1984), and ways to manage resistance to technological changes within the library environment (e.g., Weiner, 2003).

Research into the importance of ideas and their effectiveness as they diffuse in the library and information environment has been a more problematic field of endeavor because, although innovation in the form of

Advances in Library Administration and Organization, Volume 23, 1–57
Copyright © 2006 by Elsevier Ltd.
ISSN: 0732-0671/doi:10.1016/S0732-0671(05)23001-8

discrete items of information has long been a topic of interest (e.g., Chatman, 1986), the diffusion of ideas themselves is clearly much harder to study. Day's (2002) exemplary work on the diffusion of the "most influential" ideas in the library literature is indicative of the difficulty of tracing the influence of particular theories, both LIS (Library and Information Science)-oriented and more generally managerial, through the interlocking arenas of scholarship and practice. Recently, however, interest in the problem has grown substantially, as it has been noted that libraries represent one of the few remaining bastions of the so-called "public sphere" in which a democratic discourse about ideas can take place: "libraries as democratic public spheres, holding out the possibility of communicative reason, truth verification, rational argumentation, and the providing of alternatives and alternative public spaces" (Buschman, 2003, p. 179).

This interest has taken even more concrete form in the health sciences librarianship field, as an outgrowth of the practice of what is termed "evidence-based" medicine, which was originated by the late Archie L. Cochrane (1972) and popularized by Jonathan Eldredge (2000, 2002) in the United States, and Andrew Booth (Booth, 2003; Booth & Brice, 2004a, b) in the United Kingdom. Its utility for the library field, moreover, has been strengthened by the application of "evidence-based" evaluation techniques to other areas of the social sciences, a revival of the "experimenting society" movement that was originally proposed by the late Donald T. Campbell in his celebrated "Reforms as Experiments" (Campbell, 1969b), and has been more recently promulgated by the organization of the Campbell Collaboration (Boruch et al., 2004). "Evidence-based" practice advocates the utilization of "the best available evidence, moderated by user needs and preferences,...applied to improve the quality of professional judgment" (Booth & Brice, 2004b, p. 7), which is ideally held to be the meta-analysis of results from randomized clinical trial and field experiments wherever possible. The evidence-based movement tends to focus on the results of innovative practices that are the outgrowth of theory rather than on the theories themselves. However, without theories, evidence itself is largely uninterpretable. Both theories and evidence are a part of the larger research culture, which Donald Campbell (1969a) famously termed the "fish-scale model of omniscience."

This chapter, therefore, offers a different perspective both on the diffusion of ideas as innovations and the nature of evidence as shown by theories, based on empirical work on the functional characteristics of theories that may promote their diffusion into communities of scholarship and communities of practice.

THE DIFFUSION OF INNOVATIONS

Everett Rogers, the doyen of diffusion studies, once wrote that, "It should not be assumed, as it has sometimes been in the past, that all innovations are equivalent units of analysis" (Rogers, 1995a, p. 15). The most important forms of innovation, arguably, are ideas in general and theories in particular, as the diffusion of theory is indispensable to the construction of knowledge of any kind. Indeed, it has been suggested that "theorization" of an innovation (Strang & Meyer, 1993) promotes its diffusion. Like technologies, which have been shown to have "trajectories" over time and space (Dosi, 1982), theories too appear to have "cognitive trajectories" (Bucchi, 1998). Do theories have shared characteristics that may help to determine the course of these trajectories? Do these characteristics and trajectories differ from those of other innovations?

Although scientific ideas were one of the first examples discussed in early treatments of innovations and their attributes (Fliegel & Kivlin, 1966; Katz, Levin, & Hamilton, 1963), there have been relatively few investigations of the diffusion of ideas in comparison with research on the diffusion of more material innovations. These exemplary works on theory diffusion include studies from science (Oreskes, 1999) and social science (Cole, 1975), law (Posner, 1990) and literature (Lamont, 1987), mathematics (Carley, 1990) and medicine (Fennell & Warnecke, 1988). None of these, however, examined the attributes of the theories themselves as part of the problem. This is somewhat puzzling, as research on both technological and political ideas have often focused on theory attributes. Studies of technical ideas as innovations now indicate that their key attributes differ markedly from those that influence the diffusion of other innovations (e.g., Dearing & Meyer, 1994; Gatignon, Tushman, Smith, & Anderson, 2002), and studies of policy ideas as innovations indicate that their sociopolitical aspects are critical diffusion drivers (e.g., Hays, 1996a, b). Research on the essential elements of scientific or scholarly theories, however, has not similarly advanced beyond the acceptance of Rogers's early typology of innovation attributes in Crane's classic study (1972) of the diffusion of scientific ideas within "invisible colleges." Even such sophisticated advances as "constructuralism," a unified theory of the communicative interaction cycle, including simulation of the diffusion process, neglects theory attributes as part of the model of "engineered reach" (Kaufer & Carley, 1993).

On the other hand, while philosophers have found the characteristics of theories to be of great importance, the attributes that interest them tend to be more prescriptive than descriptive, and the subsequent diffusion of theories is of only minor interest. For example, Kuhn (1972) offered "accuracy, consistency, simplicity and fruitfulness" as the "shared basis for theory choice" in science, while Popper suggested "autonomy": the extent to which a theory takes on a life of its own, with previously invisible consequences (Popper & Eccles, 1981). Nozick (1981) proposed that an ideal theory should be egalitarian (encompassing all possibilities), fecund (privileging no possibility a priori), self-subsumptive (capable of explaining itself as part of the phenomena), and ultimate (permitting no deeper explanatory regress). Longino (1990) has urged the importance of "novelty," "ontological heterogeneity," and "mutuality of interaction."

James McAllister (1996) found that certain aesthetic characteristics appeared significant in the initial acceptance of the "grand" theories he analyzed, such as Einstein's theory of relativity, but more mundane theories are difficult to compare on the basis of such largely aesthetic criteria. These more mundane theories, however, clearly make up the majority of theories in use, so the diffusion of mundane theories may in fact be more informative than that of grander theories.

The question of why the work of theories has not been of more general interest as a topic of investigation, especially since the dawn of the so-called "knowledge society" is of particular interest in itself, especially given the emergence of the "new" sociology of knowledge with its emphasis on the constitution of systems of knowledge rather than Mannheim's classic individualist and ideological orientation (Swidler & Arditi, 1994). According to philosopher David Hull (1975), the primary reason appears to be methodological. Ideas lack those spatio-temporal properties that would allow them to be easily treated as "central subjects" (that is, historical entities functioning as the core of a historical narrative). More often than not, ideas change as they are communicated, so their intellectual histories generally end up either decontextualized from the actual communities that espoused the ideas or disarticulated from the competing or complementary ideas that preceded and followed them.

In addition to the difficulties involved in studying ideas themselves, a related problem appears to be the inherent complexity of studying the communication process itself, which has been termed "the cognitive dynamics" of knowledge production and/or knowledge application as exemplified within any particular knowledge system (Dunn & Holzner, 1988, p. 17). At present, citation analytic techniques remain the primary method of studying knowledge systems and their dynamics. The diffusion of theories has been one of several strands in citation analysis research from the beginning (e.g., Mullins, 1973), although in recent years the emphasis has been largely on investigating the "invisible college" networks of theorists (e.g., White, Wellman, & Nazer, 2004) and their use of rhetoric in academic attribution (e.g., Hyland, 1999) rather than any attributes of the theories themselves. The work of theories in categorizing and conceptualizing the possibilities of meaningful causation, correlation, and covariation in a modern social world rife with potential connections is, as Steve Fuller has termed it, the context of "hot pursuit" (Fuller, 1988, p. 65). This context, therefore, includes both non-systematic theories (generally lumped together as "lay epistemics" or "folk wisdom") and systematic theories such as those in science, philosophy, mathematics, and law. The primary difference between systematic and non-systematic theories is, of course, their status as knowledge systems (Curry, 1984). The troublesome, transparent question of power relations both within knowledge systems and between knowledge systems has only recently become of interest to researchers (Watson-Verran & Turnbull, 1995).

THEORIES AND TRUTH

All theories, however, purport to represent some system of reality, whether ideal or empirical and, thus, their truth-valence is of considerable moment. As Lin (2001)points out in his comparative study of the concept of certainty in different cultures at different historical time periods, "It is intersubjective validity that forms the basis of social norms, collective consensus, and the order of social interaction. ...People are compelled to accept intersubjective validity as the universal criterion by which our knowledge system, moral code, and social regulation are organized or arranged. ...[T]he cognitive and social dimensions of intersubjective validity are inseparable; both are conjoined in an identical process of the social formation of knowledge-based human activities in which the cognitive and social order are intermingled" (pp. 26–27).

The nature of these systems in terms of "truth" and their justification of beliefs as "true" have formed the central question of ontology in Western philosophy since the time of Plato, and is as yet decidedly undecided. While there are a number of rather recondite systems of ontological categorization, this discussion will focus on several established and emerging theories of truth: correspondence, coherence, consensus, and, most recently, several attempts at synthesizing aspects of all the three.

The "correspondence theory of truth" (or "foundationalism") is founded on the idea that there is a unilinear connection between empirical reality, any "basic" belief, which acquires epistemic priority through being grounded in that empirical reality, and that basic belief's justification of any other non-empirically based belief. The strength of this system is inherent in the basic belief's purported congruence with a certain state of affairs, presumably that of reality, rather than in any connections among the beliefs themselves. This classic foundationalism, in which the basic beliefs are taken as infallible and incorrigible, has been the topic of much philosophical debate since the time of Descartes, especially in regard to the "regress" problem, in which there appears to be no way that the holder of "basic" beliefs can justify holding them without reference to additional beliefs about the nature of truth (Sosa, 1991, p. 173).

The coherence theory of truth relates to the strength with which the system's theoretical propositions are mutually supportive, as epistemic priority is not granted to any particular empirically grounded "basic" belief but rather justifies itself in the network of beliefs as a whole. This coherence implies a relationship among propositions or beliefs that is "more strict than logical consistency, yet less strict than logical entailment" (Kress, 1984, pp. 369–370). There are various versions of "the" coherence theory (e.g., BonJour, 1985), but the major weaknesses they all appear to share are that case histories in psychology offer numerous examples of belief systems that are complete, consistent, and quite delusional (Tolliver, 1989), and that case histories of science offer numerous instances of anomalies that succeeded in overturning well-established belief systems (Bogen, 1989).

However, the coherence theory of truth has been extremely influential in developing normative theories in areas such as law. Even though there is clearly a distinction to be drawn between the epistemic coherence of an individual's beliefs and the constitutive coherence of a set of legal doctrines (Raz, 1992), the thinking "legal subject" must be able to rationally reconstruct these particular doctrines and their interconnections in order to achieve legal understanding (Balkin, 1993). Without this form of coherence, law would be a formless collection of norms from which judges could select at will (Edmundson, 1996).

There have also been recent efforts to advance various forms of a so-called "consensus theory of truth" (e.g., Lehrer & Wagner, 1981), often based on assessments of probability assigned by observers. This type of approach, no matter how statistically sophisticated, cannot be logically supported, as it is certainly conceivable that a particular truth exists regardless of whether anyone at all believes it or that a particular widely and stably believed truth may in fact be quite false. Further, "consensus" itself is problematic, since it begs the question of the identity of the group whose unanimity is accepted as definitive of agreement (Graham, 1984, p. 91).

Various attempts at a new synthesis of coherence, correspondence, and consensus theories are also underway. For example, Nicholas Rescher (1993) suggests a pragmatic approach that advocates "evaluative pluralism," in which he subordinates the unattainable ideal of "cognitive consensus" to the importance of the individual quest for truth and the concomitant importance of a community that recognizes the value of such quests and evaluates their cumulative contributions. Susan Haack (1993) offers an integration of correspondence and coherence theories that she terms "foundaherentism." Her work incorporates the insights from coherentism that there are no indubitable truths and that beliefs are justified by the extent to which they fit with other beliefs, and from empiricist foundationalism the insights that not all beliefs make an equal contribution to the structure of justification, while sense experience deserves a special though not completely privileged role. "Foundaherentism" therefore allows empirical evidence additional weight in her coherence network, but does not make it foundational. The work of Miriam Solomon (2001) on the varying importance of different "decision vectors," with empirical success providing the presumably least subjective but not the sole criterion for theory choice, contributes what she terms "social empiricism" to this tradition.

And, finally, James Blachowicz (1998) proposes what he calls "reciprocal justification," by developing a "logic of correction" by which observation and theory justify each other reciprocally and repeatedly until, as he says, knowledge represents experience and those representations are well-formed. This approach too is an attempt to combine the strengths of the major epistemological traditions.

Although the structure of justification (Audi, 1993) is obviously still under construction, theories of truth within contemporary Western society can be considered to be more or less "commodified." While classification systems explicitly facilitate the origination and organization of ideas and theories (Kwasnik, 1999), citation systems implicitly facilitate their association and recombination. The next section will consider citation systems in various epistemic communities, how they have been studied, and what they may reveal about the individual theories of which they are comprised. While both classification and citation practices define what is accepted as "reliable knowledge" within particular social worlds, the citation itself also plays a symbolic role as "boundary object" in intersecting social worlds with disparate epistemic standards. The next section discusses specifics of this modern "commodification of justification."

THE COMMODIFICATION OF JUSTIFICATION

In an earlier publication (Martens, 2001), I suggested that citation systems represent "commodified" theories of truth, and that the citation functions as a so-called "boundary object" (Star & Griesemer, 1989) that can be used to define those ways in which the epistemic communities of science, law, and technology represent their disparate theories of truth. This, of course, was much too simple, and the following is intended to explore the issue in more detail.

While theories of truth play indispensable explanatory roles in any culture, their modern commodification in the United States into separate citation systems offers important insights into today's taken-for-granted solutions of the problem of reliable knowledge representation. Although there has been much argument of late regarding the role of citations, the journal system, and the efficacy of peer review (Weller, 2001), all three remain central to what most observers consider the most currently reliable approach to assuring the overall quality of research. Science, as the dominant claimant to "reliable knowledge," has of course attracted the most research interest, while law and technology have only recently begun to be studied in depth. However, it is not widely known that postmodern philosophy too, an important epistemic community, can be analyzed by its citing practices. The research perspectives taken by scholars in each of these areas of inquiry can themselves be considered as parts of the problem, and the following sections offer a comparative analysis of the macrodynamics of belief (Hernnstein-Smith, 1997). Based on recent developments in epistemological theory and advances in domain visualization, citation systems should rather be considered as evolving maps of the macrodynamics of belief: visible surrogates for the underlying social structure of justification.

Citation systems all reify "reliable knowledge" or "truth" in a similar way: through the intricate connections of particular ideas accepted as legitimate within a social world. A scandalously different approach, which has its origins in postmodern philosophy, is that of deconstruction, which is best known, if not notorious, from the writings of Jacques Derrida. Derrida treats philosophical writings not as statements of positions but as texts, and uses the notion of truth as what is validated by accepted methods of validation to criticize what passes for truth (Hartman, 1981, p. 4). Deconstruction centers around the paradox that truth is both what can be demonstrated within an accepted framework and what simply is the case, whether or not anyone might believe it or validate it. Rather than developing a new philosophical framework or solution, however, deconstruction works in and around philosophical discourse, seeking to produce reversals and displacements in order to yield truth from those very contradictions at the margins (Cullen, 1982, pp. 151–155). This too can be considered a theory of truth, but one that owes its existence to a continuous interrogation of what is accepted as credible and, more importantly, as the incredible that seemingly defines, differentiates, and defers to it.

CITATIONS AS BOUNDARY OBJECTS

The critical importance of legitimation processes in rapidly changing social worlds such as law, science, and technology has been well established (Gerson, 1983; Strauss, 1982). Star and Griesemer's exemplary study of ordering and legitimation of scientific work within a complex institutional setting introduced a taxonomy of "boundary objects" consisting of abstract or concrete objects which are plastic enough to adapt to local informational needs, yet robust enough to maintain a common identity in several intersecting social worlds (Star & Griesemer, 1989). This taxonomy includes standardized forms "...devised as methods of common communication across dispersed work groups" (Star & Griesemer, 1989, p. 441). These standard forms clearly consist of what Michael Buckland (1991) has termed "information as thing," facilitating "the representation of evidence," especially in cases where the situational relevance of the information is yet to be determined (p. 358). "Information as thing," therefore, is an ideal type of the boundary object and is mundanely manifested in the citation as concept symbol (Small, 1978).

"Boundary objects...have different meanings in different social worlds but their structure is common enough to make them recognizable, a means of translation" (Bucchi, 1998, p. 30). In the case of the citation as a boundary object, this translation is enabled by a particular type of "concept symbol": the symbolic reference to an idea previously (and, presumably, authoritatively) communicated in a specified form. The origin of this type of concept symbol is unknown, but the anthropological significance of so-called "standard symbols" predates the invention of any form of writing (Leach, 1976). The use of the concept symbol in its modern sense (a written reference citing a previous writing as warrant) in religion and in law preceded its use in other forms of scholarship, as Talmudic scholars pioneered what might be termed the explicit or postdictive use of the citation (Weinberg, 1997, p. 328).

This postdictive use of citations became an integral part of both legal practice in the form of case law precedents (Ogden, 1993) and historiographic practices in the form of footnotes (Grafton, 1999) as early as the sixteenth century. Similarly, this postdictive use was the first to appear in scientific publications during the seventeenth century, as members of the Royal Society collected their correspondence as the Society's Transactions (Shapin, 1994). The performance of experiments and their replication was facilitated by explicit reference to the work of others as the scientific article took its modern form (Bazerman, 1988). Finally, patents and their citations became established during the eighteenth century as a hybrid of descriptive and proscriptive invocations of previous inventions, influenced by both scientific and legal considerations (MacLeod, 1991).

The citation as concept symbol can be considered on three levels: the micro, meso, and macro; each level translating into a different view of the relevant theory of truth. At the micro-level, the citation is used by individuals to identify past ideas or innovations that have been previously accepted as legitimate. At the middle range, citation clusters are used to identify a group's current view of reliable knowledge. At the macro-level, the entire structure of a citation system can be used to identify knowledge processes. The next sections explore these levels for science, law, technology, and philosophy, as shown in Fig. 1.

Micro-Level Citation

The micro-level usage of citation as concept symbol centers on the legitimization of ideas through positioning them in relation to the past knowledge of a particular group. Indices to such postdictive citations are primarily useful for group members in determining the location of previously legitimated concepts, as is apparent in such specialized uses as that of rabbinical scholars of the *En misphat* embedded in the Talmud. However, even at the micro-level, the "theories of truth" embodied as the nomological nets of science, law, technology, and philosophy begin to evidence themselves.

Difficulties encountered by students of the so-called "citation behavior" in science suggest that it can only be grossly described by such constructs as "citation norms" (Kaplan, 1965), but in general it does seem to "promote some degree of legitimacy and authority to the citing author through association with the cited work" (Case & Higgins, 2000, p. 643). Since there are clearly rhetorical aspects to the use of citations in scholarly writing (Cozzens, 1989), it should be noted that the intended audience considers citations as merely another form of internal evidence to be considered in conjunction with external evidence for the author's proposed addition to the corpus of knowledge about the nature of reality. Robert Connors (1998,

KNOWLEDGE DOMAIN	LEVEL OF ANALYSIS	UNIT OF ANALYSIS	USE OF ANALYSIS	PURPOSE OF ANALYSIS	THEORY OF TRUTH
SCIENCE	Micro	Individual Papers	Postdictive	Information Retrieval	CORRESPONDENCE
	Meso (Microscopic)	Invisible College	Present Indicative	Sociology of Science	
	(Telescopic)	Research Fronts	Present Indicative	Citation Analysis/ Domain Visualization	
	Macro	Map of Science	Predictive	Scientometrics	
LAW	Micro	Individual Decisions	Postdictive	Legal Research	COHERENCE
	Meso: (Precedents)	Courts, Judges	Present Indicative	Political Science	
	(Legal citations)	Legal Scholars	Present Indicative	Citation Analysis/ Legal Studies	
	Macro	Body of Law	Predictive	Social Science	
TECHNOLOGY	Micro	Individual Patents	Postdictive	Patent Research	CONSENSUS
	Meso: (Stock)	Intellectual Capital	Present Indicative	Investment Research	
	(Flow)	Knowledge Dispersion	Present Indicative	Policy Analysis	
	Macro	Patent Systems	Predictive	Information Economics	
POSTMODERN PHILOSOPHY	Micro	Individual Texts	Postdictive	Textual Interpretation	DECONSTRUCTION
	Meso:	Science as Text	Present Indicative	Social Studies of Science	
		Law as Text	Present Indicative	Legal Criticism	
		Technology as Text	Present Indicative	Social Studies of Technology	
	Macro	???	???	???	

Fig. 1. Citation Systems as Theories of Truth.

1999) has explored in detail the rhetorical ramifications of citation systems and their impact on specific epistemic communities of scholars beginning in the late nineteenth century and continuing into the present day.

Micro-level usage of citations in law is far more structured. Learning to select the most relevant citations (Dunn, 1993) and to place explicit introductory signals that serve specific semiotic purposes in indicating the role of the indicated reference (Robbins, 1999) is central to legal education. It would be considered as bizarre for a lawyer not to carefully choose and use her citations based solely on the authority of published precedents, as it would be for a scientist to do so. Thus, the coherence theory of truth is embodied within the corpus of common law.

Citation in technology takes a middle ground, as both inventors and law-yers are involved in patent strategy (e.g., Myers, 1995). The scientist or lawyer, therefore, making patent claims must be especially careful in their "transla-tion" of citations across these boundaries (Packer & Webster, 1995, 1996). Generally, patent citation focuses on the recognition of "prior art" and a defensible "engineering around" of those aspects of an existing innovation that have been currently conceded protection by the patent system (Rivette & Kline, 2000). Patents are also unique as texts in that their citations can be arbitrarily enlarged or excised during the patent examination process: the front page of an approved patent reflects a final consensus regarding the legitimacy of an innovation in reference to the claims of existing patents (Meyer, 2000).

Within postmodern philosophy, the deconstruction of citations at the micro-level is text-based, and based on a more extensive level of quotation than is seen in the other instances, as the intent is to give such a close reading that "traces" of all influences, acknowledged and otherwise, become ap-parent, leading some to speak of "echoing" and "ghost citations" as part of this practice (Wolfreys, 2002). Like other citation approaches, the intent is to identify the ideas that are considered "legitimate." In deconstruction, however, the stated goal is to problematize that very legitimacy and explore its submerged aspects. Derrida's own works, such as *Glas*, thematize the problematic of quotation by confronting two texts in parallel, in an attempt to take into account what is inevitably left out, excluded, and repressed by hermeneutic systems of interpretation (Sartiliot, 1993, p. 32).

Meso-Level Citation

The second primary usage of the citation as concept symbol is what might be termed the present indicative: that is, the use of relationships between various citations as a purported measure of influence. This presupposes an external group primarily interested in the connections between the citations of an internal group or groups. The term "invisible college" elegantly high-lights this particular distinction, as it would be used not by members of the group itself but rather by those attempting to study it (e.g., Crane, 1969). Similarly, while members of a specific "invisible college" might find a par-ticular citation index useful for practical information retrieval, especially as the group's body of knowledge grows, there would be little interest by members in the citations as presently indicative of the connections denoting their "invisible college" itself, as that information is already available through routine interactions which are only partially mapped through ci-tations, acknowledgements, and the other apparatus of scholarship.

The increase in this use of concept symbols at the middle range is clearly an outgrowth of the original purpose of citation indices (enhancing access to documents of various groups, particularly those not easily retrievable through standard monographic cataloging practices). The development of standardized disciplinary citation indices by such organizations as the Institute for Scientific Information (ISI) and West Group has both framed and facilitated the use of citations as measurements. This is emphasized by the fact that the study of such similar practices as footnoting is far from equally advanced (Hartley, 1999).

For example, the ISI indices include as original entries only those articles that are published in a selective list of peer-reviewed journals and their accompanying citations. Legal citators publish only judicial opinions from the relevant jurisdictions and those citations that they may contain. Patents and their accompanying citations are published only after a lengthy review process by the U.S. Patent & Trademark Office.

It is this process of reification that makes the citation such a potent concept symbol, focusing attention on authorial or institutional identity rather than any intrinsic qualities of the article itself. The widespread use of the "Harvard system" of citation (as used throughout the present chapter, for example) supports the utility of Science Citation Index practices in listing references and consequently the use of the citation as "a pointer, a symbol of value or authority within a larger system" (Curry, 1997, p. 100).

Meso-level concept symbols as measurements include the citation of a previous paper by another, or "direct citation" (Garfield, 1955), the citation of a previous paper by two others, or "bibliographic coupling" (Kessler, 1963), the citation of two previous papers by a third, or "co-citation" (Small, 1973), and various other forms of "multiple citation" (Small, 1974). These relationships, which originally obtained among documents rather than their authors, were also extended to authors through the development of the technique of "author co-citation analysis" (White & Griffith, 1981, 1982). ACA has led to a variety of techniques for mapping the "intellectual space" of individual disciplines (McCain, 1990).

Small aptly dubbed co-citation clusters "consensual networks of concepts" (Small, 1985, p. 85). However, the study of these meso-level concept symbols has been controversial from the beginning. The external group by definition lacks complete access to the meanings of the concept symbols as used by the members of the internal groups who produce them. While some citation analyses are done by members of disciplines themselves as a way of understanding their fields, as only a few, in Cohn's monograph on criminological research, the bulk of the citation analysis has been performed by members of that emergent "citation community" to examine and evaluate these new techniques (Cohn, Farrington, & Wright, 1998).

Critics of citation analysis, the term by which the practice of this type of meso-level concept symbolism is known, have pointed to possible purely rhetorical functions of individual citations in their particular context (Gilbert, 1977), objected to the use of scattered and separate information patterns as surrogates for actual scientific communication (Edge, 1979), listed various sources of potential random and systemic error in citation data sets (MacRoberts & MacRoberts, 1989), and lamented both the disregard of the possible propagation of scientists' individual interests through citation practices (Luukonen, 1997) and the general inattentiveness to differences observable through deconstructing both information-theoretic and sociological interpretations of citation (Leydesdorff, 1998). Defenders of citation analytic techniques, however, maintain that empirical analysis of specific citation networks result in findings very similar to those obtained by more direct research approaches to members of the invisible colleges involved (Baldi, 1998).

The citation community plays a key role in the library and information science field, as citation analysis is perhaps the only disciplinary method that has been widely "exported" for use by other disciplines (Cronin & Pearson, 1990). Meso-level citation studies of the sciences and social sciences usually draw on the database resources of the Institute for Scientific Information and fall into two major categories, which might be termed the "microscopic" and the "telescopic."

The microscopic category focuses on those fields closely associated with the researcher's own, such as communication (e.g., Paisley, 1990) or information science (e.g., Van Raan & Tijssen, 1993) or a combination of several of the above (Karki, 1996). Presumably, the intent in the selection of these particular fields is to furnish a validity check of citation findings through the researcher's own access to internal information about the subject field where matched case controls or comparable cohorts are not obtainable.

The telescopic category for research focuses on those fields that presumably promise clearly identifiable clusters of association in terms of "coherent groups" (McCain, 1990, p. 433), "rapidly developing literature" (Bierbaum & Brooks, 1995, p. 531), or "competing paradigms" (Chen, Paul, & O'Keefe, 2001, p. 6). Again, both the microscopic and telescopic approaches suggest a view of "the literature" that purports to reflect a larger reality.

Within the literature of law, the meso-level study of legal citations also bifurcates into two distinct fields of research interest, which might be termed the "visible college" and "invisible college" of law. The "visible college" is that of judges, who in the common law system, both author the judicial opinions that subsequently serve as legal precedents and cite earlier judicial precedents within those opinions. In contrast, the "invisible college" which produces citations as legal scholarship may include judges, but is a much broader community that also includes lawyers, law professors, law students, and scholars from other disciplines. Citations as legal scholarship include the entire so-called "hierarchy of authority" that governs legal citation (Neumann, 1990, pp. 129–131).

The highest rank of authorities within that hierarchy are those sources, such as the Constitution, statutes, and decisions of the highest court in the controlling jurisdiction, which are binding on courts below. Well below these precedents in the hierarchy are what are called primary persuasive authorities, which consist of relevant rulings from inferior or extra-jurisdictional courts, which can be further subdivided by such factors as the closeness of the facts of the cited case to the instant case. After primary persuasive authorities come secondary persuasive authorities, which include the restatements of law, scholarly treatises, and law review articles.

"Visible college" researchers are usually political scientists, while "invisible college" researchers are largely drawn from legal librarianship. One focus of both research fields, however, is on the reputation or subsequent influence of a particular piece of legal authorship. The best-known exemplars of this common focal point are studies of most-cited law review articles (e.g., Shapiro, 1985, 1996) and judicial opinions (e.g., Landes, Lessig, & Solimine, 1998; Posner, 1990).

While the citation of legal precedent is an inherently conservative practice, it can be either widely or narrowly construed, introducing an inevitable level of uncertainty into the process. For example, the "reliance interest" strongly linked with precedent (that is, that citizens come to rely on previous Court decisions to inform their own subsequent actions) played an important role in the 1992 decision by the Supreme Court not to overrule the central holding in Roe v. Wade (Banks, 1999, p. 239), even though that court is theoretically unconstrained by precedent. Similarly, the citation of persuasive authorities might be viewed as inherently progressive, but that is not necessarily the case. Citing the Federalist Papers in support of originalist interpretations of the Constitution is a conservative usage of persuasive authority that has become common only during the past half-century (Lupu, 1998).

Once a persuasive authority becomes embedded in a judicial opinion, whether directly cited or not, it has a much better chance of being transmitted through the corpus of legal citation and influencing future judicial interpretations and consequent societal interactions (Schauer & Wise, 2000). The right to privacy, which began as an article in the *Harvard Law Review* in 1890, is a celebrated example of this process (Robison, 1993, p. 26). In general, however, there appears to be extremely limited and lagging citation convergence between the two types of colleges (Merritt & Putnam, 1996).

Meso-studies of patent citations, like those of legal citations, are at an early stage and have been driven by the informetric insight that simple patent counts are less informative than their citation by subsequent patents in indicating innovation importance (Trajtenberg, 1990). This research area may be usefully divided into two related fields of interest which might, to borrow accounting terms, be labeled "intellectual capital" as "stock" and "flow" (Jaffe & Trajtenberg, 2002).

Researchers who view patent citations as measurements of a firm's or industry's intellectual inventory have focused on them with reference to financial performance (Deng, Lev, & Narin, 1999), technological portfolio (Thomas, 1999), and competitive position (Hicks, Breitzman, Olivastro, & Hamilton, 2001). Researchers who view patent citations as indicators of national or international "knowledge flow" are more likely to be concerned with patent policy implications (Jaffe, 2000), information diffusion or so-called "knowledge spill-over" (Jaffe, Trajtenberg, & Henderson, 1993) and the relationships of applied science to basic science (Tijssen, 2001). As in science and law, these related research interests have a common thread: in this case, the economic value of innovation as reflected by patents (Mazzoleni & Nelson, 1998).

Regardless of deconstruction's foundational claim not to have an approach that can be applied systematically or that, being applied, cannot be deconstructed in turn (McQuillan, 2001), it is clear that deconstructive citation can be considered at the meso-level, as there are recognized groups of theorists who have applied deconstruction to other areas, whose own foundational claims appear worthy of investigation for a variety of reasons. Interestingly and ironically, those areas appear to center around law, science, and technology, as leading representatives of the commodization of theories of truth in Western society (Fuchs & Ward, 1994).

Meso-level deconstructive citation analysis started in the 1970s in elite institutions such as Yale, Johns Hopkins, and Cornell. Originally confined to departments of literature, it quickly spread to other disciplines (Lamont, 1987). The Critical Legal Studies movement began at Yale, and its adherents have deconstructed a variety of legal icons, ranging from contract doctrine (Dalton, 1985) to constitutional rights (Tushnet, 1984). The use of legal precedents is central to this type of deconstruction (Balkin, 1998).

Science studies, another famously controversial arena, has also often used deconstructive techniques to examine such issues as the performance of experiments (Latour & Woolgar, 1986), the development of scientific taxonomies (Gross, 1990), and even the solving of equations in theoretical physics (Merz & Knorr-Cetina, 1997). As mentioned earlier, deconstruction of scientific citations too has recently become a focus of attention (Latour, 1987) as well as the deconstruction of technology itself, exemplified by the examination of patents as texts (Bowker, 1992) and texts as patents (Madison, 2003). All of these meso-level deconstructive practices are employed in "a work of resistance, a vigilant counter-interpretation" of what Derrida (1994) suggests actuality is always and already made: "artifactuality."

Macro-Level Citation

These empirical investigations of citation analysis lead to the third or macro-level of citations as concept symbol: the predictive. Probability distributions form the empirical underpinning of any informetric distribution (Egghe & Rousseau, 1990). At the macro-level, probability also provides the theoretical underpinnings for the study of the various metrics of science. For example, Price's (1965, 1970) seminal work on indicators of research fronts and disciplinary boundaries in networks of scientific papers is founded on comparative statistical analysis of previously substantiated research advances and hypothesizes a virtual structure of science that can be visually "mapped" (Small, 1999). Much work in scientometrics employs similar quantitative techniques in attempts to identify particularly important research endeavors (e.g., Ashton & Oppenheim, 1978; Garfield, 1990). The current "Holy Grail" in scientometrics is the development of indicator theories rather than citation theories (Wouters, 1999). Positivism's predilection for prediction as the necessary condition for scientific knowledge is clearly implicit in this perspective.

At this level, the corpus of literature becomes a body of objective, public knowledge which can itself be treated as an existent entity. Popper (1979) termed this "World 3": distinct from his so-called "World 1" of physical reality and "World 2" of individual subjective knowledge and experience. Indeed, both Herbert Simon's project of re-creating specific scientific discoveries through artificial intelligence algorithms (Langley, Simon, Bradshaw, & Zytkow, 1987) and Donald Swanson's project of discovering novel facts through improved information retrieval of previously published scientific literature (Swanson, 1986, 1987, 1989) appear to be contingent upon the existence of "World 3."

Law as a system is quite different. Without indeterminacy and the possibility of persuasion, legal doctrine would resemble religious doctrine far more closely than it does (Stone, 1993) while, without deontic logic and the stability of precedents, legal reasoning would resemble scientific reasoning far more closely than it does (Edwards, 1998). These practices enable the legal system to position its "limits of judicial creativity" (Traynor, 1977) between the axiological gaps produced by legal change and the normative gaps produced by social change. This judicial creativity and constraint, which Hart (1961) famously termed "the open texture of the law," provide the inner workings of law as a coherent system of truth, while its external workings serve to legitimize the social knowledge system.

Law as a knowledge system can also be viewed as two complementary models: the first is a case-processing model in which the law is used to resolve actual disputes, and the second is a law-articulation model in which the cases are used to enrich the existing supply of legal rules (Shuldberg, 1997, p. 548). Essential to the process is the physical manifestation of this knowledge system or what Berring calls "the legal publication universe" (Berring, 1994). He notes that this physical manifestation has decidedly impacted the law itself, demonstrated by Langdell's famous comment that "the library is the laboratory of the law," as legal information grew far beyond the working memory capacity of any individual jurist.

Macro-level analysis of the legal citation system has only become a possibility within the past decade and new ways of looking at precedents are still to be developed (Brenner, 1990). But the synthesis of earlier "visible college" studies, such as the so-called vertical precedents set by higher or controlling courts (e.g., Caminker 1994a, b), horizontal precedents set by the court itself at an earlier date or by other courts at the same level or from extra-jurisdictional courts (e.g., Kornhauser, 1995) and the unique functioning of rulings by the Supreme Court (e.g., Kelso & Kelso, 1996) or all of these at once (e.g., Talley, 1999), suggest that precedents are in fact often invoked. However, the standard "system" explanations of efficiency-maximization and error-minimization have so far failed to supply a more satisfactory explanation for their prevalence than political scientist Martin Shapiro's early conclusion that their use as expressed in the doctrine of *stare decisis* ("let the decision stand") simply signals redundancy in information transmission throughout the court system and that it is the disregard of precedent which signals novel information to which the system as a whole should attend (Shapiro, 1972).

This explanation reduces to an essentially content-free legal coherence system, since the details of the precedents in question, the thought processes of the individual judges involved, the specifics of the communication networks of the larger court system, and other environmental influences regarding the case or cases at hand are seldom factored into these analyses. What it does support, however, is the existence of an overarching legal "web of belief" that relies strongly on established precedents but that may also gradually change with the introduction of new information. Teubner says, "Law as a communicative network produces legal communications [that are] the cognitive instruments by which the law as social discourse is able to 'see' the world... There is no instruction of the law by the outside world; there is only construction of the outside world by the law" (Teubner, 1989, p. 740). Walsh's empirical study of "weak" and "strong" citations also supports the conjecture that the use of citations serves both to signal the flow of influence and ideas and to legitimate decisions in particularly problematic cases (Walsh, 1997).

Interestingly, the common if controversial claim that legal retrieval systems actually constrain legal reasoning by suggesting and supplying certain system-analytic categories (e.g., Berring, 1987, 1997) is the corollary of this critique. Thus, the separate fields of citation analysis of legal precedent and legal scholarship at the meso-level converge again with this possibility of unanticipated or unacknowledged changes in the legal web of belief that might be detected only at the macro-level.

One of the first findings at the macro-level indicates the informetric distribution of legal precedents represents a fractal structure (Post & Eisen, 2000). By definition, this fractal structure shows self-similarity at all levels created by a recursive branching process. This "crystalline structure of legal thought" (Balkin, 1986) implies that the postdictive and predictive functions of legal citation reinforce each other in a way in which the scientific citation system with its research frontiers does not. But, importantly, the influence of the larger "invisible college," however lagging and limited, cannot be totally discounted. In particular, Fred Shapiro contends that analysis of legal scholarship citation "can form the basis for generalizations about the nature of innovation in legal thought" (Shapiro, 1996, p. 778). Presumably, therefore, the "map of law," if it were to be attempted, would not show areas of predicted knowledge growth similar to that of Price's suggested mapping of science, but rather areas of particularly acute social contest. Another way of expressing this is that novel thought in science urges that earlier readings must be supplanted to achieve present accuracy: novel thought in law suggests that earlier rulings might be supplemented to increase future harmony.

Again, this supports the notion that the law resembles a coherent system of truth, entirely dissimilar to science as a correspondence system of truth. Within the legal world, legal citations signal to the initiate that substantive justice is being done; outside, they signal to the layman that procedural justice is being done. The ongoing concern over timely and appropriate publication of judicial opinions (Field, 1996), the controversies surrounding the so-called "depublication" (Kloppenberg, 1996), and the issues of copyright in their compilation (Tussey, 1998) are obvious indications of the importance of these boundaries to the legitimacy of the state.

Because patent citations function across the boundaries of both law and science, their use at the macro-level of analysis to explore the structure of innovation would necessarily have to take those linkages into account (Narin, Olivastro, & Stevens, 1994, p. 69). Possibly because of this complexity, evolutionary economists interested in studying the dynamics of technological change as the drivers of business cycles have generally chosen to use long-range aggregate patent counts rather than detailed networks of patent citations (e.g., Andersen, 1999).

However, one recent patent citation study at the macro-level has made the controversial claim that the present U.S. patent system makes no real attempt to determine patent novelty, that patent citations convey little usable information, and that the real value of technological innovation cannot accurately be ascertained through any rigorous analysis of the entirety of its patents and their interconnections (Aharonian, 2000). The study also suggests, the reason for these findings is that the Patent & Trademark Office unobtrusively manages the system to respond to the needs of the largest of what it calls its "customers": those 250 corporations that receive approximately half of all patents granted each year. Skillful use of patents in registration, negotiation, and litigation by these organizations add to the value of the patent system and to those who employ and are employed by it.

If Aharonian's speculations regarding the irregularities to be revealed in a potential patent citation macro-map are warranted, this would seem to suggest a consensus system at work. As Mandeville notes, "The patent system has always had the dual purpose of making information proprietary while still allowing some to spill over into the public domain. While these twin goals have conventionally been regarded as contradictory, they are consistent in an information-theoretic perspective" (Mandeville, 1996, p. 104). A macro-level analysis of the patent system through patent citation would, presumably, reveal those areas showing most contemporary consensus (if such a term can be applied to the cooperation, competition, coercion, and collusion inherent in all economic activities) regarding the potential economic value of various innovations.

A macro-level deconstructive analysis has yet to be undertaken of any specific field, such as law, science or technology, no doubt due to the difficulties posed by identifying and interpreting those very aspects of texts that are by definition not legitimate "concept symbols" of the specific epistemic community. Moreover, deconstruction's tenets mandate that such a macro-level deconstructive analysis would itself be subject to repeated deconstruction (Wolfreys, 1998, p. 53). A deconstructive macro-system, therefore, could not be predictive: it would continue to be recursive and relativistic in accordance with Derrida's theory of truth. It does, however, perform the essential "critical" function of highlighting how the other citation systems do in fact operate as commodified theories of truth within modern knowledge systems.

Citation systems, therefore, form the underpinnings of "reliable knowledge" today. The next section presents a comparative case study of the diffusion and non-diffusion of eight "ordinary" theories in several areas of the social sciences over the course of approximately a dozen years, and focuses on identifying the functionality of actual theory characteristics in facilitating particular "cognitive trajectories" as defined by citation histories within the citation system of science.

THE THEORIES

This study developed a typology of theory characteristics that was used in conjunction with the actual diffusion patterns of particular theories to create a model of theory functions. The units of analysis consisted of the eight individual theories shown in Fig. 2. The first cohort of theories attempts to explain at various levels of analysis the processes of internal exchange, while the second attempts to explain processes of external exchange. Possible antecedents and determinants of discretionary exchange behaviors as enacted by entire organizations, formal and informal groups within the organization, and individual employees form the subject matter of the first group of theories described below.

(1) "Institutional Isomorphism" grew out of sociological neo-institutionalism, which views organizations as evolving social constructs or rule systems rather than economic entities rationally engineered for maximum effectiveness. This theory suggested that organizations within a particular industry become increasingly similar over time due to normative, coercive, and mimetic forces within their immediate environment or "organizational field" (DiMaggio & Powell, 1983).

(2) "Leader–Member Exchange" was originally conceptualized as "Vertical Dyad Linkage," with roots in Chester Barnard's management classic

Theory Cohort 1: (Internal Exchange)	Theory Cohort 2: (External Exchange)
Institutional Isomorphism (DiMaggio and Powell, 1983) *citation count: 671*	Channel Retreat Hypothesis (English, 1985) *citation count: 0*
Leader-Member Exchange (Graen, Novak, and Sommerkamp, 1982) *citation count: 147*	Electronic Markets & Hierarchies (Malone, Yates, and Benjamin, 1987) *citation count: 143*
Organizational Citizenship Behavior (Smith, Organ, and Near, 1983) (Bateman and Organ, 1983) *citation count: 190*	Pseudo-Community Hypothesis (Beniger, 1987) *citation count: 23*
Whistleblowing (Miceli and Near, 1984) *citation count: 42*	Social Information Processing (Fulk, Steinfield, Schmitz, and Power, 1987) *citation count: 57*

Fig. 2.   List of Theories.

Functions of the Executive, which posited a cooperative equilibrium between "inducements" and "contributions" for each unique supervisor–employee dyad (Dansereau, Graen, & Haga, 1975). Building on the idea that a workgroup is an interlocking network of dyadic "interacts," the subsequent concept of "Leader–Member Exchange" suggested that the role-making system within complex organizations necessitates various stages of social exchange between managers and employees that facilitate overall organizational effectiveness over time (Graen, Novack, & Sommerkamp, 1982). Interestingly, however, one of the three theorists has continued to maintain the utility of the original dyadic concept in preference to the revised version (Dansereau, 1995).

(3) "Organizational Citizenship Behavior" was introduced in 1983 by Dennis Organ and his colleagues in the pages of the *Journal of Applied Psychology* (Smith, Organ, & Near, 1983) and in the pages of the *Academy of Management Journal* (Bateman & Organ, 1983). *Management and the Worker*, the highly influential 1939 book by Fritz Roethlisberg and William J. Dickson on the Hawthorne experiments in organizational behavior, had described the "logic of sentiment" usually expressed as informal cooperation between workers and supervisors. "The Good Soldier Syndrome" or "Organizational Citizenship Behavior" construct suggests that this "logic of sentiment" is largely based on personal predispositions in workers that motivate them to contribute spontaneous pro-social behaviors beyond their formal organizational roles, an important element in "lubricating the social machinery of the organization" (Smith, Organ, & Near, 1983, p. 654). Organ's two seminal papers identified these specific behaviors, which have become known as "organizational citizenship behaviors."

(4) "Whistleblowing" as a theoretical construct developed as a refinement of the "voice" component of Albert O. Hirschman's "exit, voice and loyalty" framework of affiliation with organizations and Bibb Latané's work on the determinants of bystander intervention in emergencies. The "whistleblowing" hypothesis introduced by Miceli and Near in the 1980s thus indicated that signs of trouble in an organizational climate induce otherwise committed members first to voice their dissatisfaction in efforts to change the organizational culture from within and to seek outside support only when their internal efforts at "voice" are disregarded (Miceli & Near, 1984).

The second cohort of theories focuses on processes of external exchange, as the exchange relationship, including both economic and social elements, has traditionally been accepted as the conceptual foundation of marketing and, latterly, of electronic commerce. These four theories had been chosen primarily on the basis of their epistemic evolution from earlier theories predating most recent technological developments in distributed commercial computing, as well as their consistency with many different information technology innovations.

(1) The "Channel Retreat" hypothesis was introduced by Wilke English in the *Journal of the Academy of Marketing Science* (English, 1985). This hypothesis built on Wroe Alderson's application of Parsonian functionalism to marketing channels and proposed that advances in "electronic technology" will ultimately collapse the traditional marketing channel,

empowering the end-consumer and forcing the suppliers and retailers to compete in a backward evolution to set up and service the new channel.

(2) The "Electronic Markets and Hierarchies" hypothesis was developed by MIT Sloan School colleagues Thomas Malone, JoAnne Yates, and Robert Benjamin, and published in the *Communications of the ACM* (Malone, Yates, & Benjamin, 1987). This hypothesis extended economist Oliver Williamson's transaction-cost theory to information technology innovation, proposing that the reduction of coordination costs made possible by advanced information technology will result in an inevitable shift towards markets rather than hierarchies, based on reduction in transaction costs.

(3) The "Pseudo-Community" hypothesis was propounded in 1987 in a review essay by James Beniger in *Communication Research*. It expands on sociologist Robert Merton's concept of the role of *pseudo-Gemeinschaft* in mass persuasion through mass communication. Beniger suggests that advanced information technology also brings with it an "unintended infrastructure" of "pseudo-community, a hybrid of interpersonal and mass communication – born largely of computer technology – that will mean both more intimate and more effective social control" easily exerted by sophisticated information marketers (Beniger, 1987, p. 369).

(4) The "Social Information Processing" hypothesis (later renamed the "Social Influence Model") was first published by Janet Fulk and colleagues at the Annenberg School of Communications in the pages of *Communication Research* (Fulk, Steinfield, Schmitz, & Power, 1987). Its authors called it an integration of "social influences with elements of traditional media use theory." Drawing from the work of management theorists Salancik and Pfeffer on the importance of social influences on individual attitudes and behavior in the organizational environment, the hypothesis suggested that an individual's technological media activities will be based partially both on objective and subjective elements.

METHODOLOGY

The method of analysis combined citation analysis, citation context analysis, interviews with the theorists and their peers, and surveys of publishing editors and editorial review boards. The case study design is shown in Fig. 3.

After the selection of the original theoretical publications, a citation analysis was performed to identify those articles published between 1975 and 1999 that cited them, and the documents (approximately 1,280) were

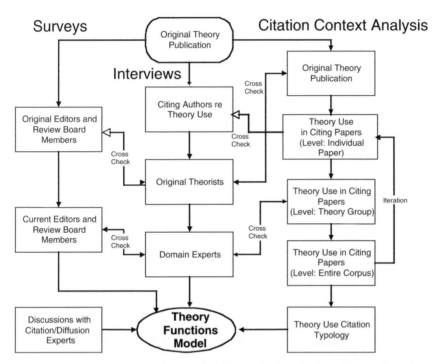

Fig. 3. Use of Convergent Lines of Evidence in Developing Theory Functions Model.

then collected. Articles that contained citation errors (i.e., were incorrectly reported as having cited the original paper) were removed from the corpus. In addition, some articles could not be located and used (usually these documents were published in languages other than English). An estimated 5 percent of the original citations belonged to this "unavailable" category. In addition, certain other documents were added to the corpus because they cited the original paper but were not included in the Institute for Scientific Information database from which the original data-set was drawn.

The next phases employed citation context analysis. Henry Small has recently called for a resumption of the project of developing a metatheory of citation, which he notes "must encompass the spectrum of observed behaviors from the most common forms such as ceremonial or perfunctory citation to the less common deviant cases, such as negative citation, self-citation, and misattribution. The empirical heart of such a theory is the comparison of the cited text with its context of citation in the citing texts"

Step 1	Initial construction of corpus through use of Institute for Scientific Information databases supplemented by additional information sources
Step 2	Preliminary analysis of all documents (initial reading of entire corpus to identify citation location and correctness of inclusion in corpus)
Step 3	Identification of additional documents for corpus through citation analysis of previously selected documents
Step 4	Preliminary construction of citation function categories through citation context analysis of individual documents
Step 5	Separation of documents into appropriate theory-groups
Step 6	Second analysis of documents and preliminary assignment of citation function categories to documents
Step 7	Citation context analysis of documents in each theory-group
Step 8	Interviews with selected theorists regarding theory usage and citation function typology
Step 9	Modification of citation function categories
Step 10	Analysis of citation anomalies
Step 11	Development of codebook for assignment of citation functions
Step 12	Final assignment of citation functions to entire corpus
Step 13	Final development of citation function typology

Fig. 4.   Corpus Analysis of Citing Documents.

(Small, 2004, p. 76). This "empirical heart" is what Small himself named "citation context analysis" over two decades ago (Small, 1982) and which is only now enjoying a revival in popularity among researchers (e.g., Hargens, 2000).

This study focused on what Small terms the "theory-use" aspect of citation context analysis (Small, 1982, p. 288). The study's first phase utilized citation context analysis on the entire corpus to determine citation correctness and the presence or absence of additional text related to the theory in each individual paper. In the second phase, citation context analysis was employed on the corpus of citing papers to develop the "theory-use" categories, and content analysis was used to develop and delimit the specific categories that comprised the final typology. The methodology for the analysis of the corpus of citing papers is shown in Fig. 4.

THE FUNCTIONS OF THEORIES

Although a fairly extensive literature exists on the functions of citations in general, none of the existing classifications were constructed specifically to

Theory Acknowledgement	Theory Analysis	Theory Application	Theory Assimilation
Positive (57%)	Empirical (71%)	Explanatory (94%)	Existing Framework (76%)
Neutral (39%)	Theoretical (29%)	Proposed (6%)	Novel Framework (24%)
Negative (4%)			
46% of all cites	*32% of all cites*	*16% of all cites*	*6% of all cites*

Fig. 5. Typology of Citation Functions for Theories.

map the uses of theory. The typology shown in Fig. 5, although bearing some resemblance to classic (e.g., Chubin & Moitra, 1975; Moravcsik & Murugesan, 1975; Murugesan & Moravcsik, 1978) and contemporary (e.g., Budd, 1999; Rice & Crawford, 1993) categorizations of cited references, is unique in its focus on theories-in-use. Particularly important in the development of this typology was the process of iterative analysis of the citing documents in the corpus. This process attempted to identify commonalities among the various functions of theory use while simultaneously considering their specificity in the context of actual citation use. This iterative analysis is a development of what Susan Leigh Star has named "grounded classification" (Star, 1998).

One problem endemic to citation context research efforts is that of category "fuzziness," as this type of research by definition considers papers in their entirety rather than by simply analyzing the individual sentence or paragraph in which a particular citation is located. The primary cause of "fuzziness" in the current study was the common case in which a paper analyzed empirical data as an integral part of a theoretical discussion. This "fuzziness" was handled by the following rule: to move beyond assignment to the preliminary category of "acknowledgement," the citing paper was analy'ed to see if it further assessed the theory in either empirical or theoretic l terms. Any empirical work was placed in the "application" category if it n ade use of the theory to explain existing empirical data, or in the "analysis-empirical" category if empirical or simulated data were collected or constructed to test the theory or any of its hypotheses. Any paper without such empirical elements were placed in the "assimilation" category if it attempted to locate the theory in a new or existing theoretical framework, or in the "analysis-theoretical" category if it discussed the theory without attempting such location.

This purely pragmatic rule was formulated in full awareness that "one could argue that citers do not think in mutually exclusive categories and that such an interpretation does violence to the cognitive processes that generate different types of references" (Chubin & Moitra, 1975, p. 439). However, since this project was intended to study the actual use of theories in specific contexts rather than to add to the extensive literature on "citation behavior" (see Case & Higgins, 2000 for a review), such simplification appeared to be warranted. The four major categories constructed from the iterative analysis of theory citations are those of theory acknowledgement, theory application, theory analysis, and theory assimilation. Figure 5 presents the typology of citation functions for theories.

Functions of Acknowledgement

The category of "theory acknowledgement" occurred with the greatest frequency, comprising 46 percent of all citations in the corpus. This category has often been dismissed as "perfunctory" or "ritual" citation, or perhaps a combination of both (e.g., Paul, 2000), but a closer examination of the specific contents of each citation indicates that "acknowledgement" may be further categorized as "positive," "negative," and "neutral," which indicates that even perfunctory citations can be evaluated thus exhaustively (see Hyland, 2004, p. 28 for a somewhat similar categorization). Among these three subcategories, "positive" was the largest, accounting for 57 percent of all "acknowledgement" citations, while "neutral" accounted for 39 percent, and "negative" accounted for only 4 percent. It should be noted that the very small percentage of negative citations is consistent with Chubin and Moitra's (1975) findings. However, it should also be noted that the "negative" acknowledgement category in this study does not include papers that analyze the theory in detail. Those papers are found under the "analysis-empirical" category.

The following describes and gives examples of each category of acknowledgement.

Acknowledgement-Neutral

The citing paper acknowledges the original paper as previous research but does not positively accept its conclusions, discuss, or analyze the theory. Example from Carley (1997, p. 25): "Literature on organizational adaption suggests that organizations change over time (DiMaggio & Powell, 1983)."

Acknowledgement-Positive
The citing paper accepts the original theory's conclusions as applicable but does not discuss or analyze the theory further. Example from Crow (1998, p. 257): "Organizations tend to imitate others considered similar, but more successful (DiMaggio & Powell, 1983)."

Acknowledgement-Negative
The citing paper rejects the original theory's thesis as applicable, but does not discuss or analyze the theory further. Example from Argyris and Liebeskind (1999, p. 53): "Institutional theory also implies that certain types of contractual arrangements can become...mimicked in a search for various types of 'legitimacy' (DiMaggio & Powell, 1983. ...Habits, pressures for legitimacy and mimicry do not play a role in our argument."

Functions of Analysis

The analytic category is the second most frequent, comprising 32 percent of the total citations in the corpus. The two subcategories ("analysis-empirical" and "analysis-theoretical") are roughly equivalent to Chubin and Moitra's categories of "experimental" and "theoretical," with the difference that this study, involving theories in the social sciences, expands the "experimental" category to include empirical non-experimental work such as surveys, case studies, trend analysis, and statistical analysis, and collapses the "theoretical" category to exclude work whose primary purpose is to situate the theory within a particular framework or typology, which is categorized below under the "functions of assimilation." Seventy-one percent of the analytic category was empirical, while the remaining twenty-nine percent were theoretical. The following examples from the corpus show the distinction between the two subcategories.

Analysis-Empirical
The primary goal of the citing paper is to test the original theory with data gathered for that purpose. Example: Bruderer and Singh's (1996) simulation study of the success of imitative strategies versus adaptive strategies by organizational agents. "The mimetic or DiMaggio and Powell routine variation model...does not adapt as well to the environment as the Schumpeterian transmission model (Bruderer & Singh, 1996, p. 1337)."

This category is not subdivided further into confirming or disconfirming subcategories, however, as due to the diversity of the nature of the theories and the analytic methods employed, such an assessment could not be performed consistently across all papers within the time limitations of this study. However, in principle, such an assessment could be performed in the future.

Analysis-Theoretical
The primary purpose of the citing paper is to critique the original theory without the use of additional empirical data. Example: Paul Hirsch's essay on reconciling "old" and "new" institutional theory. "Institutional explanations that involve the building up of structures by individual actors…are at odds with explanations that rely on action as determined by institutional structures (DiMaggio & Powell, 1983). Certainly, the former are related more to the old institutional attention to agency, whereas the latter is how the founders of this field would like to frame all future institutional discourse. …Approaches to the study of institutions should not be arbitrarily limited to some structurally determined paradigm or restricted to the study of action. What is needed instead is attention to ongoing sociological debates regarding the construction of more complex and complete forms of explanation that make lines from the micro to the macro and account for the ways in which various levels of explanation interpenetrate (Hirsch & Lounsbury, 1997, p. 415)."

Functions of Application

The application category includes both actual and suggested fields of application for the theory. This category comprises 16 percent of the total, with 94 percent of the category purporting to explain existing data and the remaining 6 percent offering proposed explanations of data that had not been collected. As noted earlier, the primary difference between the "application-explanatory" and "analysis-empirical" categories is that data were not collected to test the theory: the theory was used to explain existing data. "Application-proposed," therefore, bridges the gap between the two other categorizations. There is no equivalent for this type of subcategorization in previous citation context analytic studies. The following examples show the distinction between the two.

Application-Explanatory
The citing paper uses the theory to explain existing empirical evidence. Example: Sutton's use of DiMaggio and Powell's theory of institutional

isomorphism to explain the diffusion of the juvenile court system in the United States at the turn of the century. "The juvenile court is an institutional organization whose formal structure (or lack thereof) derives more from the need to enact a legitimacy myth than from the technical requirements of judging and disposing of delinquents. ...Societies of charity organizations helped standardize the normative structure of the court and propagated it nationwide, and states adopted it through a process of institutional modeling or 'mimesis' (DiMaggio & Powell, 1983)" (Sutton, 1985, p. 109).

Application-Proposed
The citing paper suggests that the theory be used to explore or explain a particular phenomenon, but does not introduce specific empirical evidence. Example: Iyer's suggestion that institutional isomorphism be used to study comparative marketing systems. "Some impact of the institutional environment on marketing systems may be coercive, normative, or mimetic (DiMaggio & Powell, 1983). ...Successful patterns of structure, functions, and processes will be replicated within the marketing system and innovation-imitating activities may contribute to wider patterns of organization and interactions within the marketing system" (Iyer, 1997, p. 550).

Functions of Assimilation

The assimilation category is the smallest of the four primary categories, representing only 6 percent of the total citations within the corpus. Again, there is no comparable category in previous citation context studies. The two assimilation categories are distinguished by whether or not the theoretical framework had been constructed previously to the publication of the current paper.

Assimilation-Existing
The primary purpose of the citing paper is to incorporate the theory into an existing theoretical framework. Example: Barley and Tolbert's presentation of a model of institutional isomorphism as a structuration process. "Structuration theory and institutional theory...share the premise that action is largely organized by institutions, widely held definitions of the behavior and relationships appropriate for a set of actors. Both acknowledge that institutions are created, maintained and changed through action. Structuration theory, however, explicitly focuses on the dynamics by which

institutions are reproduced and altered, an issue that has been largely neglected by institutional theorists. Our aim has been to develop the implications of structuration theory for the interplay between actions and institutions and to address the practical problem of how to study institutional maintenance and change in organizations" (Barley & Tolbert, 1997, pp. 112–113).

Assimilation-Novel
The primary purpose of the citing paper is to incorporate the theory into a new theoretical framework. Example: Deephouse's development of an "integrative theory of strategic balance" that incorporates both DiMaggio and Powell's institutional isomorphism and Porter's conceptualization of competitive advantage through the development of attractive niches. "This paper...began developing a theory of strategic balance by integrating strategic management and organizational theories. Strategic management and organizational ecology contributed the idea that competition reduces the benefits of institutional isomorphism. Institutional and resource dependence theories contribute the idea that legitimacy activates the flow of resources that energizes a firm. The theory of strategic balance directs our attention to intermediate levels of differentiation where a firm benefits from reduced competition while maintaining its legitimacy" (Deephouse, 1999, p. 162).

THE THEORY FUNCTIONS MODEL

To develop the final theory functions model, a dozen theorists who had been identified during the citation context analysis stage of the study as having been interested primarily in theoretical development were interviewed in depth. These interviews focused specifically on how they viewed and used the theories. Data from these interviews and from discussions with various members of editorial review boards and other knowledgeable observers of these theories were also used to inform particular aspects of the typology shown in Fig. 6 as the "theory functions" of citation. Specifically, the meta-categories of "applicability," "constructivity," "accessibility," "connectivity," and "generativity" were developed to capture both the original categories developed from the earlier citation context analysis stages and the insights from theorists themselves. The categories from Fig. 5 are rearranged to reflect the larger functions of theories in context.

EMPIRICAL FACTORS	SOCIO-COGNITIVE FACTORS	THEORETICAL FACTORS
APPLICABILITY application-explanatory *15% of all citations*		CONNECTIVITY acknow-negative assimilation-existing *7% of all citations*
	ACCESSIBILITY acknow-neutral acknow-positive *44% of all citations*	
CONSTRUCTIVITY analysis-empirical *23% of all citations*		GENERATIVITY analysis-theoretical application-proposed assimilation-novel *11% of all citations*

Fig. 6. Typology of Theory Functions Based on Citation Functions.

This typology highlights those empirical, socio-cognitive, and theoretical factors that appear to be most important to a theory's trajectory over time. The specific factors are described in detail in the following sections, detailing how the basic categories from the citation context analysis were further enriched by interview and survey data.

Applicability

As mentioned above, the category of "application-explanatory" comprised 15 percent of all citations within the entire corpus. "Applicability" is the general term for what a number of theorists have described as "problem-solving" and appears to be a fruitful source of innovation. Several theorists indicated that their initial research activity was not driven by the need to apply a particular theory to a particular problem, but rather originated from a problem that piqued their interest enough to provoke a search for a po-tential explanation, resulting in the application or creation of a theory. A less creative variant of this is what has been called "inference to the best ex-planation" (Lipton, 1991) in which the researcher examining a particular phenomenon selects a particular theory as the most relevant or most likely explanation of that phenomenon. The applicability of a theory tends to promote its wider diffusion, as shown by the "institutional isomorphism" case, in which the theory was often quite "loosely coupled" to the empirical data, resulting in some dismay on the part of theorists DiMaggio and Powell.

Of course, the more applicable the theory appears to be to a variety of phenomena, the more likely it is to be of interest to a variety of researchers. "Applicability," therefore, appears to promote diffusion outside a well-defined "invisible college," making methodological rigor more difficult to enforce. The less applicable a theory is to a variety of salient phenomena, the less likely it is to provoke interest on the part of others, as is most clearly shown in the case of English's "Channel Retreat." A related case is that of Beniger's "Pseudo-Community" which, although potentially applicable to highly salient phenomena, was originally presented in such a way that it reached only a circumscribed audience of communication theorists rather than the wider audience of electronic commerce practitioners.

Constructivity

"Constructivity," a term borrowed from mathematics, is intended to denote that a theory is "capable in principle of being proven" rather than to focus on constructs and variables per se. As defined, the subcategory of "analysis-empirical" accounts for 23 percent of all citations within the corpus. Empirical evidence and methodological issues are the twin poles around which "invisible colleges" seem to converge.

During the course of the interviews, it also became obvious that these are the issues most controversial in "theory work." It appears that focusing on methodological questions can be counter-productive if it leads theorists to concentrate more on refining their methods than their ideas. While periodic critical reviews of the literature by senior scholars appear to be helpful in focusing attention on central problems, it appears that methodological strictures can be internalized by reviewers to the extent of excluding otherwise promising lines of research, either unintentionally or intentionally. This corresponds to the findings of several studies of the peer review process that have indicated methodological criticisms are the primary form of so-called "gatekeeping" in the journals studied (e.g., Gilliland & Cortina, 1997).

Connectivity

"Connectivity" is defined by a particular theory's linkage to other theoretical frameworks. While the specific categories that define the meta-category of "connectivity" (acknowledgement-negative and assimilation-existing framework) in the citation context analysis accounted for only 7% of all citations within the corpus, it is also true that all documents in the corpus were initially identified through their connection to a particular theory or theories. Therefore, "connectivity" may be considered a taken-for-granted element of theory diffusion that is perhaps clearer in more standard citation analyses.

Generativity

The categories of "analysis-theoretical," "application-proposed," and "assimilation-novel" accounted for 11 percent of all citations in the corpus. They are here combined in the meta-category of "generativity" to denote their particular contribution towards the development of new theoretical frameworks. This meta-category includes the development of new theories, the suggestion of new fields for investigation and application, and the subsumption of rival theories into new theoretical frameworks.

As mentioned above, the initial citation context analysis had identified a number of theorists who had developed the theories in novel ways. Interviews with these theorists in particular underscored the value of theories that can be propagated in ways perhaps not foreseen by the original theorists. In fact, interviews with the original theorists did not reveal nearly as much interest in the subsequent "generativity" of these theories as in their "constructivity."

The combined value of "generativity" and "constructivity" was neatly summarized by one of the editorial review board respondents: "This article, subsequently reprinted in an important edited volume, helped to define a major theoretical perspective in the study of organizations and social movements – one of the most empirically fruitful, in my view." Thus, certain theory functions may best be appreciated by observers over time rather than by the contemporary theorists themselves.

Accessibility

"Accessibility" here defines the broader function of what was initially identified in the citation context analysis phase of the study as "acknowledgement." This meta-category includes 44 percent of all citations in the corpus. Much previous emphasis on the "social turn" in citation analysis, including "referencing as persuasion" (Gilbert, 1977), "captation" (Latour, 1987), and the "rhetoric-first model" (Cozzens, 1989), has been on the subjective rather than the objective side of these citations. Lately, however, there has been a renewed appreciation of citations as "knowledge claims" (Budd, 1999). As Blaise Cronin has aptly put it: "citations have multiple articulations in that they inform our understanding of the socio-cultural, cognitive, and textual aspects of scientific communication" (Cronin, 1998, p. 45).

The "accessibility" function, therefore, when considered collectively rather than individually, appears to reflect the evolution of a discipline's consensus regarding each theory's potential importance over time. "Accessibility" is a socio-cognitive measure of how visible a theory may become both inside and outside a particular discipline.

Importantly, the role of journal editors, peer reviewers, and senior scholars in the process of citation development became more obvious during the course of the interviews than was readily apparent from the citation context analysis itself. Most of the junior theorists interviewed said that their initial interest in particular theories was due to the fact that those theories were the ones that were introduced to them during their doctoral studies, either by their professors or during the course of their reading. Additionally, there was a strong personal connection in that the junior scholars were often students or former students of the original theorists or at least had had some personal contact with them. Further, in three of the eight cases studied the "seminal" paper for the theories relied on empirical support from several dissertation research projects supervised by the senior theorists. However, the interviews also revealed that "accessibility" is mediated by the other factors of "constructivity," "applicability," "connectivity," and "generativity" in ways that are not readily apparent merely by reading those articles that achieved published status.

For instance, the centrality of "constructivity" was shown not only by the large proportion of empirically oriented papers in the corpus, but was also reflected in interviews with Miceli, Near, and Dansereau, all theorists who described difficulties in receiving acceptance for their non-standard methodologies and who resorted to publishing outside the standard journal system. The characteristic of "applicability," which is often assumed only to play a role in "trickle-down" to practitioner journals in fact appeared to help make "Institutional Isomorphism" a so-called classic citation, as a large number of authors publishing in non-sociological journals used it to explain organizational phenomena of interest in their own fields, ranging from social work to education to health care. Conversely, the lack of "applicability" of English's "Channel Retreat" to any actual empirical phenomena at the time, clearly played a part in the neglect his paper received, while the salience of various information technology advances in the late 1980s and early 1990s, beginning with advances in electronic data interchange and culminating in the commercialization of the Internet, is obvious in the prevalent use of anecdotal evidence in a number of subsequent papers citing Malone's "Electronic Markets and Hierarchies."

The importance of "connectivity" to dominant theories, already apparent in the convention of the literature review required by scholarly articles, was addressed by both senior and junior theorists in their interviews, all of whom appeared to have an excellent grasp of the literature that related to their own publications. It should be noted, however, as several did, that the journal review and revision process sometimes made the theoretical connections more prominent in the article than was warranted by the author's original intentions. Thus "connectivity" was probably both over represented as a factor (in that most papers in the corpus were in fact identified through their explicit citation connections with the theories being studied) and underrepresented (in that most interviewees preferred to focus discussion on what was novel in their own work).

"Generativity," one of the smallest categories in terms of absolute numbers, however, may eventually be found to play a critical role in the careers of theories over a longer period of time than that of the current study. The ease with which a theory is able to suggest new empirical and theoretical paths is presumably central to a long and, by definition, "fruitful" career.

In summary, this issue of how theoretical and empirical factors relevant to specific theories do in fact mediate their "accessibility" has been somewhat neglected in recent studies of scholarly communication, which have emphasized its networking and discursive aspects. While both co-citation analysis (Rousseau & Zuccala, 2004) and rhetorical analysis (White, 2004) are now considered essential tools of investigation, they have tended to obscure other potentially fruitful approaches to theoretic communication, especially in regard to what has been variously termed the "integral," "substantive," or "organic" citation of theories that has been emphasized here. It is our contention that theories, as the most important form of innovation, are at the heart of "organic" citation, and an examination of their perceived attributes can help to provide an explanation of why "most scientific innovations fail to diffuse widely" (Crane, 1972, p. 76). Figure 7 compares the "theory characteristics" typology to Everett Rogers's classic "characteristics of innovations that promote diffusion" (Rogers, 1962).

The characteristics that promote diffusion of even "ordinary" theories as shown appear to be similar to but distinct from those previously defined in innovation diffusion research in that the so-called "context of justification" (Reichenbach, 1938) in scientific communication requires considerably more empirical and epistemological support by potential adopters than that

Theory Characteristics Typology	Accessibility	Applicability	Connectivity	Constructivity	Generativity
Rogers's Innovation Characteristics	Observability/ Complexity	Relative Advantage	Compatibility	Trialability	Reinvention

Fig. 7. Theory Characteristics Compared to General Innovation Characteristics.

required for the adoption of other artifacts and ideas. This is, of course, in full accordance with exemplary historical case studies of the growth of scientific consensus around particular theories even prior to the development of the formalized gatekeeping processes inherent in the contemporary journal system (e.g., Rudwick, 1985).

"Accessibility" incorporates all those socio-cognitive factors that lead to the publication of a theory. This corresponds to and combines Rogers's categories of "observability" and "complexity:" that is, with what ease or difficulty the results of an innovation may be observed and understood by other potential adopters. This characteristic is essential to any further theoretic communication, as a theory that is not somehow communicated beyond its originator cannot diffuse.

"Applicability" resembles Rogers's "relative advantage" (the degree to which an innovation is perceived as better than the idea it supersedes) in that it describes the extent to which a theory may be used to explain a variety of phenomena. Generalizability promotes wider diffusion to scholarly communities. It may also promote a more superficial use of the theory as it is applied to explain a broader range of evidence without an accompanying increase in rigor.

"Connectivity" corresponds to Rogers's "compatibility" (the degree to which an innovation is perceived as being consistent with the existing values, past experiences, and needs of potential adopters) but is more specific in that it describes the extent to which a theory connects to or is built on existing theory. In general, connectivity with existing theory promotes diffusion to current theorists through the common process of "citation chaining" (that is, following the citations in an article of interest to uncover additional related articles).

"Constructivity" is similar to Rogers's "trialability" (the degree to which an innovation may be experimented with on a limited basis) in that it is the extent to which a theory may be tested. Unlike "trialability," however, which was meant to convey whether an innovation might be adopted on a temporary basis, "constructivity" conveys the extent to which the theory has been constructed so as to facilitate testing or replication, and the potential relevance of empirical data.

"Generativity" does not correspond to any of Rogers's original categories, but it does relate to his and Ronald Rice's work on "re-invention" of innovations (Rice & Rogers, 1980; Rogers, 1995b), in that it describes the extent to which a theory can generate new ideas. Generativity of theory promotes diffusion to later theorists through the potential for new publications, as novelty is a desired, though not defining, characteristic of publishable theoretic contributions (Whetten, 1989).

The use of these categories allows the theories to be analyzed as shown in Fig. 8. This figure is ordered by a normalized diffusion ratio (total number of citations for each theory divided by number of years since its original date of publication) and shows the percentages within each category for each individual theory. It is apparent from this figure that the various theories did not accrue their citations equally across all categories.

While all theories (except "Channel Retreat") received a third or more of all of their citations through "accessibility" (that is, by ritual or perfunctory citation), the remaining percentages of citations for each theory indicate interesting differences. "Applicability" is seen to be below 5 percent for most of these theories. "Institutional Isomorphism," however, earned more than a quarter of all its citations in that category, indicating that the theory has been widely employed outside what is in comparison (though not in absolute terms) a much smaller "invisible college" that focuses on "constructivity" (13 percent of the citations). Relatedly, another analyst of the diffusion of this theory has also commented on its unusual citation pattern and identified it as a problem in terms of maintaining theoretical rigor (Mizruchi & Fein, 1999).

The absence of any "constructivity" citations for "Pseudo-Community" indicates that no "invisible college" has crystallized, and that this paper is usually cited as part of another theory's framework. The "Whistleblowing," "Social Influence," "Leader-Member Exchange," and "Organizational Citizenship Behavior" theories, however, all received more than a third of their citations in this category, indicating the presence of an active group testing the theory's constructs. The "invisible colleges" of the last two theories named, however, are substantially larger than those of the first two. The smaller percentage of "constructivity" citations for "Electronic Markets and Hierarchies" probably reflects the fact (not apparent in the figure) that this particular theory has now been overshadowed by a more comprehensive "coordination theory" (Malone & Crowston, 1994).

THEORY	Accessibility	Applicability	Connectivity	Constructivity	Generativity	Total Citations	Diffusion Ratio
Channel Retreat						0	0
Pseudo-Community	87%		13%			23	2.09
Whistle-blowing	33%	2%	17%	41%	7%	42	2.80
Social Influence	49%	2%	4%	36%	4%	55	4.58
Leader-Member Ex.	29%	4%	7%	50%	10%	147	8.65
Organiz. Cit. Behav.	32%	4%	10%	35%	19%	190	11.87
Electronic Markets	57%	7%	3%	19%	14%	143	11.91
Institutional Isomorphism	47%	26%	9%	13%	5%	671	41.94

Fig. 8.   Functional Characteristic Percentages for Theories.

The "Electronic Market and Hierarchies" theory's relatively high percentage in the "generativity" category is also an indicator of these ongoing theoretical discussions involving new permutations of theory in the electronic commerce arena. Similarly, the high percentage in this category for "Organizational Citizenship Behavior" shows that it has become a seminal theory for the emerging field of "prosocial behavior." Though not obvious from the figure, the relatively low percentage in the "generativity" category for "Institutional Isomorphism" is more a reflection of its unusually high "applicability," as in fact the absolute number of "generativity" cites for this theory is far higher than for the others.

Finally, all these attributes were combined to create the "theory functions model" shown in Fig. 9, which represents how various empirical and theoretical factors mediate and are mediated by socio-cognitive factors central to the scholarly communication system. The questions are those that are asked, implicitly or explicitly, about any theory as it is considered for inclusion within the system.

The theory functions model represents a new framework for the investigation of scientific communication. This model suggests that a theory that collects the majority of its citations in particular functional categories is likely to diffuse in particular directions and have particular strengths and weaknesses. A theory attracting more "applicability" than "constructivity" citations in its early stages may never develop sufficient rigor to withstand competing theories, while a theory with a preponderance of "constructivity" citations may be of limited practical use. A theory lacking "generativity" citations may be less likely to persist over time than one with many such citations. A theory lacking "connectivity" citations may fail to attract necessary support from the surrounding research community. A theory that has many "accessibility" citations but fails to accrue citations in other functional categories is unlikely to survive over time.

Obviously, in the theory cases studied here, none of the eight theories represent an "ideal type," but more of a continuum, with the "Channel Retreat" theory showing the most common outcome for theories (non-diffusion), the "Pseudo-Community" and "Whistleblowing" theories showing limited diffusion largely due to their methodological limitations, the "Social Influence," "Electronic Markets and Hierarchies," "Leader-Member Exchange," and "Organizational Citizenship Behavior" theories all showing aspects of the normal diffusion expected in "invisible college" clusters, and the "Institutional Isomorphism" theory showing the explosive diffusion characteristic of a disciplinary paradigm in the making.

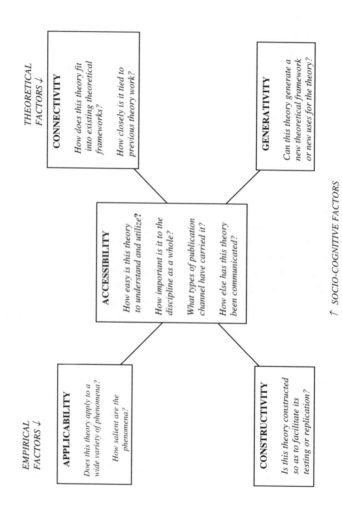

Fig. 9. Theory Functions Model.

The theory functions model presented here is preliminary, based on a very small set of recent theories from areas that may not be representative of theoretic communication. However, it does provide a basis for further research on the functions of theories in general, as well as an initial set of factors for theorists themselves to ponder.

There is, depending on one's view of the purpose of theory, a number of ways in which a theory may be said to have a "successful" career, whether that success is in application to a broad variety of practical or theoretical problems, in explicating an overarching theoretical framework, in generating new approaches to a field or in generating new fields themselves, or simply in becoming widely known in a number of different fields.

THE THEORY FUNCTIONS MODEL AND COMMUNITIES OF PRACTICE

The most practical use of this model, however, is to point out some potential linkages between "applicability" and "constructivity" that also relate to recent work on "critical appraisal" and "applicability" by practitioners (Booth & Brice, 2004a, pp. 105–106). The theory functions model was developed from data collected from theorists and their theoretical writings, as the purpose of the original study was to study the diffusion of theory among theorists. Notably, the model as it exists shows no direct link between the testing of theory and the application of theory. All connections appear to be mediated through the journal system studied.

This is entirely consistent with the observation that "two distinct and separate cultures exist – that researchers carry out their work without regard for practical value, and that practitioners have a deep resistance to reading research based on a perception that theory is unlikely to assist them with day-to-day decision making in their workplace. This is the view supported by the majority of commentators on the subject." (Genoni, Haddow, & Ritchie, 2004, p. 56). However, the model also shows that two of the main questions regarding "accessibility" are as oriented towards practitioners as they are towards theorists: "How easy is this theory to understand and utilize?" and "How else has this theory been communicated?" These two questions indicate that, ideally, the travels of theory should extend well beyond the boundaries of the journal system and into the communities of practice. It is recognized that practitioners, in fact, both read about research and do research. However, they don't choose to use theory in the same way as do theorists, so their work is seldom published and valued in the same way (Powell, Baker, & Mika, 2002). However, theories without applications and theories tested in a vacuum appear equally lacking as sources of evidence. The well-known "file drawer" problem of difficulty in publishing both the findings of apparently less significant results (Rosenthal, 1979) and replication studies also contribute to the inconclusiveness of much theory.

The issues of "doing research that is useful for theory and practice" (Lawler III, Mohrman, Mohrman, Ledford, & Cummings, 1985) and "the reciprocal transfer of learning from journals to practice" (Latham, 2001) are of long standing that have yet to be satisfactorily addressed in many fields. For library and information science, however, a community of practice is coming into existence that is unusually well positioned and increasingly motivated to assist in bridging the gaps between the construction of theories, their testing, and their application. One of the primary differences between the tenure-track academic and the tenure-track librarian is the reward system for scholarly publication. An academic in a research-intensive institution must publish in refereed scholarly journals, preferably prestigious ones, to achieve tenure; it is not mandatory for a librarian seeking tenure at the same institution to publish at the same level (Cubberley, 1996, pp. 13–14).

However, an increasing number of librarians, especially in academic libraries, are being encouraged to enter the field with Ph.Ds in addition to the M.L.S. (Macauley, 2004). These tenure-track librarians are well prepared to publish in peer-reviewed scholarly journals or to present in a variety of public forums, and are presumably eager to do so. Although there has been little or no discussion in published advice for prospective tenure-track librarians as to the utility of testing or applying particular theories in practice as a possible subject for scholarly publication or presentation, such an endeavor would clearly assist in bridging these "two cultures." For example, one of the theories discussed above as part of the development of the theories function model is that of "organizational citizenship behavior." An intriguingly "generative" use of that theory has been work on the so-called "customer citizenship behavior" that examines the voluntary helping behaviors performed by customers in the retail environment, such as returning shopping carts or notifying employees of potential hazards in the aisles (Bettencourt, 1997). While there has been studies of organizational citizenship behaviors enacted by library employees, there has been no similar theoretical extension into possible "library patron citizenship behaviors," which would presumably be equally useful to both theory and practice.

Librarians without doctorates are also being encouraged to consume research findings more critically and creatively (Eldredge, 2004; Winning, 2004) and to employ evidence-based practices both for their own work

(Clyde, 2004; Koufogiannis & Crumley, 2004) and for that of their clients (Booth, 2003; Booth & Brice, 2004a, b). Andrew Booth notes that, "it is important to preserve evidence-based practice as fundamentally pragmatic. ...Its focus on everyday decision-making, as carried out by information practitioners, sees research as a tool to enlighten and inform practical decisions and policy. ...A culture of evidence-based information practice is evidenced by both 'well-informed practitioner behavior and well-informed research directions'" (Booth, 2003, p. 66). Relatedly, Bill Crowley notes that, "it is possible to use the LIS practitioner-generated literature as a point of entry for generating theory regarding the tacit knowledge of working professionals. However, such efforts should be guided by a superficially simple yet ultimately complex question: 'What are the implications for practice?'" (Crowley, 1999, p. 288).

In his discussion of developing such communities of practice, Etienne Wenger urges the importance of what he terms "the duality of participation and reification" (Wenger, 1998, p. 63). This duality implies the necessity of the social negotiation of meaning around particular artifacts to develop communal practices. Further, he underscores the importance of the 'boundary object" as an artifact (Star & Griesemer, 1989) around which communities of practice may organize and the role of the "brokers" who connect elements of one practice into another (Wenger, 1998, p. 105). The role of citations as boundary objects has been discussed above. The potential participation of librarians as "brokers" or intermediaries between the community of scholarship and the community of practice may provide the other part of Wenger's duality. He notes that "reificative connections" (such as citations) and "participative connections" (such as developing "critical appraisals," "systematic reviews," and "evidence-based librarianship") provide distinct but complementary channels of communication. He points out also that as communities of practice "differentiate themselves and also interlock with each other, they constitute a complex social landscape of shared practices, boundaries, peripheries, overlaps, connections, and encounters" (Wenger, 1998, p. 118). It is not enough that librarians critically consume research and then apply it selectively and effectively: it is also important for the growth and development of theories as potential sources for and explanations of evidence that librarians contribute to the research culture by responding in the form of systematic reviews and published papers to the theorists' claims. Wenger's so-called "landscape of practice" could therefore provide a much-needed relief map to what is often barren theoretical terrain as well as providing more applicable and reliable theoretical direction to practice in return.

As the theory functions model continues to be revised and as both the journal system and the library environment continue to evolve, future efforts may well explore these potential changes in how theories diffuse.

REFERENCES

Aharonian, G. (2000). U.S. patent examination system is intellectually corrupt. Accessed September 12, 2003 at http://www.bustpatents.com/corrupt.html
Andersen, B. (1999). The hunt for S-shaped growth paths in technological innovation: A patent study. *Journal of Evolutionary Economics, 9*, 487–526.
Argyris, N. S., & Liebeskind, J. P. (1999). Contractual commitments, bargaining power, and governance inseparability: Incorporating history into transaction cost theory. *Academy of Management Review, 24*, 49–63.
Ashton, S. V., & Oppenheim, C. (1978). A method of predicting Nobel Prizewinners in chemistry. *Social Studies of Science, 9*, 341–348.
Audi, R. (1993). *The structure of justification.* New York: Cambridge University Press.
Baldi, S. (1998). Normative versus social constructivist processes in the allocation of citations: A network-analytic model. *American Sociological Review, 63*, 829–846.
Balkin, J. M. (1986). The crystalline structure of legal thought. *Rutgers Law Review, 39*, 1–110.
Balkin, J. M. (1993). Understanding legal understanding: The legal subject and the problem of legal coherence. *Yale Law Journal, 103*, 105–176.
Balkin, J. M. (1998). Deconstruction's legal career. Accessed September 1, 2005 at http://www.yale.edu/lawweb/jbalkin/writings.htm#deconlegalcareer
Banks, C. P. (1999). Reversals of precedent and judicial policy-making: How judicial conceptions of *Stare Decisis* in the U.S. Supreme Court influence social change. *Akron Law Review, 32*, 233–258.
Barley, S. R., & Tolbert, P. S. (1997). Institutionalization and structuration: Studying the links between action and institution. *Organization Studies, 18*, 93–117.
Bateman, T. S., & Organ, D. W. (1983). Job satisfaction and the good soldier: The relationship between affect and employee 'Citizenship'. *Academy of Management Journal, 26*, 587–595.
Bazerman, C. (1988). *Shaping written knowledge: The genre and activity of the experimental article in science.* Madison: University of Wisconsin Press.
Beniger, J. R. (1987). Personalization of mass media and the growth of pseudo-community. *Communication Research, 14*, 352–371.
Berring, R. C. (1987). Legal research and legal concepts: Where form molds substance. *California Law Review, 75*, 15–27.
Berring, R. C. (1994). Collapse of the structure of the legal research universe: The imperative of digital information. *Washington Law Review, 69*, 9–34.
Berring, R. C. (1997). Chaos, cyberspace and tradition: Legal information transmogrified. *Berkeley Technology Law Journal, 12*, 189–212.
Bettencourt, L. A. (1997). Customer voluntary performance: Customers as partners in service delivery. *Journal of Retailing, 73*, 383–406.
Bierbaum, E. G., & Brooks, T. A. (1995). The literature of acquired immunodeficiency syndrome (AIDS): Continuing changes in publication patterns and subject access. *Journal of the American Society for Information Science, 46*, 530–536.

Blachowicz, J. (1998). *Of two minds: The nature of inquiry.* Albany, NY: State University of New York Press.

Bogen, J. (1989). Coherentist theories of knowledge don't apply to enough outside of science— and don't give the right results when applied to science. In: J. W. Bender (Ed.), *The current state of the coherence theory* (pp. 142–159). Dordrecht, The Netherlands: Kluwer Academic Publishers.

BonJour, L. (1985). *The structure of empirical knowledge.* Cambridge, MA: Harvard University Press.

Booth, A. (2003). Where systems meet service: Towards evidence-based information practice. *VINE: The Journal of Information and Knowledge Management Systems, 33,* 65–71.

Booth, A., & Brice, A. (2004a). Appraising the evidence. In: A. Booth & A. Brice (Eds), *Evidence-based practice for information professionals: A handbook* (pp. 104–118). London: Facet Publishing.

Booth, A., & Brice, A. (2004b). Why evidence-based information practice? In: A. Booth & A. Brice (Eds), *Evidence-based practice for information professionals: A handbook* (pp. 1–12). London: Facet Publishing.

Boruch, R., May, H., Turner, H., Lavenberg, J., Petrosino, A., De Moya, D., Grimshaw, J., & Foley, E. (2004). Estimating the effects of interventions that are deployed in many places: Place-randomized trials. *American Behavioral Scientist, 47,* 608–633.

Bowker, G. (1992). What's in a Patent? In: W. E. Bijker & J. Law (Eds), *Shaping technology, building society* (pp. 52–74). Cambridge, MA: MIT Press.

Brenner, S. W. (1990). Of publication and precedent: An inquiry into the ethnomethodology of case reporting in the American Legal System. *DePaul Law Review, 39,* 461–542.

Bruderer, E., & Singh, J. V. (1996). Organizational evolution, learning, and selection: A genetic algorithm-based model. *Academy of Management Journal, 39,* 1322–1349.

Bucchi, M. (1998). *Science and the media: Alternative routes in scientific communication.* London: Routledge.

Buckland, M. K. (1991). Information as thing. *Journal of the American Society for Information Science, 42,* 351–360.

Budd, J. M. (1999). Citations and knowledge claims: Sociology of knowledge as a case in point. *Journal of Information Science, 25,* 265–274.

Buschman, J. E. (2003). *Dismantling the public sphere: Situating and sustaining librarianship in the age of the new public philosophy.* Westport, CT: Libraries Unlimited.

Caminker, E. H. (1994a). Precedent and prediction: The forward-looking aspects of inferior court decisionmaking. *Texas Law Review, 73,* 1–82.

Caminker, E. H. (1994b). Why must inferior courts obey superior court precedents? *Stanford Law Review, 46,* 817–873.

Campbell, D. T. (1969a). Ethnocentrism of disciplines and the fish-scale model of omniscience. In: M. Sherif & C. W. Sherif (Eds), *Interdisciplinary relationships in the social sciences* (pp. 328–348). Xenia, OH: Aldine Publishing.

Campbell, D. T. (1969b). Reforms as experiments. *American Psychologist, 24,* 409–429.

Carley, K. M. (1990). Structural constraints on communication: The diffusion of the homomorphic signal analysis technique through scientific fields. *Journal of Mathematical Sociology, 15,* 207–246.

Carley, K. M. (1997). Organizational adaptation. *Annals of Operations Research, 75,* 25–47.

Case, D. O., & Higgins, G. M. (2000). How can we investigate citation behavior? A study of reasons for citing literature in communication. *Journal of the American Society for Information Science, 51*, 635–645.

Chatman, E. (1986). Diffusion theory: A review and test of a conceptual model in information diffusion. *Journal of the American Society for Information Science, 37*, 377–386.

Chen, C., Paul, R. J., & O'Keefe, B. (2001). Fitting the jigsaw of citation: Information visualization in domain analysis. *Journal of the American Society for Information Science and Technology, 52*, 315–330.

Chubin, D. E., & Moitra, S. (1975). Content analysis of references: Adjunct or alternative to citation counting? *Social Studies of Science, 5*, 423–441.

Clayton, P. (1997). *Implementation of organizational innovation: Studies of academic and research libraries.* San Diego, CA: Academic Press.

Clyde, L. A. (2004). Evaluating the quality of research publications: A pilot study of school librarianship. *Journal of the American Society for Information Science and Technology, 55*, 1119–1130.

Cochrane, A. L. (1972). *Effectiveness and efficiency: Random reflections on health services.* London: Nuffield Provincial Hospitals Trust.

Cohn, E. G., Farrington, D. P., & Wright, R. A. (1998). *Evaluating criminology and criminal justice.* Westport, CT: Greenwood Press.

Cole, S. (1975). The growth of scientific knowledge: Theories of deviance as a case study. In: L. A. Coser (Ed.), *The idea of social structure: Papers in honor of Robert K. Merton* (pp. 175–220). New York: Harcourt Brace Jovanovich.

Connors, R. J. (1998). The rhetoric of citation systems: Part I. The development of annotation studies from the Renaissance to 1900. *Rhetoric Review, 71*, 6–49.

Connors, R. J. (1999). The rhetoric of citation systems: Part II. Competing epistemic values in citation. *Rhetoric Review, 17*, 219–246.

Cozzens, S. E. (1989). What do citations count? The rhetoric-first model. *Scientometrics, 15*, 437–447.

Crane, D. (1969). Social structure in a group of scientists: A test of the "Invisible College" hypothesis. *American Sociological Review, 34*, 35–352.

Crane, D. (1972). *Invisible colleges: Diffusion of knowledge in scientific communities.* Chicago: University of Chicago Press.

Cronin, B. (1998). Metatheorizing citation. *Scientometrics, 43*, 45–55.

Cronin, B., & Pearson, S. (1990). The export of ideas from information science. *Journal of Information Science, 16*, 381–391.

Crow, M. (1998). Personnel in transition: The case of Polish women personnel managers. *Personnel Review, 27*, 243–261.

Crowley, B. (1999). Building useful theory: Tacit knowledge, practitioner reports, and the culture of LIS inquiry. *Journal of Education for Library and Information Science, 40*, 282–295.

Cubberley, C. W. (1996). *Tenure and promotion for academic librarians: A guidebook with advice and vignettes.* Jefferson, NC: McFarland Publishing.

Cullen, J. (1982). *On deconstruction: Theory and criticism after structuralism.* Ithaca, NY: Cornell University Press.

Curry, M. R. (1997). Shelf length zero: The disappearance of the geographical text. In: G. Benko & U. Strohmeyer (Eds), *Space and social theory: Interpreting modernity and postmodernity* (pp. 88–112). Oxford: Blackwell Publishers.

Curry, P. M. (1984). Theories as systems. *Behavioral Science, 29*, 270–273.

Dalton, C. (1985). An essay in the deconstruction of contract doctrine. *Yale Law Journal, 94*, 997–1114.

Damanpour, F. (1985). The adoption of innovations in public libraries. *Library and Information Science Research, 7*, 231–246.

Damanpour, F. (1988). Innovation type, radicalness, and the adoption process. *Communication Research, 15*, 545–567.

Damanpour, F., & Evan, W. M. (1984). Organizational innovation and performance: The problem of organizational lag. *Administrative Science Quarterly, 29*, 392–409.

Dansereau, F. (1995). A dyadic approach to leadership: Creating and nurturing this approach under fire. *Leadership Quarterly, 6*, 479–490.

Dansereau, F., Graen, G., & Haga, W. J. (1975). A vertical dyad linkage approach to leadership within formal organizations: A longitudinal investigation of the role making process. *Organizational Behavior and Human Performance, 13*, 46–78.

Day, M. T. (2002). Discourse fashions in library administration and information management: A critical history and bibliometric analysis. In: F. D. Lynden (Ed.), *Advances in librarianship* (pp. 231–298). San Diego, CA: Academic Press.

Dearing, J. W., & Meyer, G. (1994). An exploratory tool for predicting adoption decisions. *Science Communication, 16*, 43–57.

Deephouse, D. L. (1999). To be different, or to be the same? It's a question (and theory) of strategic balance. *Strategic Management Journal, 20*, 147–166.

Deng, Z., Lev, B., & Narin, F. (1999). Science and technology as predictors of stock performance. *Financial Analysts Journal, 55*, 20–32.

Derrida, J. (1994). The deconstruction of actuality: An interview with Jacques Derrida. *Radical Philosophy, 68*, 28–41.

DiMaggio, P., & Powell, W. (1983). The iron cage revisited: Institutional somorphism and the collective rationality in organizational fields. *American Sociological Review, 48*, 147–160.

Dosi, G. (1982). Technological paradigms and technological trajectories. *Research Policy, 11*, 147–162.

Dunn, D. J. (1993). Why legal research skills declined, or when two rights make a wrong. *Law Library Journal, 85*, 49–69.

Dunn, W. N., & Holzner, B. (1988). Knowledge in society: Anatomy of an emergent field. *Knowledge in Society, 1*, 3–26.

Edge, D. O. (1979). Quantitative measures of communication in science: A critical review. *History of Science, 17*, 102–134.

Edmundson, W. A. (1996). The antimony of coherence and determinism. *Iowa Law Review, 82*, 1–20.

Edwards, C. N. (1998). In search of legal scholarship: Strategies for the integration of science into the practice of law. *Southern California Interdisciplinary Law Journal, 8*, 1–37.

Egghe, L., & Rousseau, R. (1990). *Introduction to informetrics: Quantitative methods in library, documentation and information science.* Amsterdam: Elsevier.

Eldredge, J. D. (2000). Evidence-based librarianship: Formulating EBL questions. *Bibliotecha Medica Canadiana, 22*, 74–77.

Eldredge, J. D. (2002). Evidence-based librarianship: Levels of evidence. *Hypothesis, 16*, 10–13.

Eldredge, J. D. (2004). How good is the evidence base? In: A. Booth & A. Brice (Eds), *Evidence-based practice for information professionals: A handbook* (pp. 36–48). London: Facet Publishing.

English, W. D. (1985). The impact of electronic technology upon the marketing channel. *Journal of the Academy of Marketing Science*, *13*, 57–71.

Fennell, M. L., & Warnecke, R. B. (1988). *Diffusion of medical innovations: An applied network analysis*. New York: Plenum Press.

Field, T. F. (1996). Judicial information policy: Whose responsibility is it, anyway? In: T. L. Coggins (Ed.), *The national conference on legal information issues: Selected essays* (pp. 215–221). Littleton, CO: Fred B. Rothman & Co.

Fliegel, F. C., & Kivlin, J. E. (1966). Attributes of innovations as factors in diffusion. *American Journal of Sociology*, *72*, 235–248.

Fuchs, S., & Ward, S. (1994). What is deconstruction, and where and when does it take place? Making facts in science, building cases in law. *American Sociological Review*, *59*, 481–500.

Fulk, J., Steinfield, C. W., Schmitz, J., & Power, J. G. (1987). A social information processing model of media use in organizations. *Communication Research*, *14*, 529–552.

Fuller, S. (1988). *Social epistemology*. Bloomington, IN: University of Indiana Press.

Garfield, E. (1955). Citation indices for science. *Science*, *122*, 109–110.

Garfield, E. (1990). Who will win the Nobel Prize in economics? *Current Contents*, *11*, 3–7.

Gatignon, H., Tushman, M. L., Smith, W., & Anderson, P. (2002). A structural approach to assessing innovation: Construct development of innovation locus, type, and characteristics. *Management Science*, *48*, 1103–1122.

Genoni, P., Haddow, G., & Ritchie, A. (2004). Why don't librarians use research? In: A. Booth & A. Brice (Eds), *Evidence-based practice for information professionals: A handbook* (pp. 49–60). London: Facet Publishing.

Gerson, E. M. (1983). Scientific work and social worlds. *Knowledge*, *4*, 357–377.

Gilbert, G. N. (1977). Referencing as persuasion. *Social Studies of Science*, *7*, 113–122.

Gilliland, S. W., & Cortina, J. M. (1997). Reviewer and editor decision making in the journal review process. *Personnel Psychology*, *50*, 427–452.

Graen, G. B., Novack, M. A., & Sommerkamp, P. (1982). The effects of leader-member exchange and job design on productivity and satisfaction: Testing a dual attachment model. *Organizational Behavior and Human Performance*, *30*, 109–131.

Grafton, A. (1999). *The footnote: A curious history*. Cambridge, MA: Harvard University Press.

Graham, G. J. (1984). Consensus. In: G. Sartori (Ed.), *Social science concepts* (pp. 89–124). Beverly Hills, CA: Sage Publications.

Gross, A. G. (1990). The origin of species: Evolutionary taxonomy as an example of the rhetoric of science. In: H. W. Simons (Ed.), *The rhetorical turn: Invention and persuasion in the conduct of inquiry* (pp. 91–111). Chicago: University of Chicago Press.

Haack, S. (1993). *Evidence and inquiry: Towards reconstruction in epistemology*. Cambridge, MA: Blackwell Publishers.

Hargens, L. L. (2000). Using the literature: Reference networks, reference contexts, and the social structure of scholarship. *American Sociological Review*, *65*, 846–865.

Hart, H. L. A. (1961). *The concept of law*. Oxford: Clarendon Press.

Hartley, J. (1999). What do we know about footnotes? Opinions and data. *Journal of Information Science*, *25*, 205–212.

Hartman, G. H. (1981). *Saving the text: Literature, Derrida, philosophy*. Baltimore, MD: Johns Hopkins University Press.

Hays, S. P. (1996a). Influences on reinvention during the diffusion of innovations. *Political Research Quarterly*, *49*, 631–650.

Hays, S. P. (1996b). Patterns of reinvention: The nature of evolution during policy diffusion. *Policy Studies Journal, 24*, 551–566.

Hernnstein-Smith, B. (1997). *Belief and resistance: Dynamics of contemporary intellectual controversy*. Cambridge, MA: Harvard University Press.

Hicks, D., Breitzman, T., Olivastro, D., & Hamilton, K. (2001). The changing composition of innovative activity in the U.S.: A portrait based on patent activity. *Research Policy, 6*, 199–240.

Hirsch, P. M., & Lounsbury, M. (1997). Ending the family quarrel: Toward a reconciliation of 'Old' and 'New' institutionalisms. *American Behavioral Scientist, 40*, 406–418.

Hull, D. L. (1975). Central subjects and historical narratives. *History and Theory, 14*, 253–274.

Hyland, K. (1999). Academic attribution: Citation and the construction of disciplinary knowledge. *Applied Linguistics, 20*, 341–367.

Hyland, K. (2004). *Disciplinary discourses: Social interactions in academic writing*. Ann Arbor: University of Michigan Press.

Iyer, G. R. (1997). Comparative marketing: An interdisciplinary framework for institutional analysis. *Journal of International Business Studies, 28*, 531–561.

Jaffe, A. B. (2000). The U.S. patent system in transition: Policy innovation and the innovation process. *Research Policy, 29*, 531–557.

Jaffe, A. B., & Trajtenberg, M. (2002). *Patents, citations and innovations: A window on the knowledge economy*. Cambridge, MA: MIT Press.

Jaffe, A. B., Trajtenberg, M., & Henderson, R. (1993). Geographic localization of knowledge spillovers as evidenced by patent citations. *Quarterly Journal of Economics, 108*, 577–598.

Kaplan, N. (1965). The norms of citation behavior: Prolegomena to the footnote. *American Documentation, 16*, 179–184.

Karki, R. (1996). Searching for bridges between disciplines: An author co-citation analysis on the research into scholarly communication. *Journal of Information Science, 22*, 323–324.

Katz, E., Levin, M. L., & Hamilton, H. (1963). Traditions of research on the diffusion of innovation. *American Sociological Review, 28*, 237–252.

Kaufer, D. S., & Carley, K. M. (1993). *Communication at a distance: The influence of print on sociocultural organization and change*. Hillsdale, NJ: Lawrence Erlbaum Associates.

Kelso, R. R., & Kelso, C. D. (1996). How the Supreme Court is dealing with precedents in constitutional law. *Brooklyn Law Review, 62*, 973–1037.

Kessler, M. M. (1963). Bibliographic coupling between scientific papers. *American Documentation, 14*, 10–25.

Kloppenberg, L. A. (1996). The public interest in the work of the courts: Opinions and beyond. *Oregon Law Review, 75*, 49–256.

Kornhauser, L. A. (1995). Adjudication by a resource-constrained team: Hierarchy and precedent in a judicial system. *Southern California Law Review, 68*, 1605–1629.

Koufogiannis, D., & Crumley, E. (2004). Applying evidence to your everyday practice. In: A. Booth & A. Brice (Eds), *Evidence-based practice for information professionals: A handbook* (pp. 119–126). London: Facet Publishing.

Kress, K. (1984). Legal reasoning and coherence theories: Dworkin's Rights thesis, retroactivity, and the linear order of decisions. *California Law Review, 72*, 369–402.

Kuhn, T. S. (1972). *The structure of scientific revolutions*. (2nd ed.). Chicago: University of Chicago Press.

Kwasnik, B. H. (1999). The role of classification in knowledge representation and discovery. *Library Trends, 48*, 22–47.

Lamont, M. (1987). How to become a dominant French philosopher: The case of Jacques Derrida. *American Journal of Sociology*, *93*, 584–622.

Landes, W. M., Lessig, L., & Solimine, M. E. (1998). Judicial influence: A citation analysis of federal Courts of appeals judges. *The Journal of Legal Studies*, *27*, 271–332.

Langley, P., Simon, H. A., Bradshaw, G. L., & Zytkow, J. M. (1987). *Scientific discovery: An account of the creative process*. Cambridge, MA: MIT Press.

Latham, G. P. (2001). The reciprocal transfer of learning from journals to practice. *Applied Psychology: An International Review*, *50*, 201–211.

Latour, B. (1987). *Science in action: How to follow scientists and engineers through society*. Cambridge: Harvard University Press.

Latour, B., & Woolgar, S. (1986). *Laboratory life: The social construction of scientific facts* (2nd ed.). Princeton NJ: Princeton University Press.

Lawler III, E. E., Mohrman, A. M., Mohrman, S., Ledford, G. E., & Cummings, T. G. (1985). *Doing research that is useful for theory and practice*. San Francisco: Jossey-Bass Publishers.

Leach, R. (1976). *Culture and communication: The logic by which symbols are connected*. Cambridge: Cambridge University Press.

Lehrer, K., & Wagner, C. (1981). *Rational consensus in science and society: A philosophical and mathematical study*. Dordrecht, The Netherlands: D. Reidel Publishing Co.

Leydesdorff, L. (1998). Theories of citation? *Scientometrics*, *43*, 5–25.

Lin, M. (2001). *Certainty as a social metaphor: The social and historical production of certainty in China and the West*. Westport, CT: Greenwood Press.

Lipton, P. (1991). *Inference to the best explanation*. London: Routledge.

Longino, H. (1990). *Science as social knowledge: Values and objectivity in scientific inquiry*. Princeton: Princeton University Press.

Lupu, I. C. (1998). Textualism and original understanding: Time, the Supreme Court, and the Federalist. *George Washington Law Review*, *66*, 1324–1336.

Luukonen, T. (1997). Why has Latour's theory of citations been ignored by the bibliometric community? Discussion of sociological interpretations of citation analysis. *Scientometrics*, *38*, 27–37.

Macauley, P. (2004). Challenging librarians: The relevance of the doctorate in professional practice. Paper presented at the 2004 ALIA Conference in Gold Coast, Queensland, Australia. Accessed 9/2/2005 at http://conferences.alia.org.au/alia2004/pdfs/macauley.p.paper

MacLeod, C. (1991). The paradoxes of patenting: Invention and its diffusion in 18th and 19th-century Britain, France, and North America. *Technology & Culture*, *32*, 885–910.

MacRoberts, M. H., & MacRoberts, B. R. (1989). Problems of citation analysis: A critical review. *Journal of the American Society for Information Science*, *40*, 342–349.

Madison, M. (2003). Reconstructing the software license. *Loyola University Chicago Law Review*, *35*, 275–340.

Malinconico, S. M. (1997). Librarians and innovation: An American viewpoint. *ASLIB Proceedings*, *31*, 47–58.

Malone, T. W., & Crowston, K. (1994). The interdisciplinary study of coordination. *ACM Computing Surveys*, *26*, 87–119.

Malone, T. W., Yates, J., & Benjamin, R. (1987). Electronic markets and electronic hierarchies. *Communications of the ACM*, *30*, 484–497.

Mandeville, T. (1996). *Understanding novelty: Information, technological change, and the patent system.* Norwood, NJ: Ablex Publishing Co.

Marshall, J. G. (1990). Diffusion of innovation theory and end user searching. *Library and Information Science Research, 12,* 55–69.

Martens, B. (2001). Do citation systems theories represent theories of truth? *Information Research, 6.* Accessed August 26, 2005 at http://www.inforesearch.org

Mazzoleni, R., & Nelson, R. R. (1998). Economic theories about the benefits and costs of patents. *Journal of Economic Issues, 32,* 1031–1052.

McAllister, J. W. (1996). *Beauty and revolution in science.* Ithaca: Cornell University Press.

McCain, K. W. (1990). Mapping authors in intellectual space: A technical overview. *Journal of the American Society for Information Science, 41,* 433–443.

McQuillan, M. (2001). Introduction: Five strategies for deconstruction. In: M. McQuillan (Ed.), *Derrida: A reader* (pp. 1–43). New York: Routledge.

Merritt, D. J., & Putnam, M. (1996). Judges and scholars: Do courts and scholarly journals cite the same law review articles? *Chicago–Kent Law Review, 71,* 871–899.

Merz, M., & Knorr-Cetina, K. (1997). Deconstruction in a 'Thinking' science: Theoretical physicists at work. *Social Studies of Science, 27,* 73–111.

Meyer, M. (2000). What is special about patent citations? *Scientometrics, 49,* 93–123.

Miceli, M. P., & Near, J. P. (1984). The relationships among beliefs, organizational position, and whistle-blowing status: A discriminant analysis. *Academy of Management Journal, 27,* 687–705.

Mizruchi, M., & Fein, L. (1999). The social construction of organizational knowledge. *Administrative Science Quarterly, 40,* 653–683.

Moravcsik, M. J., & Murugesan, P. (1975). Some results on the function and quality of citations. *Social Studies of Science, 5,* 86–92.

Mullins, N. C. (1973). *Theories and theory groups in contemporary American sociology.* New York: Harper & Row.

Murugesan, P., & Moravcsik, M. J. (1978). Variation of the nature of citation measures with journals and scientific specialties. *Journal of the American Society for Information Science, 20,* 141–147.

Myers, G. (1995). From discovery to invention: The writing and rewriting of two patents. *Social Studies of Science, 25,* 57–105.

Narin, F., Olivastro, D., & Stevens, K. A. (1994). Bibliometrics: Theory, practice and problems. *Evaluation Review, 18,* 65–76.

Neumann, R. K. (1990). *Legal reasoning and legal writing: Structure, strategy, and style.* Boston, MA: Little, Brown.

Nozick, R. (1981). *Philosophical Explanations.* Cambridge, MA: Belknap Press of Harvard University Press.

Ogden, P. (1993). Mastering the lawless science of our law: A story of legal citation indexes. *Law Library Journal, 85,* 1–47.

Oreskes, N. (1999). *The rejection of continental drift: Theory and method in American earth science.* New York: Oxford University Press.

Packer, K., & Webster, A. (1995). Inventing boundaries: The prior art of the social world. *Social Studies of Science, 25,* 107–117.

Packer, K., & Webster, A. (1996). Patenting culture in science: Reinventing the scientific wheel of credibility. *Science, Technology & Human Values, 21,* 427–453.

Paisley, W. (1990). An oasis where many trails cross: The improbable cocitation networks of a multidiscipline. *Journal of the American Society for Information Science, 41*, 459–568.

Paul, D. (2000). In citing chaos: A study of the rhetorical uses of citation. *Journal of Business and Technical Communication, 14*, 185–222.

Popper, K. R. (1979). *Objective knowledge: An evolutionary approach*. (Revised ed.). Oxford: Oxford University Press.

Popper, K. R., & Eccles, J. C. (1981). *The self and its brain*. Berlin: Springer International.

Posner, R. (1990). *Cardozo: A study in reputation*. Chicago: University of Chicago Press.

Post, D. G., & Eisen, M. B. (2000). How long is the coastline of the law? Thoughts on the fractal nature of legal systems. *Journal of Legal Studies, 29*, 545–584.

Powell, R. R., Baker, L. M., & Mika, J. J. (2002). Library and information science practitioners and research. *Library and Information Science Research, 24*, 49–72.

Price, D. J. (1965). Networks of scientific papers. *Science, 149*, 510–515.

Price, D. J. (1970). Citation measures of hard science, soft science, technology, and nonscience. In: C. E. Nelson & D. K. Pollock (Eds), *Communication among scientists and engineers* (pp. 3–22). Lexington, MA: Heath Lexington Books.

Pungitore, V. L. (1995). *Innovation and the library: The adoption of new ideas in public libraries*. Westport, CT: Greenwood Press.

Raz, J. (1992). The relevance of coherence. *Boston University Law Review, 72*, 273–320.

Reichenbach, H. (1938). *Experience and prediction*. Chicago: University of Chicago Press.

Rescher, N. (1993). *Pluralism: Against the demand for consensus*. Oxford: Clarendon Press.

Rice, R. E., & Crawford, G. A. (1993). Context and content of citations between communication and library and information science articles. In: J. R. Schement & B. D. Ruben (Eds), *Between communication & information* (pp. 189–217). New Brunswick, NJ: Transaction Publishers.

Rice, R. E., & Rogers, E. M. (1980). Reinvention in the innovation process. *Knowledge, 1*, 499–514.

Rivette, K. G., & Kline, D. (2000). *Rembrandts in the attic: Unlocking the hidden value of patents*. Boston: Harvard Business School Press.

Robbins, I. P. (1999). Semiotics, analogical legal reasoning and the *Cf.* citation: Getting our signals uncrossed. *Duke Law Journal, 48*, 1043–1079.

Robison, W. L. (1993). The constitution and the nature of law. *Law and Philosophy, 12*, 5–32.

Rogers, E. M. (1962). *Diffusion of innovations*. New York: Free Press of Glencoe.

Rogers, E. M. (1995a). *Diffusion of innovations* (5th ed.). New York: Free Press.

Rogers, E. M. (1995b). Diffusion of drug abuse prevention programs: Spontaneous diffusion, agenda setting, and reinvention. In: T. E. Backer, S. L. David & G. Saucy (Eds), *Reviewing the behavioral science knowledge base on technology transfer* (pp. 90–105). Rockville, MD: U.S. Dept. of Health and Human Services, National Institute on Drug Abuse.

Rosenthal, R. (1979). The "File Drawer Problem" and tolerance for null results. *Psychological Bulletin, 86*, 638–641.

Rousseau, R., & Zuccala, A. (2004). A classification of author co-citations: Definitions and search strategies. *Journal of the American Society for Information Science and Technology, 55*, 513–529.

Rudwick, M. J. S. (1985). *The Great Devonian Controversy: The shaping of scientific knowledge among gentlemanly specialists*. Chicago: University of Chicago Press.

Sartiliot, C. (1993). *Citation and modernity: Derrida, Joyce, and Brecht*. Norman, OK: University of Oklahoma Press.

Schauer, F., & Wise, V. J. (2000). Nonlegal information and the delegalization of law. *Journal of Legal Studies*, *29*, 451–494.

Shapin, S. (1994). *A social history of truth*. Chicago: University of Chicago Press.

Shapiro, F. R. (1985). The most-cited law review articles. *California Law Review*, *73*, 1540–1554.

Shapiro, F. R. (1996). The most-cited law review articles revisited. *Chicago–Kent Law Review*, *71*, 751–779.

Shapiro, M. (1972). Towards a theory of stare decisis. *Journal of Legal Studies*, *1*, 125–134.

Shuldberg, K. (1997). Digital influence: Technology and unpublished opinions in the federal courts of appeals. *California Law Review*, *85*, 541–575.

Small, H. G. (1973). Co-citation in the scientific literature: A new measure of the relationship between two documents. *Journal of the American Society for Information Science*, *24*, 265–269.

Small, H. G. (1974). Multiple citation patterns in scientific literature: The circle and hill models. *Information storage and Retrieval*, *10*, 393–402.

Small, H. G. (1978). Cited documents as concept symbols. *Social Studies of Science*, *8*, 327–340.

Small, H. G. (1982). Citation Context Analysis. In: B. Dervin & M. J. Voight (Eds), *Progress in communication sciences*, (Vol. 3, pp. 287–310). Norwood, NJ: Ablex Publishing Co.

Small, H. G. (1985). The lives of a scientific paper. In: K. S. Warren (Ed.), *Selectivity in information systems: Survival of the fittest* (pp. 83–97). New York: Praeger Publishers.

Small, H. G. (1999). Visualizing science by citation mapping. *Journal of the American Society for Information Science*, *50*, 799–813.

Small, H. G. (2004). On the shoulders of Robert Merton: Towards a normative theory of citation. *Scientometrics*, *60*, 71–79.

Smith, C. A., Organ, D. W., & Near, J. P. (1983). Organizational citizenship behavior: Its nature and antecedents. *Journal of Applied Psychology*, *68*, 653–663.

Solomon, M. (2001). *Social empiricism*. Cambridge, MA: MIT Press.

Sosa, E. (1991). *Knowledge in perspective: Selected essays in epistemology*. New York: Cambridge University Press.

Star, S. L. (1998). Grounded classification: Grounded theory and faceted classification. *Library Trends*, *47*, 218–232.

Star, S. L., & Griesemer, J. R. (1989). Institutional ecology: 'Translations' and boundary objects: Amateurs and professionals in Berkeley's Museum of vertebrate zoology, 1907–39. *Social Studies of Science*, *19*, 387–420.

Stone, S. L. (1993). In pursuit of the counter-text: The turn to the Jewish legal model in contemporary American legal theory. *Harvard Law Review*, *106*, 813–894.

Strang, D., & Meyer, J. W. (1993). Institutional conditions for diffusion. *Theory and Society*, *22*, 487–512.

Strauss, A. (1982). Social worlds and legitimation processes. In: N. Denzin (Ed.), *Studies in symbolic interaction*, (Vol. 4, pp. 171–190). Greenwich, CT: JAI Press.

Sturges, P. (1996). Conceptualizing the public library, 1850–1919. In: M. Kinnell & P. Sturges (Eds), *Continuity and innovation in the public library: The development of a social institution* (pp. 28–47). London: Library Association Publishing.

Sutton, J. R. (1985). The juvenile court and social welfare: Dynamics of progressive reform. *Law and Society Review*, *19*, 107–145.

Swanson, D. R. (1986). Undiscovered public knowledge. *Library Quarterly*, *56*, 103–118.

Swanson, D. R. (1987). Two medical literatures that are logically but not bibliographically connected. *Journal of the American Society for Information Science*, *38*, 228–233.

Swanson, D. R. (1989). A second example of mutually isolated medical literatures related by implicit, unnoticed connections. *Journal for the American Society for Information Science*, *40*, 432–435.

Swidler, A., & Arditi, J. (1994). The new sociology of knowledge. In: J. Hagan & K. S. Cook (Eds), *Annual review of sociology*, (Vol. 20, pp. 305–329). Palo Alto, CA: Annual Reviews Inc.

Talley, E. (1999). Precedential cascades: An appraisal. *Southern California Law Journal, 73*, 87–137.

Teubner, G. (1989). How the law thinks: Towards a constructivist epistemology of law. *Law & Society Review, 23*, 727–757.

Thomas, P. (1999). The effect of technological impact upon patent renewal decisions. *Technology Analysis & Strategic Management, 11*, 181–197.

Tijssen, R. J. W. (2001). Global and domestic utilization of industrial relevant science: Patent citation analysis of science-technology interactions and knowledge flows. *Research Policy, 30*, 35–54.

Tolliver, J. (1989). The St. Elizabethan world. In: J. W. Bender (Ed.), *The current state of the coherence theory* (pp. 160–167). Dordrecht, The Netherlands: Kluwer Academic Publishers.

Trajtenberg, M. (1990). A penny for your quotes: Patent citations and the value of information. *RAND Journal of Economics, 21*, 172–187.

Tran, L. A. (2005). Diffusion of community information networks in New Zealand public libraries: A case study. *New Library World, 106*, 269–283.

Traynor, R. J. (1977). The limits of judicial creativity. *Iowa Law Review, 63*, 1–13.

Tushnet, M. (1984). Critical legal studies and constitutional law: An essay in deconstruction. *Stanford Law Review, 36*, 623–647.

Tussey, D. (1998). Owning the law: Intellectual property rights in primary law. *Fordham Intellectual Property, Media & Entertainment Law Journal, 9*, 173–240.

Van Raan, A. F. J., & Tijssen, R. F. W. (1993). The neural net of neural network research: An exercise in bibliometric mapping. *Scientometrics, 26*, 169–192.

Walsh, D. J. (1997). On the meaning and pattern of legal citations: Evidence from state wrongful discharge precedent cases. *Law & Society Review, 31*, 337–360.

Watson-Verran, H., & Turnbull, D. (1995). Science and other indigenous knowledge systems. In: S. Jasanoff, T. Pinch, J. C. Petersen & G. E. Markle (Eds), *Handbook of science and technology studies* (pp. 115–139). Thousand Oaks, CA: Sage Publications.

Weinberg, B. H. (1997). The earliest Hebrew citation indexes. *Journal of the American Society for Information Science, 48*, 318–330.

Weiner, S. G. (2003). Resistance to change in libraries: Applications of communication theories. *Portal: Libraries and the academy, 3*, 69–78.

Weller, A. C. (2001). *Editorial peer review: Its strengths and weaknesses*. Medford, NJ: Information Today Publications.

Wenger, E. (1998). *Communities of practice: Learning, meaning, and identity*. New York: Cambridge University Press.

Whetten, D. A. (1989). What constitutes a theoretical contribution? *Academy of Management Review, 14*, 490–495.

White, H. D. (2004). Citation analysis and discourse analysis revisited. *Applied Linguistics, 25*, 89–116.

White, H. D., & Griffith, B. C. (1981). Author cocitation: A literature measure of intellectual structure. *Journal of the American Society for Information Science, 12,* 163–171.

White, H. D., & Griffith, B. C. (1982). Authors as markers of intellectual space: Co-citation in studies of science, technology and society. *Journal of Documentation, 38,* 255–272.

White, H. D., Wellman, B., & Nazer, N. (2004). Does citation reflect social structure? Longitudinal evidence from the globenet interdisciplinary research group. *Journal of the American Society for Information Science and Technology, 55,* 111–126.

White, M. D. (2001). Diffusion of a innovation: Digital reference service in Carnegie Foundation Master's (comprehensive) Academic Institution libraries. *Journal of Academic Librarianship, 27,* 173–187.

Wildemuth, B. M. (1992). An empirically grounded model of the adoption of intellectual technologies. *Journal of the American Society for Information Science, 43,* 210–224.

Winning, A. (2004). Identifying sources of evidence. In: A. Booth & A. Brice (Eds), *Evidence-based practice for information professionals: A handbook* (pp. 71–88). London: Facet Publishing.

Wolfreys, J. (1998). *Deconstruction, Derrida.* New York: St. Martin's Press.

Wolfreys, J. (2002). Citation's haunt: Spectres of Derrida. *Mosaic, 24,* 21–34.

Wouters, P. (1999). Beyond the holy grail: From citation theory to indicator theories. *Scientometrics, 44,* 561–580.

LEADERSHIP AND CHANGE: AN INTELLECTUAL JOURNEY

Jean Mulhern

In 2000, the author of this reflective paper had earned the proverbial 20-year service pin for directing small libraries. Her memories of being in library school decades before had faded. She was questioning why she felt bored or burned out in a field that has changed so rapidly and with such positive results for library users. Was she really embracing these ongoing changes? She wondered how she could strengthen the role of her academic library in student learning and institutional vitality. How could she change in order to be a more effective academic library administrator in this new century? In a search for answers, the author decided to return to the classroom in pursuit of an advanced degree in educational leadership. Her official goals were to obtain increased theoretical knowledge and improved research skills for personal development and improved professional practice as an educational leader/librarian. Her personal goal was to revive her passion for academic librarianship.

The author's coursework emphasized that research findings and theory development have not transferred easily to practice in academe (Willower & Forsyth, 1999). She learned how personal practice can be enhanced when (re)considered in the new or different lights of relevant theory. For example, Adrianna J. Kezar (2001), scholar and editor of the ASHE-ERIC Higher Education Report Series, values praxis, connecting theory and practice in higher education (Kezar & Eckel, 2000; Kezar, 2001). Using Kezar's guidelines for leading academic change as a meaning perspective (Mezirow, 1990,

Advances in Library Administration and Organization, Volume 23, 59–83
Copyright © 2006 by Elsevier Ltd.
All rights of reproduction in any form reserved
ISSN: 0732-0671/doi:10.1016/S0732-0671(05)23002-X

p. xvi) for this paper, the author identified six significant intellectual bridges
linking theory with her own practice as an academic administrator and
library director.

In this paper, the author discusses how the six bridges in her intellectual
journey form a foundation appropriate for better understanding and implementing academic library leadership and change. To focus the discussion,
she decided to reference two self-studies she had coordinated for her college's institutional accreditation processes in 1998 and 2003. Such projects
are familiar to many academic librarians as other duties as assigned. Since
these two projects were completed just before and just after her several years
of doctoral coursework, they provided a pair of personal benchmarks that
informed her critical self-reflection on how she had changed as an academic
administrator. This paper illustrates how her integrated learning outcomes
from the program offered the potential of refreshed library practice enhanced by broader academic perspectives.

BRIDGE 1: LEARNING TO APPRECIATE
THE DISTINCT CHARACTERISTICS OF HIGHER
EDUCATION

The author's course of graduate study was designed to increase awareness of
the distinctive characteristics of higher education. Constructing this intellectual bridge between theory and practice showed her that library administrators could obtain useful insights from research and experiences in the
broader field of educational administration and leadership. For example,
she crossed this bridge in the process of designing and implementing her
institution's 2003 accreditation progress report on student learning. Such
required self-studies are intended to drive an institution's critical self-
reflection that is so important to quality assurance and internal change
processes.

Higher education's distinctive characteristics formed two intersecting
perspectives in the report, those of the accrediting agency and of the local
institution. These same characteristics drive change in academic libraries.

From one perspective, the accrediting agency required that the progress
report evaluate the college's planning and implementing of its student
learning assessment program. The general intent of this monitoring process
is to direct local student learning programs and assessment toward identified
best practices (North Central Association of Colleges and Schools, Higher
Learning Commission (NCA-HLC), 2003a). As a form of peer mentoring,

accreditation reviews and progress monitoring help each institution set baselines for tracking teaching/learning quality and show how that is promoted by the local fiscal, physical plant, support services, human resources, and ethical environments (North Central Association of Colleges and Schools, Commission on Institutions of Higher Education (NCA-CIHE), 1997, 2003b). Those institutions successful in institutionalizing the guidelines for accreditation have developed internal feedback loops focused on mission-driven quality improvement (Alverno College as described by Mentkowski, 2000; Baldrige, 2001). Exemplar institutions typically have the characteristics of effective learning organizations (Senge, 1990) and learning communities (Helgesen, 1995; Lenning & Ebbers, 1999; Sergiovanni, 1994). Such institutions are open, inclusive, reflective, and focused on collaborative quality improvement efforts, all characteristics to be valued in academic libraries as well.

The second perspective important to the progress report depended on the college's unique characteristics that have a bearing on student learning and learning assessment. Through her studies, the author had learned that an effective institutional self-study project requires knowledge about the interplay of contextual differences in legal status, Carnegie classification, mission, and student profile (NCA-HLC, 2003b). It is important to understand how local curriculum decisions (Eisner, 1994), policy decisions (Goodchild, Lovell, Hines, & Gill, 1997), and decisions within institutions, including libraries, are complex and temporary alignments of socio-political, legal, environmental, discipline-based, and fiscal characteristics.

Two general characteristics of higher education have major impacts on implementing student learning assessment plans as well as library programs and services. One characteristic, local financial status, points toward a long-standing conflict in sources of power within any American institution of higher education (Brubacher & Rudy, 1997; Goodchild et al., 1997). The history and pervasive nature of this power conflict were not apparent to the author prior to her coursework. She learned that the fiduciary interests of an administration often clash with the discipline-focused and instructional interests of its faculty (Brubacher & Rudy, 1997; Mulhern, 2002c). Accreditors encourage local institutions to resolve these fiscal conflicts in the interest of mission-centered student learning and achievement (NCA-HLC, 2003a).

Second, in addition to academe's traditional tensions, the progress report's topic of student learning assessment tapped directly into the historic and always dramatic political subtext of curriculum choice and control (Eisner, 1994). Certainly the whole concept of assessing student-learning hinges on curriculum control. Learning assessment can be viewed as a threat to the autonomy of the faculty as well as a long-overdue shift toward accountability for the educational value added by a particular institution or its library (Ewell, 1997; Mulhern, 2002c). College administrators, faculty, librarians, students, parents, employers, and sources of funding all are actively influencing college curriculum decisions (and thus student learning) in a loosely coupled governance environment (Brubacher & Rudy, 1997; Goodchild et al., 1997). Adding to this complexity, colleges with developmental academic missions have special concerns with assessing student learning (Allen & Jewell, 2002; Freeman & Thomas, 2002). These colleges struggle to balance the need for fiscal responsibility and accountability against their mission-driven need to support and improve an ever-more-expensive teaching/learning environment where rapid results are difficult to demonstrate.

The expectation of quality assurance, the historic economic and political/governance tensions unique to higher education, and local issues were important variables for the author's progress report project. These factors signal significant considerations for library leadership as well. Based on that insight, the author vowed to examine library issues from multiple perspectives, including an institution's general fiscal, curricular, and socio-political perspectives.

BRIDGE 2: INCREASING KNOWLEDGE ABOUT EDUCATIONAL RESEARCH: DESIGN AND DATA

The author identified significant improvements in research design and data gathering in her 2003 progress report compared with her 1998 project. She attributes this improvement in practice to her coursework that focused on current educational research knowledge and skills essential for developing assessment and evaluation processes.

Prior to these courses, she had no formal exposure to educational research. Like many librarians of her generation, her library education preceded any emphasis on critical self-reflection as an administrator/researcher or on formal research design and implementation. Among the 2003 improvements were the addition of a reflective process prior to accepting the new project, the development of a research design, and the proper use of appropriate data-gathering and data analysis techniques.

Two phases of the 2003 progress report provide examples of bridging the theory and application of educational research. One phase was the author's process for determining whether she understood the research question and was appropriately equipped to address the question. The other phase involved designing the project research with appropriate data gathering and analysis activities.

In Spring 2003, the college president asked the author to consider taking on the progress report project. Unsure, she assessed her role in the institutional environment using SWOT analysis (strengths, weaknesses, opportunities, threats) (matrix analysis in Krathwohl, 1998) in order to acquire and organize information to inform her decision. She needed to determine whether she could be a tenable leader of such a project. Her coursework had emphasized the importance of having sound bases for successful leadership and recognizing when to lead and when to follow. In this case, she considered her minor position in the organizational structure and governance, the interrelationships among the administrative and faculty leaders, and the critical importance of accreditation to the institution (Brubacher & Rudy, 1997; Kezar, 2001; NCA-CIHE, 1997). The author used the SWOT analysis to clarify writing her role as the report coordinator and writer. Buoyed by the president's support of her responding project proposal, the author accepted the challenges presented by this additional assigned duty. Applying that decision process to library programs and services, one would place a high priority on broad-based preplanning and winning early and significant formal institutional support for library initiatives.

A second important decision requiring a systematic assessment approach was selecting the project's research design. Unlike the 1998 self-study, the 2003 project had a research design and gave attention to appropriate quality control. The author chose a qualitative design appropriate to the purpose of the report and developed a qualitative content analysis tool, relying on knowledge gained from coursework.

The author's design decisions acknowledged the differences between qualitative and quantitative research and their appropriate uses (Krathwohl, 1998; Newman & Benz, 1998). Assessment of student learning involves a variety of quantitative and qualitative research strategies. On the other hand, assessing the progress of implementing an assessment plan depends on an accumulation of qualitative data. Such data needs chronological organization to track and evaluate progress. Detailed data could demonstrate positive change and progress, no progress, or even negative change since 1998 for each of five required categories of characteristics (NCA-HLC, 2003a). Further, to increase the perceived truth-value of report conclusions, such changes could be measured against a set of standards or accepted norms. Based on these criteria, the author designed the assessment project to chart and match documented institutional characteristics with those described in a rubric, the NCA Levels of Implementation, Patterns of Characteristics (2000).

Newman and Benz (1998) supplied more than a dozen specific criteria for systematically elevating the truth-value of the qualitative research design of the project report. Almost all of these criteria were met through the research plan for the project. In contrast, the 1998 self-study did not even have a research plan, just miscellaneous data gathering strategies without a consistent philosophical research paradigm. The lesson learned was that the quality of academic library research can benefit from the selection of appropriate research paradigms with integrated design.

Missing in the research process for the 2003 progress report was peer debriefing by someone external to the institution but familiar with accreditation expectations and guidelines and with student learning assessment (Newman & Benz, 1998). Having a critique by such a person(s) in dialog with the major stakeholders in the academic areas would have been a valuable exercise in shared learning (Senge, 1990). Such a critique could have helped build shared understanding and internal expertise and increased the planning value of the report (Newman & Benz, 1998, pp. 51–52). Nevertheless, the accrediting agency response to the progress report would provide a third-party critique, a strategy implicit in other aspects of its accreditation processes as well (Mulhern, 2000a).

The author also bridged the theory and practice of educational research in her design choices for project data gathering and evaluation. She discovered multiple internal interpretations of what had or had not been accomplished in learning assessment in the previous five years. As cautioned in the agency documents (NCA-HLC, 2000), a college's decentralized approach to assessment often hinders development of shared understandings. To both demonstrate and resolve this common organizational communication barrier, the author designed a chronology template as a way to systematically organize the qualitative data supplied by multiple sources. This template was flexible in accommodating different types of academic programs and the different interpretations of progress. Coding the data entries in the chronology spreadsheet identified common themes and eased sorting the data for later analysis.

In summary, the author learned to value systematic, systemic educational research as an intellectual bridge because it can provide a common information base for participants in any academic change process and a baseline for cycles of evaluation. The empirical research approach practiced by scientific scholars since the Enlightenment (Boorstin, 1983) remains fundamental to research in education (Willower & Forsyth, 1999). Even so, researchers can balance quantitative research strategies with ways to acquire and evaluate qualitative information about a complex culture and its activities (interactive continuum in Newman & Benz, 1998). Constructing this intellectual bridge allowed the author to move away from using self-taught research strategies based on descriptive input/output data. Accessing professional research terminology and techniques enabled her strengthen a goal-appropriate educational research design. With increased knowledge about assessment and research, she reports increased confidence in selecting library research projects appropriate to her skill set and with higher design quality.

BRIDGE 3: DEVELOPING INFORMED SENSITIVITY TO SOCIO-POLITICAL RELATIONSHIPS

This bridge connects the theory and application of building socio-political capital for leadership and change in academe. Constructing this bridge emphasizes the importance of learning why and how to value and achieve productive socio-political relationships. Since the author admits a level of naivete with regard to socio-political relationships, this bridge required significant personal reflection and growth in order to move toward a more effective professional practice.

Increased sensitivity to human relationships was implicit in the curriculum design of the author's degree program. Likewise, Kezar's (2001) explicit guidelines assert that understanding and facilitating change in academe means that committed educators/librarians must realize that such change is a human process requiring inclusive collegiality (p. 123). This human process has been viewed from different epistemological stances: the subjective, possessive individualism perspective (where the acquisition of knowledge is personal and competitive) or the relational perspective (where knowledge is ongoing, mutual meaning making among members of a group) (Dachler & Hosking, 1995).

Constructing this bridge clarified the dominance of politics and negotiation, assertion of power, power struggles, and occasional personality clashes in the day to day activities of academe (Brubacher & Rudy, 1997; Kowalski, 2001; illustrated in Duberman, 1972; Sarton, 1961; Smiley, 1996). By acknowledging the ubiquity of political motivations in human activities, academic leaders can strive to use political strategies unapologetically to leverage constructive change through negotiation and compromise with those with varying points of view (Brubacher & Rudy, 1997; Dachler & Hosking, 1995; Hanson, 1996; Havel, 1997; Kowalski, 2001). Alternatively, leaders sometimes can encourage networking where participants enjoy equity, collective authority and responsibility, and build new meanings through consideration of their differences (Dachler & Hosking, 1995). Regardless of approach, effective academic leaders are self-aware and proactive in their approaches to change.

The following portion of this paper describes the socio-political theories that can contribute to increased sensitivity to socio-political relationships and interest in the dynamics of organizational leadership. These theories include the role of precise language in communication, cognitive resource theory (CRT), social cognition theory, and the dominance of socio-political motivators in human interactions. Exposure to these theoretical concepts can increase the number of ways to analyze a situation; agreement with the theories is not required.

First, sensitivity to socio-political context increases when one understands that words and language depend on personal context and can be a barrier in processes of leadership and change. Precisely defined terminology is essential to improved critical thinking and analysis and to communication. To illustrate, consider the following common terms. In theory, there are differences between the terms *leadership* (creating vision and setting direction in an organization) and *management* (implementing vision and sustaining direction) (Hanson, 1996; Kotter, 1990, 1995). There also can be separate leadership and management structures and processes within one organization. Then, there are differences between the terms *leader* (person who performs leadership functions) and *leadership* (functions such as creating vision and setting direction of an organization, not necessarily tied to specific individuals) (Kotter, 1990; Schruijer & Vansina, 2002). In practice, these terms often are used interchangeably, laden with unspoken assumptions and conflicting expectations that can obstruct communication. In this single illustration, understanding theory elevates the importance of precise language as a tool for improving practice.

The terms manager, management, leader, and leadership just described are important to understanding expectations and responsibilities in academic activities. For example, the author discovered that she needed multiple types of power to fulfill dual roles as manager and leader in the progress report process (Yukl, 2002). She needed positional power to manage the progress report itself. At the same time, the report process offered an opportunity to help shape or facilitate the development of assessment processes, a leadership function.

For the 2003 report process, she had almost no positional power. As the president's appointee to the task, she could claim only that tenuous political tie and some small control of the flow of information (Yukl, 2002). Without sufficient positional power, such a project would be difficult to accomplish as a high-quality process and timely product. Ultimately, she bolstered support for project management through alliances with three administrators with sufficient positional management power. To assert leadership in assessment process development, she relied on her own expert and referent power developed from previous successes with other accreditation-driven activities.

Immersion in these problems of assessing leadership and management power and authority in a specific project provided the author a personal reference point for integrating socio-political theory with library practice. This experience also informed her consideration of leadership, power, and decision-making in non-traditional organizations such as library consortia, which figure prominently in the daily practice of most academic library directors today and where relational perspectives may prevail.

Another pertinent socio-political concept studied was Fiedler's cognitive resource theory (cited in Hanson, 1996, pp. 168–175). Fiedler contends that high-stress situations, as commonly experienced in organizations enduring budget and personnel reductions, call for relationship-motivated leadership (Hanson, 1996). Wildavsky (1997) might have said that a task orientation depends too much on pure intellect (p. 27), neglects social relationships, and expends energy without gaining value for the organization (Huxham, 1993). Dachler and Hosking (1995), Fiedler (Hanson, 1996); Vangen and Huxham (2003) and Wildavsky (1997) all call for much more leadership emphasis on building and sustaining productive human relationships, especially in complex organizations operating in a turbulent environment, thus, in perpetual high stress.

The author perceived personal growth as she consciously tested in practice two additional socio-political theories introduced in her studies: the interpersonal relationship implications of the theory of social cognition and the dominance of socio-political factors in interpersonal relationships.

Interpersonal Relationships and the Theory of Social Cognition

Briefly, the theory of social cognition suggests that each person's complex environment and social experiences influence how and what they know (Henson, 2003). Language, perceptions, judgments, and influences all have social origins. Knowledge, according to this theory, is constructed at a personal level through social experiences. This general theory of social knowledge construction was developed by such influential constructivist theorists as John Dewey and Lev Vygotsky (Dewey, 1938; Henson, 2003) and informs modern education. This theory provides a basis for such current academic leadership concepts as critical self-reflection, cooperative learning, learning communities as a medium for personal and institutional change, and the importance of such personal and institutional values as caring and justice (Kezar, 2001; Lenning & Ebbers, 1999; Mayeroff, 1971; Smeyers, 1999; University of Dayton, 2004). In light of the theory of social cognition, in a multi-cultural and multi-disciplinary academic environment, one should anticipate the diversity of knowledge and viewpoints likely represented among the stakeholders. One way academic and library leaders can anticipate and work with diversity is by supporting inclusive group processes.

Failing to recognize or even denying one's own unique cognitive lens can impede the work of an educator/librarian (Fine, 1994; Kezar, 2001). The author's own lens was problematic in both her studies and in her library practice. As a student, she was an older college administrator and librarian among mostly K-12 educators. Professionally, she was a white, female, Ohio born and educated librarian with 21 years of experience working in a historically black college administered by black males, most of whom were newcomers educated in other states and countries, primarily in fields other than education. She needed to acknowledge the implications of her own perspective in order to share in and benefit from their viewpoints. At the same time, given the diversity of the environment, the opportunities were great for learning from one another, for synergy to develop (Dewey, 1938; Sergiovanni, 1994). For example, as a former junior high teacher, the author appreciated being able to reconnect with K-12 teachers and their issues and then to apply that knowledge to the college's progress report as it related to basic skills deficits and remedial skills courses.

With regard to facilitating the progress report process, the author needed to consider that each individual to be involved in the project likely had a different understanding of assessment and the accreditation process, of the subtext of local politics and curriculum control, and even of interpersonal relationships. Instead of seeing a homogeneous group of dutiful college employees, the author consciously considered that the dozen distinct individuals, all dedicated professionals, were mostly multi-tasking to fulfill multiple roles. Their individual viewpoints on assessment would be shaped by their varying lengths of service in current positions, previous positive or negative experiences with accreditation issues, levels of morale depending on their professional and financial stability, cognitive approaches honed in specialty research, and differences based on age and gender. Awareness of differences grounded in race, nationality, and economic status could be relevant. In addition, home and health issues could be active. These same or similar considerations also are relevant when facilitating internal or campus-wide library or information literacy projects. Given such diversity, the goal is to identify relevant points and to acknowledge but set aside personal issues to envision a group *hologram* of a project or problem. The varied underlying assumptions, interpretation of data, and valuing of any project always need careful examination to assure valid positioning and acceptance within the organization.

During her intellectual journey, then, the author learned to tap into the creative synergy that exists within any group of people presenting rich and varied ways of knowing and different points of view. She learned that a project created autonomously lacks organizational authenticity but that obtaining complete consensus in any project is unrealistic. Instead she now values working toward inclusiveness, broad ownership, and mutual under-standing balanced with timely decision-making and project completion.

Interpersonal Relationships Translated through Socio-Political Theory

It is on the concept of organization as social process that such authors as Dachler and Hosking (1995), Kezar (2001), Tsoukas and Chia (2002), and Wildavsky (1997) intersect. These authors assert the dominance of socio-political relationships in human endeavors. Acknowledging these socio-political relationships as a powerful force in academic organizations was a critical learning experience for the author.

The following four examples illustrate the broad range and significant impact of dominating socio-political relationships on the 2003 progress re-port process. As a first example, the author identified functional silos as a barrier to effective communication on assessment. One writer called them chimneys (Helgesen, 1995, p. 34), spewing evidence of independent, closely held operations. Various participants will view key events differently based on their position in the organization and their sources of information and knowledge (Hanson, 1996, p. 52). With skill, however, a proactive leader can direct attention and energy toward finding the common goals of the organization. Instead of allowing the academic grapevine to announce changes along with highly embellished interpretations of these changes, change leaders can use positional, expert, or referent power to communicate vision directly (see Hanson, 1996, pp. 50–52; Kezar, 2001; Yukl, 2002).

Second, cognitive differences can be revealed in the different strategies for research and problem solving offered by faculty and librarians from various academic disciplinary backgrounds (Boorstin, 1983; Brubacher & Rudy,

1997). In the progress report process, science faculty associated assessment with standardized achievement tests and enrollment and retention statistical trends. Taking a quantitative approach to learning assessment, the science faculty agreed to and implemented their assessment plan much more quickly than other areas. Faculty teaching in the social sciences and the arts connected assessment with an array of assessment tools including complex personal narratives, portfolios, and career path achievements. Their planning progress was slower because of the complexity of their assessment choices and their projected higher assessment expenses in terms of cost and time. Taking note of the variety of cognitive approaches active in academe, librarians can plan for working in an environment of intellectual diversity, whether on campus or among other librarians in consortia.

Third, any hope for modeling a learning community as part of the report process was tempered by the cautions provided by Lenning and Ebbers (1999, pp. 96–97). They concluded that learning communities at the faculty level have been given lip service but few communities have been realized given the pressures of the faculty reward systems and their focus on activities within their disciplines. For any particular institution, there also may be heavy teaching loads acting as barriers to focusing faculty interest and energy on planning for student learning assessment or collaborating with librarians.

In the final example, socio-politics need not impede change initiatives (Helgesen, 1995). The author developed a positive working relationship with a key administrator who expedited the project. In cultivating this new and essential relationship, she was guided by a study of the theory of self-fulfilling prophecy, also known as the Pygmalion effect (Mulhern, 2002d). According to this theory, one's positive expectations often are met in human relationships.

As suggested by this review of the socio-political theories that can impact practice, acknowledging their significance obviously is important to every administrator (Hanson, 1996; Kezar, 2001; Wildavsky, 1997). Especially in academe and in the field of library and information science, the rational mind is idealized and classical theory has deep cognitive roots (Boorstin, 1983). The important role of social negotiation, assertion of power (politics), and complex ethical choices in the development of academic policy or library decision-making can go unacknowledged or denied in favor of what Wildavsky termed "pure intellect" (p. 27). Instead, research demonstrates that socio-political relationships dominate over the factor of intellectual rationality in the leadership of change in academe (Dachler & Hosking, 1995; Wildavsky, 1997, p. 32). In research for a course paper, the author observed how W. E. B. Du Bois revised his doctrine of the Talented Tenth later in his life as he moved from a speculative mode to his own life experience with the power of socio-politics (Mulhern, 2000b). As a result of this intellectual journey toward better understanding of socio-political factors, the author gained access to additional broadly useful critical thinking and leadership tools.

BRIDGE 4: DEVELOPING A PERSONAL CONTEXT-BASED MODEL OF CHANGE

For the author, the fourth intellectual bridge between theory and improved practice meant developing a personal, context-based model of organizational change based on her understanding of recent theories of complex change. Constructing the previous three bridges was good preparation for this fourth bridge. Kezar (2001) insists that the model may be personal but it must be broadly inclusive. Such a model evolves from environmental scanning and systematic/systematic evaluation of diverse stakeholders. It must be both flexible and balanced. It would be incomplete without consideration of how socio-political processes are made more complex by the unique characteristics of higher education and of the local institution.

The coursework emphasized developing such a personal model of change. Plato's (1975) Socrates, Havel (1997), and Tolstoy's (1993) Ivan Ilych were studied as examples of how a personal model for understanding societal change would be strengthened by strong and clear commitment to ethical issues such as caring and justice. Change for the sake of change lacks meaning and gains undue power when it operates under the leadership radar. Having a personal model of change assures a conscious connection between leadership and change processes (Kezar, 2001).

Researchers have found considerable agreement among studies for understanding the direct relationship between organizational change and leadership (Kezar, 2001; Tsoukas & Chia, 2002). They say that change emerges from the fluid and open-ended attempts of the leaders and followers in an organization to accommodate a kaleidoscope of environmental, social, and economic change factors. They find robust research support for the concept of leaders shaping change through socio-political relationships (the social cognition/learning and political/negotiation change models in Hanson, 1996; Kezar, 2001). Forming a personal model of change for a local organization increases the likelihood that the leader's own critical self-reflection on the interrelationships among vision, purposes, and values will acknowledge ongoing change (illustrated in the study of Havel, 1997; Iacocca & Novak, 1984).

With the change model in mind as an intellectual bridge, the author determined that her own contextual model for change would acknowledge her institution's irregular pattern of subtle incremental changes. Not atypical, these sporadic changes historically have occurred in response to narrow windows of opportunity opened by the stimulus of a new program chairperson or director, a grant proposal, or an NCA requirement. Given that pattern, evidence of student learning assessment progress and change would best be tracked at Tsoukas and Chia's (2002) microchange level, the source of incremental change. For the 2003 progress report, the author needed to identify clues to assessment progress (and non-progress) in the comments of the stakeholders and in existing documents of all kinds. Since changes typically were responsive and incremental, purposeful leadership could assist the institution's stakeholders in interpreting whether and how these small changes represented a holistic effort to increase student learning. Common acknowledgment of institutional progress in student learning, almost in spite of itself, could leverage the institution's stakeholders toward identifying their implicit common vision and then establishing explicit shared goals.

Tsoukas and Chia's Theory of Change

The author's personal model of change focuses on the significance of microchanges as presented in Tsoukas and Chia (2002). Although the author used this theory to make sense of the assessment process changes discovered to be relevant to the 2003 project, this theory has significance for understanding change in libraries as well.

This section explicates Tsoukas and Chia's (2002) theory of change and change leadership, which helps with understanding complex change (Mulhern, 2002b).

Microchanges and Change

Tsoukas and Chia's (2002) unique focus is on an organization's microchanges. Microchanges are real time, practical front-line human adjustments that diverge from routines and norms. According to their theory of change, change is continuous, natural, and neutral. Analysts later may try to track an organization through its accomplished changes and may label these changes as positive or negative depending on their cognitive lenses. Tsoukas and Chia (2002) criticize this traditional organizational research approach for failing to acknowledge the continuous motion, even commotion of change processes. Librarians can certainly identify with the image of commotion in the library field today. Tsoukas and Chia say that traditional organization researchers ignore the thousands of lost microchanges, the dead ends and missed opportunities, as well as the non-linear and openly fluid nature of change processes. They call on researchers to conduct more sensitive studies of microchanges, the overlooked fuel of change. Without this information, the authors contend that change in organizations continues to be reported as a predictable event, rather than as the non-linear, complex, and unpredictable process that it is (see also Mulhern, 2002b). This is certainly a postmodern analytical method, looking for what did not change, what changes died out, as well as what changes did become institutionalized (Carlson, 1997; Giroux, 1997).

Especially in the complex, loosely coupled organizations in higher education, including libraries, purposefully effecting major change goals is difficult. Instead, change is incremental. If a series of related microchanges gains common use in a library or among librarians and becomes institutionalized as a norm, only then has that organization changed. The only norms that emerge from change processes are those that naturally stabilize the organization within a given environment (Hall & Hord, 2001; Kezar, 2001; Tsoukas & Chia, 2002). Announcing change is easy; achieving an announced change is rare because of the power of established institutional norms. Postmodern theorists such as Giroux (1997) have explicated the highly conservative power of traditional norms in schooling. In colleges and universities, the strongest barriers to developing a learning assessment program (which implies change toward increased emphasis on the student) have been such traditional norms as faculty autonomy, instructional delivery by lecture, the faculty reward system, and the student grading system. Today, in a similar way, librarians can consider the strength of the norms for cataloging, bibliographic instruction, building design, and even library etiquette in the face of pressures for change driven by technology and students (De Rosa, Dempsey, & Wilson, 2004).

Replacement norms that may emerge from a change process are not always anticipated or desired by those within an organization. In addition, because of external environmental changes over time, existing norms may become ineffective or counter-productive, stimulating improvisation and informal microchanges even without leadership (Tsoukas & Chia, 2002). The 1995 NCA deadline for the development of student learning assessment plans in all its member institutions is a relevant example of one such external change that placed pressure to change on each college (NCA-CIHE, 1997). Certainly, in libraries, Google is exerting an external pressure that is driving change.

The Organization and Change

Rather than defining organization as a stable object as in classic organizational theory (Hanson, 1996), Tsoukas and Chia (2002) present it as an open, complex, and continuous social process that emerges because of change (p. 570). The authors define organizations as "situation-specific webs of social relations in which technology [or some other new factor] enters and modifies and, in turn, is modified" (p. 568). They see organization as a response to change. In its historical context, the academic library itself developed in response to change.

According to the Tsoukas and Chia (2002) theory of organizational change, change happens with or without facilitation. Change is ongoing and cannot be stopped. Leadership is the energy that shapes change toward a shared goal. Leadership can leverage further change by harnessing the momentum of change. Tsoukas and Chia's concept of leadership in an organization parallels the role of an attractor in increasing the chances of a chaotic state achieving stability in the physical sciences (Mulhern, 2002b; Wheatley & Kellner, 1996). An attractor works like a magnet, drawing together relevant factors. Organizational chaos theorists find intriguing the idea that effective leadership ncreases the chances of an organization coming together for periods of useful, relative stability between its natural periods of instability (Fullan, 1999; Mulhern, 2002b). The author thought that the 2003 progress report process could be an attractor capable of drawing diverse campus stakeholders together to strengthen horizontal socio-political relationships (Helgesen, 1995).

Some researchers have found a role for leadership in destabilizing an organization in order to release creative or reorganizing processes. This interesting view of leadership comes from a secondary concept derived from chaos theory, that change emerges only from periods of instability (Fullan, 1999; Merry, 1995; Wheatley & Kellner, 1996). Likewise, Hanson (1996) describes conflict (instability) as often very constructive and "inevitable" (p. 71) under the assumptions of social system or open system theories. Sources of conflict within an academic organization range broadly from collegial debate and competitive silo-based initiatives to allocation of scarce resources and ideas from new key administrators or faculty. An institutional accrediting agency, through its requirement for institutions to assess student learning, offers assessment as a means to destabilize the institution by decreasing complacency and encouraging purposeful and cyclical responses to self-identified weaknesses (NCA-HLC, 2004).

Classical organizational theory celebrates stability, suppresses conflict, and assumes that change, if it is to occur, can be planned and controlled by the leaders (Hanson, 1996). In contrast, open systems theory finds that constructive change grows out of conflict (Hanson). In turn, Tsoukas and Chia (2002) contend that while leaders can influence and shape the socio-political or human processes of organization and change, they cannot know or control the radiating consequences of change over time (Hanson). They do support purposeful, rational planning for short-term organizational objectives (the teleological/rational model of change, Kezar, 2001). In contrast, they contend that long-range planning to control change is unlikely to be successful. They conclude that leaders lead when they work to create social environments hospitable to selected types of improvisation and to micro-changes in selected areas (nudging) (see also Mulhern, 1999b). Compared to edicts, incremental nudging of the type and direction of change is more likely to be successful in complex organizations such as academic institutions, libraries, or consortia (see also Fullan quoted by Hanson, 1996, p. 307; Fullan, 1999; Kezar, 2001).

Model of Change for the Progress Report

As Kezar (2001) has indicated, leading change requires developing a personal context-based model of change (also Hanson, 1996, p. 307). At the time of the 1998 self-study project, the author had formed no local model for change nor had she considered change processes. She based the localized model for the 2003 progress report on Tsoukas and Chia's (2002) theory emphasizing the importance of microchanges. Based on that model, she verified how microchanges in assessment contributed incrementally to positive institutional change that might stimulate further improvisation and microchanges. She also included evidence of failed microchanges since these revealed areas of risk taking and an assessment interest or need.

The author's change model for the progress report included a vision of its potential to influence the direction of organizational change. Of Hanson's (1996) change agent functions of catalyst, solution giver, process helper, or resource linker, she considered herself a process helper (p. 307). The report itself had the potential to become a catalyst to improve the student learning assessment process. One way to increase the likelihood of achieving longer-term assessment goals was to expand the assessment process web of inclusion (Helgesen, 1995), beginning with the progress report process itself. Strategies to increase stakeholder inclusion would increase the likelihood of broader ownership of the process. Potentially, the learning assessment process could become institutionalized over time.

The author's coursework suggested that educational leaders need to acknowledge organizational change directly, reflectively, and intentionally.

Such an approach assures that the change leader has considered the dynamics and ethics of the change process and assumes responsibility for leadership strategies that will have the greatest positive influence on an envisioned direction for change.

Flake and Williams (1999) offer insights on the responsibilities of a leader similar to those just described. They move beyond Kezar (2001) with change leadership guidelines that fight the drag of inertia and compel change. They recommend two steps to intentionally destabilize the status quo. With these two steps, take the lead and stretch, they anticipate the practical application of Tsoukas and Chia's (2002) theory of change that depends on proactive human improvisation. Other writers focus on the role of personal values as a leadership driver, motivating a leader to take a stand, take the lead, stretch, and even withdraw (see especially Giroux, 1997; Carlson, 1997). Leading at any level requires an active exploration of the environment with the intent of facilitating ethical problem-solving changes, regardless of existing norms. To evaluate leadership with integrity in practice, the author read Lee Iacocca's autobiography (with Novak, 1984) and shadowed Tom Sanville, head of the library consortium OhioLINK, for insights about leading with stretch and risk (Mulhern, 1999b). Other proactive leaders studied in the program included Jesus (Jones, 1995), Vaclav Havel (1997), and Helgesen's (1995) inclusive leaders.

Based on learning about leadership and change as a student and through continued reading, the author gave greater attention to change processes in the 2003 progress report compared to the 1998 self-study. She considered how conflict affected the participants and their motivation to selectively embrace change processes.

In summary, to construct this intellectual bridge related to developing a personal model of change, one must integrate learning from a focused study of organizational change, leadership, and ethics. Crossing this bridge enabled the learner to accept the concept of complex change processes being shaped but not necessarily controlled by leadership in our institutions and in our libraries.

BRIDGE 5: STRIVING FOR FLEXIBILITY AND CREATIVITY

During her intellectual journey, the author learned of the importance for those leading change processes in academe to be open to surprises and to focus on creativity (Kezar, 2001). Given the dominance of the power of socio-political relationships, it is imperative to anticipate impact of the various motivations and complex social interactions involved in any activity and still be ready to be surprised.

Proactive creativity also is important for effective change leadership. Even minor initiatives can contribute to achieving the organization's greater vision. To illustrate, the natural sciences faculty in the author's college brainstormed a list of expected common learning outcomes for science majors. Senior-level students, in turn, used the list to reflect on their own learning experiences and then pointed out a lack of course emphasis on certain outcome topics. Faculty used the student critiques to make changes in the curriculum. In this case, cyclic curriculum revision, one of the most important goals of student learning assessment, began with minimum effort and maximum effect. The next step would be to review the learning expectation list with students new to the majors. Ethically, clear delineation of learning expectations to new and prospective students is one strategy for making good matches between students and programs and motivating their active participation in their own learning (NCA-HLC, 2003a). Library information literacy and bibliographic instruction learning objectives that correlate explicitly with institutional and field-specific learning goals can reinforce such active learning (Calderhead, 2000). Ultimately, active and successful student learners are important to the long-term vitality of the institution through student retention and student-to-student recruitment (Levine & Cureton, 1998).

BRIDGE 6: LEARNING TO BALANCE ETHICAL LEADERSHIP AND FOLLOWERSHIP

The author learned about purposeful balance from courses on institutional culture, leadership ethics, and organizational theory. Building the intellectual bridge between the theory and practice of ethical leadership prompted a review of examples of the types of balance important to facilitating the progress report or leading change in libraries. It is important to maintain a balance between one's internal, personal, and professional lives, especially in terms of determining ethical priorities and ethically fulfilling the role of leader or follower.

Ethical Priorities

At several points in the 2003 progress report project, the author was forced to balance conducting the business of education with sustaining caring social and professional relationships for the benefit of both the participants and the institution (Mayeroff, 1971; Mulhern, 2000b). Two classic ethical dilemmas (present good vs. future good, individual vs. the community) commonly confront educational leaders. These dilemmas that became relevant to the assessment project grew out of sharp differences in professional opinion and a competitive assertion of authority, part of the daily interplay of diversity in all academic organizations.

Achieving and sustaining balance is becoming ever more important in any workplace. The educational leader, whether a general administrator or a library director, can attain a sense of ethical balance and proportion from a combination of study, reflection, and practical experience.

Leadership/Followership

As a second example of the importance of balance, effective followership is essential to effective leadership. Joseph C. Rost (1995) analyzed the relationships between leaders and followers and between leaders and managers. He describes how one individual can find himself/herself alternately leading, managing, and following, always sensitive to the situation (see also Chaleff, 1995; Gardner, 1995; Havel, 1997). According to Rost, and very much in concert with the human processes described by Kezar (2001) and Tsoukas and Chia (2002), "followers and leaders do leadership" (p. 192). The effectiveness of leadership depends on skillful socio-political negotiation and the construction of shared meanings (Dachler & Hosking, 1995). For example, an administrator who met Chaleff's definition of a courageous follower supported the author's progress report project. He was very active in working with her in a shared meaning process. As a courageous follower, he also was implementing the college president's vision in other campus venues. Observing the dynamics of these two key administrators was a good illustration of the leadership–followership process since administrators such as academic library directors effectively lead as they follow.

CONCLUSION

Prompted by her graduate studies, the author's intellectual journey featured the construction of six bridges between theory and practice in educational leadership and academic librarianship. It has been and continues to be a valuable journey to the author as library director in a small college. Constructing each of these bridges required tests in practice of the speculative or theoretical knowledge attained through an academic program focused on leadership and change in higher education. The author learned to distinguish between leading (really influencing) the process of change and reacting to change. To participate more effectively in change leadership in academe, she learned how to select, design, and implement educational research and information gathering to obtain appropriate truth-value. She learned to recognize in herself and in others how complex variations in cognitive viewpoints affect social and political relationships. She learned to examine personal and professional choices, relationships, and potential actions reflectively and critically.

Throughout the process of working on her 2002 institutional report project, the author kept a reflective journal of her thoughts and behaviors. She used the 1998 project as a prior benchmark for self-assessing personal learning. From that comparative analysis, enriched by knowledge gained from her formal course of study, she reached several conclusions relevant to professional library practice. These conclusions form an intellectual foundation for research and for practice. First, an aspiring library leader and change agent needs to know about organizations in higher education and how their unique characteristics impact leadership and change processes. Second, to support change processes through ongoing assessment and evaluation, one needs technical skills in the areas of research and critical evaluation. Third, to be proactive in influencing the direction of change processes, leaders must draw on informed critical self-awareness and reflection, flexibility, and creativity, especially in order to negotiate productive socio-political relationships. Finally, appropriate balance must be achieved in terms of ethics and the responsibilities of leadership/followership.

With such knowledge and skills identified and developed through her recent experience as a graduate student, the author has assumed greater leadership risks in practice. She approaches challenges with greater confidence, greater patience, and more realistic expectations based on her personal and customized model of change leadership. Her studies have helped her develop greater social capital as well as intellectual capital (Weidman, Twale, & Stein, 2001).

This paper has demonstrated how library practice can be been affected positively by integrating important theoretical concepts of academic leadership and leadership for change. The identification of six learning outcomes/bridges between theory and practice was grounded in research reported by Kezar (2001) and Tsoukas and Chia (2002), and supported by many other sources (especially Carlson, 1997; Eisner, 1994; Fullan, 1999; Hall & Hord, 2001; Hanson, 1996; Helgesen, 1995; Yukl, 2002). This paper concludes with the author's personal statement on the broad function of leadership in higher education, appropriate to leadership in academic libraries. Implicit in the statement is her renewed passion for her profession. This emerging personal definition of leadership bears the marks of theory and the scars of experience obtained during a productive intellectual journey that continues:

> Essentially transformational in vision, leadership in loosely coupled educational institutions is a social process that purposefully establishes and strengthens the web of socio-political relationships necessary to accomplish a common purpose. The goal of leadership is increased capacity within an institution to capitalize on change to better accomplish the common purpose. As a part of the leadership process, leaders help members of an organization define and focus on vision – a holistic sensemaking of the goals and purposes of the organization or of one of its departments or projects. Leaders use such tools as critical self-reflection, rational analysis, and open communication to help locate and privilege opportunities for change. While administrative leaders certainly have a responsibility for leadership, others within the organization are key players as well, being both committed leaders in their own right and courageous followers.

REFERENCES

Allen, W. R., & Jewell, J. O. (2002). A backward glance forward: Past, present, and future perspectives on historically black colleges and universities. *The Review of Higher Education, 25,* 241–261.

Baldrige, B. (2001). *Education criteria for performance excellence (brochure).* Gaithersburg, MD: Baldrige National Quality Program.

Boorstin, D. (1983). *The discoverers: A history of man's search to know his world and himself.* New York: Random House.

Brubacher, J. S., & Rudy, W. (1997). *Higher education in transition: A history of American colleges and universities* (4th ed.). New Brunswick, NJ: Transaction.

Calderhead, V. (2000). Reflections on information confusion in chemistry information learning: The meaning of the shift from library instruction to information literacy. *Research Strategies, 16*(4), 285–299.

Carlson, D. (1997). *Making progress: Education and culture in new times.* New York: Teachers College Press.

Chaleff, I. (1995). *The courageous follower: Standing up to and for our leaders.* San Francisco, CA: Berrett-Koehler Publishers.

Dachler, H. P., & Hosking, D. (1995). The primacy of relations in socially constructing organizational realities. In: D. Hosking, H. P. Dachler & K. J. Gergen (Eds), *Management and organization: Relational alternatives to individualism* (pp. 1–28). Aldershot, England: Avebury.

De Rosa, C., Dempsey, L., & Wilson, A. (2004) *The 2003 OCLC environmental scan: Pattern recognition, a report to the OCLC membership.* Research report. OCLC Online Computer Library Center, Inc., Dublin, OH.

Dewey, J. (1938). *Experience and education.* New York: Macmillan.

Duberman, M. (1972). *Black mountain: An exploration in community.* New York: W. W. Norton.

Eisner, E. W. (1994). *The educational imagination: On the design and evaluation of school programs* (3rd ed.). Upper Saddle River, NJ: Prentice-Hall.

Ewell, P. (1997). The role of states and accreditors in shaping assessment practice. In: L. F. Goodchild, C. Lovell, E. R. Hines & J. I. Gill (Eds), *Public policy and higher education* (pp. 305–314). Needham Heights, MA: Simon & Schuster.

Fine, M. (1994). Working the hyphens. In: N. K. Denzin & Y. S. Lincoln (Eds), *Handbook of qualitative research* (pp. 70–82). Thousand Oaks, CA: Sage.

Flake, F. H., & Williams, D. M. (1999). *The way of the bootstrapper: Nine action steps for achieving your dreams.* San Francisco, CA: Harper.

Freeman, K., & Thomas, G. E. (2002). Black colleges and college choice: Characteristics of students who choose HBCUs. *The Review of Higher Education, 25,* 349–358.

Fullan, M. (1999). *Change forces: The sequel.* Philadelphia, PA: Falmer Press.

Gardner, J. N. (1995). Leaders and followers. In: J. T. Wren (Ed.), *The leader's companion: Insights on leadership through the ages* (pp. 185–188). New York: Free Press.

Giroux, H. A. (1997). *Pedagogy and the politics of hope: Theory, culture, and schooling; a critical reader.* Boulder, CO: Westview Press.

Goodchild, L. F., Lovell, C. D., Hines, E. R., & Gill, J. I. (Eds) (1997). *Public policy and higher education.* Needham Heights, MA: Simon & Schuster.

Hall, G. E., & Hord, S. M. (2001). *Implementing change: Patterns, principles, and potholes.* Boston, MA: Allyn & Bacon.

Hanson, E. M. (1996). *Educational administration and organizational behavior.* Boston, MA: Allyn and Bacon.

Havel, V. (1997). *The art of the impossible: Politics as morality in practice.* New York: Knopf.

Helgesen, S. (1995). *The web of inclusion: A new architecture for building great organizations.* New York: Currency/Doubleday.

Henson, K. T. (2003). Foundation for learner-centered education: A knowledge base. *Education, 124,* 5–16.

Huxham, C. (1993). Collaborative capability: An intraorganizational perspective on collaborative advantage. *Public Money and Management, 13,* 21–28.

Iacocca, L. A., & Novak, W. (1984). *Iacocca, an autobiography.* New York: Bantam.

Jones, L. B. (1995). *Jesus, CEO: Using ancient wisdom for visionary leadership.* NY: Hyperion.

Kezar, A. J. (2001). *Understanding and facilitating organizational change in the 21st century: Recent research and conceptualizations.* San Francisco, CA: Jossey-Bass.

Kezar, A. J., & Eckel, P. (Eds) (2000). *Moving beyond the gap between research and practice in higher education.* San Francisco, CA: Jossey-Bass.

Kotter, J. P. (1990). *A force for change: How leadership differs from management.* New York: Free Press.

Kotter, J. P. (1995). What leaders really do. In: J. T. Wren (Ed.), *The leader's companion: Insights on leadership through the ages* (pp. 114–123). New York: Free Press.

Kowalski, T. J. (2001). *Case studies on educational administration* (3rd ed.). New York: Longman.

Krathwohl, D. R. (1998). *Methods of educational and social science research* (2nd ed.). New York: Longman.

Lenning, O. T., & Ebbers, L. H. (1999). *The powerful potential of learning communities: Improving education for the future.* Washington, DC: The George Washington University, Graduate School of Education and Human Development.

Levine, A., & Cureton, J. S. (1998). *When hope and fear collide: A portrait of today's college student.* San Francisco, CA: Jossey-Bass.

Mayeroff, M. (1971). *On caring.* New York: Harper Collins.

Mentkowski, M. (2000). *Learning that lasts: Integrating learning, development, and performance in college and beyond.* San Francisco, CA: Jossey-Bass.

Merry, U. (1995). *Coping with uncertainty: Insights from the new sciences of chaos, self-organization, and complexity.* Westport, CN: Praeger.

Mezirow, J. (Ed.) (1990). *Fostering critical reflection in adulthood: A guide to transformative and emancipatory learning.* San Francisco, CA: Jossey-Bass.

Mulhern, J. (1999b). *Tom Sanville, Executive Director of the Ohio Library and Information Network (OhioLINK): Making it up as "we" go.* Unpublished project portfolio. University of Dayton, Dayton, OH.

Mulhern, J. (2000a). Facing (and listening) to the music: Effective use of the third party comment process. In: S. E. Van Kollenburg (Ed.), *A collection of papers of self-study and institutional improvement* (pp. 384–387). Chicago, IL: North Central Association-CIHE.

Mulhern, J. (2000b). *From talented tenth to guiding hundredth: Tracing the evolution of W.E.B. Du Bois' race leadership concept in his writings related to Wilberforce University* [research paper]. Unpublished Manuscript. University of Dayton, Dayton, OH.

Mulhern, J. (2002b). *Chaos theory: Is this butterfly causing a flap in organization theory?* Unpublished paper. University of Dayton, Dayton, OH.

Mulhern, J. (2002c). Current issues in higher education quality assurance – An overview for academic library administrators. In: E. D. Garten & D. E. Williams (Eds), *Advances in library administration and organization* (Vol. 19, pp. 137–164). Amsterdam: JAI/Elsevier.

Mulhern, J. (2002d). *Self-fulfilling prophecy or the Pygmalion effect: An overview for school librarians.* Unpublished paper. Syracuse University, Sysracuse, NY.

Newman, I., & Benz, C. R. (1998). *Qualitative–quantitative research methodology: Exploring the interactive continuum.* Carbondale, IL: Southern Illinois University Press.

North Central Association of Colleges and Schools, Commission on Institutions of Higher Education (NCA-CIHE). (1997). *Handbook of accreditation* (2nd ed.). Chicago: NCA-CIHE.

North Central Association of Colleges and Schools, Higher Learning Commission. (NCA-HLC). (2000). *Levels of implementation – patterns of characteristics: Addendum to the handbook of accreditation* (2nd ed., pp. 8–13). Chicago: NCA-HLC.

North Central Association of Colleges and Schools, Higher Learning Commission (NCA-HLC). (2003a). *Commission statement on assessment of student learning* (Adopted February 21, 2003). Chicago: NCA-HLC. Retrieved July 7, 2004, from www.ncahigherlearningcommission.org/resources/positionstatements/assessment/

North Central Association of Colleges and Schools, Higher Learning Commission (NCA-HLC). (2003b). *Handbook of accreditation* (3rd ed.). Chicago: NCA-HLC.

North Central Association of College and Schools, Higher Learning Commission (NCA-HLC). (2004). *Assessment resources.* Retrieved February 21, 2004, from www. ncahigherlearningcommission.org/resources/assessment/index.html

Plato (1975). *The trial and death of Socrates.* Indianapolis, IN: Hackett (G. M. A. Grube, Trans).

Rost, J. C. (1995). Leaders and followers are the people in this relationship. In: J. T. Wren (Ed.), *The leader's companion: Insights on leadership through the ages* (pp. 189–192). New York: The Free Press.

Sarton, M. (1961). *The small room*. New York: W. W. Norton.

Schruijer, S. G. L., & Vansina, L. (2002). Leader, leadership and leading; from individual characteristics to relating in context. *Journal of Organizational Behavior, 23*, 869–874.

Senge, P. (1990). *Fifth discipline*. New York, NY: Doubleday.

Sergiovanni, T. J. (1994). Organizations or communities? Changing the metaphor changes the theory. *Educational Administration Quarterly, 30*, 214–226.

Smeyers, P. (1999). "Care" and wider ethical issues. *Journal of Philosophy of Education, 33*, 233–251.

Smiley, J. (1996). *Moo*. New York: Ballentine Books.

Tolstoy, L. (1993). The death of Ivan Ilych. In: G. Gibian (Ed.), *The portable nineteenth-century Russian reader* (pp. 440–489). New York: Penguin.

Tsoukas, H., & Chia, R. (2002). On organizational becoming: Rethinking organizational change. *Organization Science, 13*, 567–582.

University of Dayton (2004). *Mission statement for the Ph.D. program in educational leadership*. School of education and allied professions. Retrieved July 7, 2004, from www.soeap.udayton.edu/doctoral/index.htm

Vangen, S., & Huxham, C. (2003). *Nurturing collaborative relations: Building trust in interorganizational collaboration*. Working paper. Glasgow, UK.

Weidman, J. C., Twale, D. J., & Stein, E. L. (2001). *Socialization of graduate and professional students in higher education: A perilous passage?* San Francisco, CA: Jossey-Bass.

Wheatley, M. J., & Kellner-Rogers, M. (1996). *A simpler way*. San Francisco, CA: Berrett-Koehler.

Wildavsky, A. (1997). Between planning and politics: Intellect vs. interaction as analysis. In: L. F. Goodchild, C. D. Lovell, E. R. Hines & J. I. Gill (Eds), *Public policy and higher education* (pp. 26–45). Needham Heights, MA: Simon & Schuster Custom Publishing.

Willower, D. J., & Forsyth, P. B. (1999). A brief history of scholarship on educational administration. In: J. Murphy & K. L. Seashore (Eds), *Handbook of research on educational administration* (2nd ed., pp. 1–24). San Francisco, CA: Jossey-Bass.

Yukl, G. (2002). *Leadership in organizations* (5th ed.). Upper Saddle River, NJ: Prentice-Hall.

COUNTING PERFORMANCE: PERCEPTIONS AND RESOURCES OF PERFORMANCE ASSESSMENT IN FLORIDA PUBLIC LIBRARIES

Larry Nash White

INTRODUCTION

There have been many challenges and uncertainties in determining the future direction(s) for performance measurement (PM) in Florida public libraries over the years. Social pressures for establishing increased accountability and community needs combined with the library administrators need to respond to these pressures served as the catalysts for the need to evolve PM processes in Florida public libraries.

The need to determine the current status of PM in Florida's public libraries is paramount before further understanding of the use and perceptions of PM could be achieved and actions to correctly promote the evolution of PM could be initiated. Under these conditions, Florida public library administrators attempting to alter or improve their reporting or utilization of PM, without a clear understanding of their individual and the overall PM environments (i.e. reporting, usage, impact, and effectiveness), could actually limit their abilities to succeed. Before public library administrators could initiate any PM initiatives to better respond to the social and political changes effecting their libraries and library service delivery, they

Advances in Library Administration and Organization, Volume 23, 85–140
Copyright © 2006 by Elsevier Ltd.
ISSN: 0732-0671/doi:10.1016/S0732-0671(05)23003-1

would first need an assessment of the current status of PM in public libraries. Reviewing the costs and resources used to conduct PM in Florida public
libraries was also needed to determine if the PM process was viably funded
by libraries to produce the desired positive results.

STATEMENT OF PROBLEM

In 2002, the public libraries in the State of Florida began experiencing a
series of challenges to the traditional accountability of public library service.
The most dramatic challenge was the significant statewide growth in the
service population (SP). The total population of the state of Florida grew
at a rate of 23.5% from 1990 to 2000 (U.S. Census Bureau, 2000). In FY
1999–2000, public library administrative units (LAUs) in Florida provided
information access and services to approximately 16 million residents
through approximately 490 service outlets in 75 LAUs at a cost of approximately $363,901,438 (Florida Public Library Directory with Statistics,
2001, p. 153). Other population-related affects on public library services
from Florida's rapid population growth over the last five years are depicted
in Table 1.

Florida public libraries have a long history of reporting organizational
performance. Florida public library administrators began voluntarily re-
porting PM outputs to the State Library of Florida in 1947. In 1960,
Florida's public libraries were then required to report to the State Library of
Florida a collection of performance outputs as a result of the passage of
Chapter 257 of the Florida Statutes establishing State Aid for Public

Table 1. Selected Florida Libraries Statistical Information for FY
1994–1995 to FY 1998–1999.

Statistical Category	FY 1994–1995	FY 1998–1999	Difference
Library expenditure/capita	$17.34	$19.21	+ 10.78%
Staff expenditure/capita	$9.89	$11.53	+ 16.58%
Total paid staff	4,976	5,458	+ 9.69%
Circulation of materials	70,109,292	73,899,704	+ 5.41%
Circulation/capita	5.19	4.78	−7.90%
Library visits	52,189,469	49,358,853	−4.85%
Total program attendance	3,785,765	2,955,823	−21.92%
Web site hits	N/A	21,713,633*	N/A
Patron log ons	N/A	4,381,582*	N/A

*Statistics not kept unit FY 1998–1999.

Libraries. In 2002, reporting output measures (OM) was only required if the LAU wished to qualify to receive financial aid from the State of Florida.

Each Florida public LAU must submit an annual plan of service and a long-range plan of service to receive financial aid from the State of Florida. Both plans describe the service roles of the library. The plans provide public library administrators and stakeholders with a publicly known and agreed upon course of action for reporting organizational performance. When the annual plan of service is used in conjunction with effective PMs to evaluate and report the annual efforts of the libraries, Florida public library administrators are able to effectively report PM results to stakeholders and identify deficiencies in service provision.

In 2002, state statutes did not include an evaluation component for either plan of service in Florida. In addition, of the annual plans of service and long-range plans of service on file at the State Library of Florida Grants Office, which administers the dispersement of State Aid (SA), only 18 of the submitted strategic plans of service mentioned "performance measurement." The plans mentioning PM did not provide any details of the PM nor did the plans indicate how the results of PM would be utilized by the library administration.

A theoretical model of the PM process operating in Florida public libraries was designed by the author in order to aid the study of the problem (White, 2002, p. 11). The theoretical model used in this study is portrayed in Fig. 1. The model describes the PM process components as they reside in and interact with the Culture of Assessment, the Organizational Culture, and Organizational Boundaries. The PM process components consist of Planning and Acquisition, Resources, Activities, Outputs, Evaluation, and Information.

Theoretically, as an organization proceeds through the PM process, the results of each component's activities are used to initiate the next component's actions. When the "Information" component is completed, the resulting data and information is then utilized by library administrators to provide corrective feedback at each step of the process and to address accountability, service quality, or other stakeholder concerns, i.e. the two purposes of PM in this study. The feedback from library administrators into the PM process was directed to each component of the process in order to improve the overall effectiveness of the process.

While there has been a great deal of research in library professional literature on the first four components of the PM models: i.e. Planning and Acquisitions, Resources, Activities, and Outputs, there have been no identified research efforts in the actual usage and perceived impacts of PM, i.e.

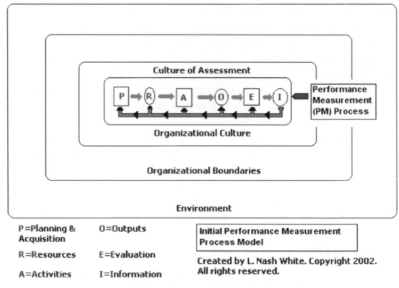

Fig. 1. Initial Performance Measurement (PM) Model.

Evaluation and Information. As of 2002, no identified studies had been conducted on how the results of PM were used to report organizational performance to public library stakeholders generally or the use and perceptions of PM in Florida public libraries. The survey instrument designed for the study focused the data collection on evaluating the "Evaluation" and "Information" components of the theoretical model in order to determine how PM was used, the perceived impact of using PM, and how the resulting information was used to address stakeholder concerns.

OVERARCHING QUESTIONS

Certain questions needed to be addressed in the study in order to conduct the evaluative study of the "Evaluation" and "Information" components of the theoretical model. These questions became the overarching questions of the study.

Question 1. What types of performance measures were used in Florida's public libraries?

Question 2. What were the current perceptions of public library administrators regarding performance measurement in Florida's public libraries?

Question 3. What resources were being allocated for performance measurement in Florida's public libraries?

Question 4. Were there any correlations between the amount of experience of head library administrators and the usage and perceptions of impact of performance measurement in Florida's public libraries?

Question 5. Were there any correlations between the amount of experience of head library administrators and the resources allocated to conduct performance measurement in Florida's public libraries?

Question 6. Did demographic factors such as the service population size or whether libraries received State Aid affect the use and perceived impact of performance measurement in Florida's public libraries? (White, 2002, pp. 14–15).

LIMITATIONS AND ASSUMPTIONS

The limitations of the study were:

- The survey population was limited to the 75 head public library administrators in the State of Florida.
- Because the work experience of the researcher provided the researcher with working relationships with many of the members of the sample population, precautions were taken to inhibit bias in the data interpretation through dealing with all data analysis and interpretation anonymously.
- The results of the study were not generalizable to other types of libraries in Florida or public libraries in other states.
- The available time and financial resources of the researcher limited the study and survey delivery designs.

The assumptions of the study were:

- Head public library administrators actively engage in the PM processes in their LAUs.
- Head public library administrators have the interest/desire to effectively report organizational PMs to stakeholders including governing bodies.

- Head public library administrators have an interest in understanding the current status, developments, and trends of PM in Florida public libraries.
- Head library administrators (HLAs) have the necessary technical skills to complete and return the survey instrument to the researcher in an electronic environment.
- Library administrators would complete this study's survey instrument in an accurate and objective manner.

DEFINITION OF TERMS

The definitions provided were considered the conceptual definitions of the survey and employed methodology. The abbreviations included with the definitions are used throughout the study.

Head Library Administrators (HLAs). The study participants were the head public library administrators of Florida. In this study, HLAs were defined as either the HLA or the assistant HLA who was primarily responsible for conducting PM in the 75 public LAUs, regardless of time of tenure. (White, 2002, p. 16)

Library Administrative Units (LAUs). An LAU was a political subdivision or geographical service area which the library was established to service and from which the library primarily derives its revenue. The LAU of Florida were further categorized into the following service areas: city, county, and regional for purposes of this study. (White, 2002, p. 17)

Performance Measurement (PM). A process of collecting organizational data on the current state of organizational achievement, resource use, and customer relationships that enables administrators to communicate organizational performance to stakeholders in terms of efficiency and accountability. (White, 2002, p. 17)

Output Measures (OM). The indicators of the quantity or quality of service(s) resulting from library activities. (White, 2002, p. 17)

REVIEW OF THE LITERATURE

A general overview of the literature of PM is provided that includes an overview of the current status of PM in public libraries and an in-depth review of the use of PM in Florida public libraries.

Overview of Performance Measurement

Evaluating business organizations was simple until the mid-18th century. Business organizations consisted mostly of families who shared the responsibilities of work and worked for the common good. Success was measured in the strict terms of financial reward and organizational survivability. However, with the advent of the Industrial Revolution, many business organizations began to grow both in size and in complexity. It was during this period of growth that Adam Smith stated that, by dividing labor into smaller, specialized tasks, efficiency would improve and production costs would decrease. In related performance literature, Robert Owen wrote in 1813 that managers should pay as much attention to the people working in a company as they did to the machinery. Owen's work was the beginning of the study of organizational dynamics and organizational administration, work designed to gauge how the (efficiency) of work contributions of individual or small specialized groups related to the overall performance of a company.

The need for organizations to harness greater amounts of efficiency from machinery and people increased due to the effects of the advances in communications and technology during the late 19th and early 20th century. Businesses began to access markets that were previously closed to their goods through the use of such devices as the telegraph and railroads. Businesses and industrial plants grew and serviced larger geographical areas of the world. The geographic reach of businesses caused organizational size and complexity to increase further. Businesses required more employees and opened new facilities with increasingly mechanized production technologies, further complicating the operation of their organizations. Obtaining greater amounts of efficiency and reducing cost in producing or providing goods and services became of paramount importance to owners and stockholders during this expansion of global markets.

From the mid-19th to the early 20th century, most administrative or performance research was based on the perception by business managers and owners that increasingly higher levels of efficiency were possible and necessary to maintain or increase profitably. Because of the broader global markets, business owners and managers found themselves in an increasingly competitive arena. Businesses that could produce large quantities of goods at the highest level of efficiency and thus an affordable cost in a highly competitive market were deemed to be the most successful, with success being measured solely on the scale of profitability for business owners and stockholders. Business owners and stockholders believed that increased profitability was to be accomplished only through increased organizational efficiency and cost reduction.

It was with the viewpoint of generating the highest efficiency and in reducing costs in the workplace that in 1885 Henry Metcalfe used his observational studies of soldiers in a military arsenal to advocate that the "science of administration" would be beneficial to managers. Work organization research led to the field of scientific management. Louis Brandeis coined the phrase "scientific management" in 1910 when he stated before the Interstate Commerce Commission that through scientific management of resources and men, the nation's railroads could save over $1 million a day (Shafritz & Ott, 1997, p. 11).

While Brandeis may have coined the term scientific management, its father is considered to be Frederick Taylor. Taylor conducted a series of scientific time and motion studies on different groups of workers in order to determine the most efficient way to accomplish tasks, thus reducing costs. It is from Taylor's work, as well as other PM researchers, that many of today's PM systems derive their scientific or analytical qualities.

Scientific management researchers such as Taylor attempted to organize workers and resources into effective, scientific patterns of operation in order to improve production and reduce costs of an industrial or commercial plant. The organizing process focused on determining the most effective size and operation of an organization to maximize the quantity of work produced, but not necessarily the quality of the work. Emphasis was placed on management's absolute control of the organization and its employees as the primary means to achieve increased productivity, efficiency, and cost reduction. In order to determine the performance of organizations under this philosophy, managers measured the efficiency, degree of control, and profitability of the organization. The high quantity-control style of operations management and PM continued through the early 20th century up through the post-World War II era.

The emphasis of scientific organizational control and optimization of the quantity of work slowly shifted to an emphasis on quality after the post-World War II era. In the late 1950s and early 1960s, advances in communications and technology were again providing the foundation for the expansion of the global economy. These advances allowed new competitors and products into older competitive markets where they had never been before. Because of increased competition, many business organizations seeking a competitive edge were forced to switch from a focus on providing and delivering large quantities of affordable, but cheaply produced goods and services, to a focus on providing and delivering high-quality goods and services.

The culture of business organizations was affected by this change in production philosophy. New organizational structures, values, and practices that supported the quality production philosophy were encouraged, created, and rewarded. New types of PM methodologies and measures were created to assist business owners and managers in evaluating the production and service quality of their organizations. It was during this period that such quality-driven, cost accountability tools as total quality control (TQC), total quality management (TQM), reengineering, and the like became prevalent. Business organizations emphasized and prioritized the quality of work. The new quality-driven, cost accountable PM tools enhanced the administrator's ability to monitor the quality of production through tight control of resources, staff, and processes to reduce costs and improve the quality of products and services by using PM information to identify problems and make corrective changes in organizational processes.

Quality-driven, cost accountable PM tools also enabled managers to address their stockholders' demands for accountability and quality performance by providing them with tangible and mutually understood performance information. Customers and stockholders began appreciating, because of increased service quality, profitability, and/or access to accountability information, the new competitive practice of quality management and began to expect such control, accountability, and quality assessment in the social and political aspects of their lives.

The quality-driven, cost accountable production culture of businesses began to encroach on the overall societal culture in the mid-1990s. The culture encroachment began in the early 1990s into government agencies, community service groups, and other nonprofit organizations that began incorporating qualitative PM methodologies and measures into their traditional quantitative PM systems. The qualitative PM was appealing to many nonprofit organizations and their stakeholders. The interest by nonprofit administrators and stakeholders in the shift from quantitative to quality-driven, cost accountable PM was due in large part to the growing number of increasingly difficult inquiries related to accountability facing administrators and stakeholders of nonprofit organizations. Nonprofit administrators found it increasingly difficult to answer public concerns about the effective or efficient delivery of public services as their stakeholders made inquiries regarding the impact of the service provided. Nonprofit administrators perceived that to more effectively respond to these impact inquiries, quality-driven, cost accountable performance measures could be used to address the question of whether the service provided was truly needed and what difference the service made for its recipients. While traditional quantitative PM could potentially demonstrate the cost-effectiveness of a nonprofit organization, these measures alone could not provide many nonprofit administrators with the necessary tools to effectively address impact.

Nonprofit organization administrators and stakeholders also perceived that just as businesses had adopted a quality-driven, cost accountable culture and system, they could do so to improve their competitive abilities. Nonprofit organizations that used the quality-driven, cost accountable performance measures could also derive a competitive advantage over other nonprofit organizations in obtaining community and funding support. As nonprofit organizations incorporated quality-driven, cost accountable PM systems, their organizational cultures, priorities, and values began to change just as they had in by business organizations. The performance measures that addressed customer satisfaction and impact or outcomes assessment were of particular interest to nonprofit organizations.

OVERVIEW OF THE LITERATURE OF PUBLIC LIBRARY PERFORMANCE MEASUREMENT

"Reliable and valid measurement in the social sciences is extremely difficult" (World Encyclopedia of Library and Information Services, p. 547). Public libraries, as a member of the social sciences community, have been attempting to demonstrate their value through PM since the inception of public libraries in this country in the early 18th century. While there were many attempts and variations in the efforts to develop performance measures, there has been little progress made in establishing a systematic, universally accepted PM system that effectively addresses all of the inquiries of quality and cost accountability.

Florida's public libraries are now facing a great deal of uncertainty in determining the future direction(s) of PM methodologies after several decades of little progress and consensus. The future of PM is important to the HLA of the public libraries of the State of Florida, whose libraries provide information service to approximately 16 million residents through approximately 490 service outlets in 75 LAUs. (Florida Library Directory with Statistics, 2001, p. 153)

While the changing nature of the delivery of library and information services and the recipients of those services are creating uncertainty in PM for HLA, another equally important source of uncertainty affecting the future of PM for Florida's public libraries is they are not insulated from the social changes in the environments they serve. Florida public libraries are interwoven into the community and the culture that they serve and reflect the changes these communities are experiencing. The communities that Florida public libraries serve are facing the same types of changes and challenges in providing the community and its residents with quality, cost-effective services as public libraries face.

The changing nature of public library service (increased population, introduction of technology, and dwindling resources) is prompting stakeholders, including governing bodies, to pose questions to HLA regarding how to meet these increasingly diverse information needs and services while maintaining or improving the accountability and quality performance of their agencies. This increased request for quality service and cost accountability is a part of a larger social development in Florida culture. Public perceptions of government and other public services (such as public libraries) are shifting from accepting the "community goodness" as evidence of quality service and cost accountability in public service to a perception that requires government/public services to adhere to the more business-based practices of quality-driven, cost accountability. While stakeholders have seldom doubted the overall "community goodness" of a public service, such as a public library, stakeholders are increasingly demanding tangible proof from HLA that the "community goodness" is being delivered through the most cost-effective methods and that service quality concerns are being effectively addressed.

HISTORY, DEVELOPMENT, AND USE OF PUBLIC LIBRARY PERFORMANCE MEASUREMENT

Today's challenges in PM (i.e. quality service, cost accountability, increasing use of technology, etc.) generate discussion in the literature of the library profession. Most public libraries have felt pressure from their stakeholders to continually redefine and improve their abilities to report performance information. However, PM is not a new development in public libraries. PM in public libraries began in 1876 with Cutter using cost–benefit analysis in a study of cataloging effectiveness. The traditional techniques of PM developed during the early history of PM in public libraries, which include interviews, input/output analysis, costs analysis, and activity analysis, are still the most popular forms of PM today.

Lubans states that Shaw was one of the earliest practioners and proponents of scientific management in the library profession, dating back to the 1930s. Shaw was an advocate of integration, using a "total system approach" and "reductions in workforce" to increase efficiency. Lubans also describes how Rider used unit cost study to maximize efficiency as early as 1934. Rider was quoted as saying that if librarians did not use scientific management or cost–benefit analysis to justify performance, nonlibrarians would come in and do it for us. This statement still bears effective warning to today's library professionals.

Stakeholder and community pressure to change and the discussion generated about PM within the profession has led to the sporadic adoption of a few new performance methodologies or measures in some public LAU. Since the late 1980s, a small percentage of public libraries have reported incorporating these new types of PM into their arsenal of evaluation. Examples of some of the new PM methodologies that have been reported utilized include: benchmarking, outcomes assessment, TQM, or other strongly quantitative measurements such as the balanced scorecard (BSC), and a variety of customer satisfaction measurement systems. Determining the actual PM methodologies used in Florida public libraries is an integral component of this study.

One cause for the lack of change in using PM in public libraries is the lack of consensus among members of the profession as to when performance measures should be used and the reasons for their use. Lancaster stated that PM consists of microevaluation, which is how a system operates and why, and macro-evaluation, which is how well a system operates. McClure, Zweizig, Van House, and Lynch suggest that the primary utility of performance measures is for internal staff diagnosis. Van House et al. stated that, "performance measurement serves several purposes in libraries: assessing current levels of performance; diagnosing possible problem areas; comparing current and desired levels of performance; and monitoring progress"(Van House et al., 1987, p. 2). Van House also cites the major benefit of PM to be, "that it provides information for planning and decision-making" (Van House et al., 1987, p. 3). Other additional benefits according to Van House include the following.

- The ability to communicate library data to external agencies and individuals
- Enhancing the library's ability to plan, evaluate, and determine effectiveness within the library
- Funding justification or other resource decisions to stakeholders
- Service enhancements or improvements
- Increasing staff ability to collect and use performance data
- The creation of a PM process that has meaning to the organization and staff

Determining whether these purported benefits of using PM exist in Florida public libraries is an integral component of the study. According to Van House, there are three types of performance measures used by libraries: inputs, outputs, and productivity. Input measures are described as the resources (human, financial, and materials) and costs of producing and delivering library services and products. OM fall within three categories: quantitative, qualitative, and timeliness. OM are geared to provide data on the overall quantities of service and products provided; the financial cost of the service and products provided; and the speed of the service provided. Kraft and Boyce (1991) determined that there are four types of library performance measures that HLA should employ to address stakeholder inquiries:

- The amounts of resources library have at their disposal.
- The efficiency in using these resources to generate services.
- The effectiveness in how alternatives are used to meet goals.
- The benefit to society and environment.

Risher and Fay (1995) suggest that PM should measure anything that is important to at least one group of stakeholders. They continue by saying that PM should illustrate the variation of service the organization is capable of providing, customer satisfaction, and timeliness. Administrators can accomplish this by ensuring that multiple performance measures originate from customer needs and provide feedback to the organization. Hernon and Altman state that performance "measures characterize the extent, effectiveness, and efficiency of library programs and services" (Hernon & Altman, 1996, p. 27).

The Public Library Association (PLA) and its parent organization, the American Library Association (ALA), have played the lead role in the use and development of standards of service and PM for public libraries throughout most of the 20th century. In 1933, the ALA published its first set of performance standards for public libraries. Standards of service were the first attempt to provide public libraries with the ability to demonstrate their level of achievement. The first standards of service simply recommended minimum levels of resources to provide library service; examples included $1 per capita as the minimum level of expenditure to support library services. These standards of service were gradually increased until 1956 when it became apparent that there were, "uneven effects of library size and mission on resource requirements and partially in recognition of the imperfect relationship between expenditure level and service quality" (Withers, 1974, pp. 322–323).

ALA introduced the first qualitative standards of service in 1933. These qualitative standards of service possessed a broad scope to allow for wide acceptance by the profession. However, qualitative standards of service were of limited benefit as a standard against which to measure quantitative performance. Initially, according to Ammons these qualitative standards of service prescribed, "appropriate levels of financial support and staff credentials" (Ammons, 2000, p. 211). The standards contained phrasing that provided little specific information to facilitate measuring performance to professionals or the community at large. Ammons states that the qualitative standards, "offered little leverage for prying resources from the city (county) treasury. In short, they (standards) failed to arm library directors with a persuasive means of demonstrating to budget makers' local shortcomings in facilities, services, and funding" (Ammons, 1996, p. 212). From these qualitative standards of service came the "formulation of qualitative library goals and, eventually, quantitative standards of service pertaining to library collection, facilities, services, and performance"(Ammons, 1996, p. 211).

These quantitative standards were appreciated by professionals who needed a set of quantitative measurements that improved their ability to report performance. The uses of quantitative standards of service alone have proven to be controversial within the library profession since their inception in the 1950s–1960s. Some of the more common negative statements made regarding the uses of quantitative standards of service are:

• They were created without considering the different service needs of individual communities.
• The quantitative standards do not support the top echelon level of libraries in their efforts to demonstrate performance. The top echelon libraries felt penalized when their performance results exceeded the standards, providing local officials with "justification" to divert library funding to other agencies.
• The quantitative standards did not systematically approach PM from the perspective of library customers or potential customers.

This was unsettling for many who were accustomed to having customer input as a part of the PM process. Customer input in the PM process in public libraries was initiated in 1939, when Wilson became the first library professional to incorporate the use of customer surveys to determine organizational performance accomplishment. Hatry et al. stated: "Most library systems lack information on: the level of citizen satisfaction with library operations, including the comfort of facilities, hours of operations, speed of service, and helpfulness of the staff; the availability of materials sought by the users; and the percentage of households using the system, with estimates of reasons for nonuse by those not using the system" (Hatry et al., 1979, p. 67). Several sets of performance measures have been issued to supplement the older standards of service for public libraries since the 1960s; i.e. Deprospo, Altman, and Beasley (1973); Altman et al. (1977); Van House, Lynch, McClure, Zweizig, and Rodger (1987); Himmel and Wilson (1998), and electronic performance measures by Bertot, McClure and Ryan (2001). Each set of performance measures took years of work to develop and varied in content and measurement techniques to allow for a wide level of application. However, the profession received many of these measures with limited enthusiasm due to the lingering lack of consensus in the use and application of PM by HLA.

The International Federation of Library Associations (IFLA) produced a consolidated collection of recommended minimal quantitative standards and measurements in 1986. Because these minimal quantitative standards were written to have the greatest application, IFLA cautioned readers that its standards were, "not likely to be universally relevant" (Guidelines for Public Libraries, p. 61). The IFLA quantitative standards were in contradiction to the direction being set by the PLA at the time.

By the late 1980s, PLA had ceased using what it saw as prescriptive quantitative standards as a national measurement tool and had been working to develop and utilize new PMs. One of the more noted new PM methodologies being used in public LAU's today is outcomes assessment. The Institute of Museum and Library Services (IMLS) states, "it believes that outcomes-based assessment, a systematic measurement of impact, holds great promise for libraries" (IMLS, 2000, p. 2). "In April 1995, UWA established an internal team charged to help United Way organizations document and improve their impact on community problems by developing and supporting approaches to measuring the outcomes of United Ways' investment in health and human services" (United Way of America's Outcome Measurement Resource Network, 1995–2002, http://www.unitedway.org/outcomes/).

The United Way outcomes assessment model for PM seeks to provide information to stakeholders about the impact, i.e. changes in knowledge, behavior, status, or condition, that an organization (in this case, public libraries) has had on clients or customers. However, in outcomes assessment, customer satisfaction is not considered an appropriate outcome, because it does not represent a change in knowledge, behavior, status, or condition. IMLS (2000) further states, "outcome based assessment is not a form of research, nor is it simple data collection. It joins both of those essential processes, however, as a powerful tool in reporting the kinds of differences libraries make among their users" (IMLS, 2000, p. 2).

The Bureau of Library Development (BLD) of the State Library of Florida is presently encouraging public libraries in Florida to implement outcomes assessment to measure library services in order to improve public libraries' abilities to report customer and community impact. The BLD has provided publications and numerous training opportunities to HLA in order to increase the awareness and implementation rates for outcomes assessment. The BLD has even made an outcomes assessment handbook available on its Web site to facilitate ease of access for HLA.

The BLD began requiring in FY 1999–2000 that all Library Service and Technology Act (LSTA) grant applications contain an outcomes assessment model in order to qualify to receive a LSTA grant award. As of 2002, approximately 35 public LAU in Florida are currently using outcomes assessment because of this requirement. However, most libraries still have not developed outcomes assessment measures to evaluate their comprehensive library services in spite of the efforts and encouragement from the BLD to local libraries to develop outcome measures.

As outcomes assessment is a relatively new PM methodology being used in public libraries, there is little evidence as to what impact it is having on its practioners. Even the UWA states that, "This question merits serious research that explores not only whether there are benefits, but also under what circumstances, for what types of programs, and other issues of applicability and whether or not results can be generalized" (UWA Outcome Measurement Resource Network, 2001, http://www.unitedway.org/outcomes/).

The change in emphasis to qualitative PM by some LAU and PLA has caused concern among those who still feel the need to have quantitative PM standards. To respond to the perceived concern among those library practioners many state library agencies have attempted to mandate the use of quantitative PM. While none of these attempts have proven successful to date, at least 23 state-level associations, including the Florida Library Association in 1993–1994, have set their own prescriptive quantitative standards for PM in public libraries. (Ammons, 1996, p. 224)

Kaplan states that administrators and stakeholders of nonprofit organizations are becoming increasingly aware that financial performance measures alone are not sufficient to evaluate organizational performance. Other libraries are looking to introduce more complex quantitative PM methodologies that consider more aspects of organizational performance than traditional library output measurements in order to respond to accountability concerns from stakeholders. BSC is one such strongly quantitative PM methodology being used in public libraries.

The BSC was originally designed for use in the private sector. BSC generates feedback on current critical performance processes and targets future performance from both within and outside an organization. Performance measures come from four general areas: financial performance, customers, internal business processes, and learning and growth. The resulting measures from these four areas align individual, unit, and organizational goals against the objectives needed to meet or exceed customer and stakeholder objectives.

In summary, the literature of librarianship suggests that there is little consensus regarding the purposes and definitions of PM in public libraries. Further, the literature suggests there is little consensus as to what types of PM methodologies should be used in public libraries or what benefits are derived from using these PM methodologies. Additionally, there has been no study to date of the use and perceptions of PM in public libraries (including Florida public libraries). However, the literature does demonstrate a consensus that public libraries, in particular Florida public libraries, have been using PM to report some form of efficiency and accountability information to stakeholders for many years without and assessment of the PM process.

Based on the literature findings, this study has been designed to determine what types of PM are being used in Florida public libraries, who receives the resulting information, and what impacts Florida public libraries are experiencing from using PM.

STUDY METHODOLOGY

The first statewide comprehensive study of the uses of PM in Florida public libraries and the perceptions of PM of HLAs in Florida was undertaken by the researcher in 2002. As a part of this comprehensive study, data was collected on all aspects of the PM process in libraries, including costs, estimated staff time and estimated staff training time in implementing PM. The researcher selected an evaluative research design to conduct the PM study due to the wide range of aspects, data, viewpoints, and themes to be covered in order to comprehensively study the use and perceived impact of PM in Florida public libraries. Information obtained on the resources, i.e. time, money, and training, expended in conducting PM in Florida public libraries was of particular interest to the researcher as no study to date (2002) had yet been conducted on this aspect of PM in public libraries.

Because of the variety of topics involved in studying the PM process in Florida public libraries, the researcher conducted the study using an evaluative research design using a mixed-methods methodology to collect and analyze data. " ...Evaluative research is generally applied, the primary objective of which is to determine the extent to which a given program or procedure is achieving some desired result" (Suchman, 1967, p. 21). Scriven states that, "Evaluation research can be defined as an autonomous discipline that refers to the study and application of procedures for doing objective and systematic evaluation" (Scriven, 1991, p. 141), and suggests that there is a distinction to be made between evaluative research and traditional empirical research. "Evaluation as a particular kind of investigative discipline is distinguished from, for example, traditional empirical research in the social sciences...partly by its multidisciplinarity. It typically requires consideration of costs, comparisons, and psychological dimensions" (Scriven, 1991, p. 141). The study of the use and perceived impact of PM processes in Florida public libraries can be defined as multidisciplinary, which requires similar considerations.

The use of evaluation research is common in the fields of organizational dynamics, business administration, public administration, social work, and educational study because of its multidisciplinary approach. Evaluative research is primarily used in organizational and administrative evaluation and includes designs to evaluate " ...program, product, personnel, performance, proposal, and policy evaluation (the big six): other applied areas include technology assessment, medical or psychological evaluation, and quality control" (Scriven, 1991, p. 143).

Another reason the researcher used an evaluative research design is that the results of the study needed to have a practical and immediate utility. "In any applied field, meaning one that services clients with real world problems (i.e. HLA), there is always one criterion for good work that is absent from the research field, namely the immediate utility of the conclusions" (Scriven, 1991, p. 143).

The study's evaluative research design requires a variety of data collection methods to effectively address the study's overarching questions. The researcher chose to use a mixed-methodology to collect and analyze data. Creswell states that a researcher employing a mixed-methodology would, "mix aspects of both qualitative and quantitative paradigms at all or many methodological steps in the design. The paradigms might be mixed in the introduction, in the literature review and theory use...and the research questions" (Creswell, 1994, p. 178) .While this added a degree of complexity to the study design, the mixed-methodology used incorporated the advantages and disadvantages of both quantitative and qualitative methods. The impact of using the mixed-methodology in the study design is discussed in each chapter of this study.

QUESTIONNAIRE AND SURVEY DESIGN

The researcher designed the study instruments to be used as self-administered questionnaires (see the appendix). The researcher used the questionnaire technique in order to reach the intended study population, which is widely dispersed throughout the state of Florida. The attitudinal survey incorporated both open-ended and closed question styles to address the mixed-method methodology of the study. Creswell (1994) suggests that closed questions are best used when determining the degree of participation or involvement, intensity of feelings, or frequency of events. All other demographic data, i.e. SP served, total expenditure, staffing, and total expenditure per capita, were obtained from the 2001 Florida Library Directory with Statistics.

During pretesting of the survey instruments, the technical considerations of completing and returning the survey were reviewed. It was determined that the technical skills required for HLA to complete and return the survey consisted of: how to read e-mail, how to open either an Excel spreadsheet or Word document received as an e-mail attachment, entering data into an Excel spreadsheet or Word document and saving the file, and how to return the files as e-mail attachments. These skills are routinely taught by libraries and have been made available to HLA for many years through the Gates Foundation, the state's multitype library cooperatives, and other providers of computer training opportunities. Other considerations of the use of electronic surveys was to minimize the logistics and resources in conducting the study and providing faster assistance and responses to respondents allowed the researcher to quickly and directly address inquiries while being able to document the researcher – respondent correspondence.

The study population consisted of either the HLA or the assistant HLA who was primarily responsible for conducting PM in each of the 75 public LAU, regardless of time or tenure. Hernon and Altman state in *Service Quality in Academic Libraries* that the HLA of each administrative unit is chosen, as they are "the driving force for PM and are essential for the success in performance. If the leader does not demonstrate understanding and willingness to use the performance measures process in a productive manner, the staff will not be able to implement the process successfully either" (Hernon and Altman, 1996, p. 24).

The 75 HLA administered the access to information and the provision of library services to all of Florida's nearly 16 million residents through approximately 490 service outlets, using over 6,000 FTE of staff, and receiving income of approximately $363,901,438 (Florida Library Directory with

Table 2. Selected Florida Libraries Statistical Information for FY
1998–1999 and FY 1999–2000.

Statistical Category	FY 1999–2000	FY 1998–1999	Difference (%)
Library expenditure/capita	$20.26	$19.21	5.5
Staff expenditure/capita	$11.80	$11.53	2.3
Total paid staff	6,016	5,458	10.2
Circulation of materials	75,292,057	73,899,704	1.9
Circulation/capita	4.79	4.78	0.2
Library visits	53,993,881	49,358,853	9.4
Total program attendance	3,004,792	2,955,823	1.7
Web site hits	39,145,609	21,713,633	80.3
Patron log ons	7,328,204*	4,381,582	67.3
Service population	15,721,729	15,466,152	1.7

*Estimated from weekly average.

Statistics, 2001, p. 153) to deliver information access and services. Further
details of the level of accomplishment of Florida's public libraries are provided in Table 2.

GENERAL SURVEY ANALYSIS

There were 75 possible survey respondents. Of these 75 possible respondents, 40 returned useable, completed surveys, for a response rate of 53.3%
and an estimated survey error rate of ± 5.4%. Twenty-six respondents were
"City" LAUs, 31 were "County" LAU, and eight were "Regional" LAU.
Survey respondents did not represent 23 of Florida's 67 counties. Of the 23
counties not represented by survey respondents, nine were represented by
three HLA who did not respond to the survey.

Of the 35 nonrespondents: two HLAs were currently unavailable (one
position was vacant, one library administrator was on active military duty,
and neither had a backup administrator in place who could answer the
survey questions); four nonrespondents returned incomplete surveys or in-
sufficient or inappropriate responses or data, rendering their surveys unus-
able; two nonrespondents stated that they did not have the technical skills
necessary to return the survey; and twenty-seven nonrespondents either did
not respond to any inquiries from the researcher or stated they did not have
the time to or interest in participating in the study.

The LAU of the 40 study respondents provided information access and
library service to approximately 7,239,547 Florida residents in FY 1999–2000

(Florida Library Directory with Statistics, 2001, pp. 153–202). The total population of the state of Florida during FY 1999–2000 was approximately 15,947,240, thus 45.4% of all Florida residents receiving public library service in Florida are provided service by the survey respondents (White, 2002, p. 122). The study respondents expended approximately $150,436,543 to deliver library service, which was approximately 41.4% of the State total expenditure for public library service (Florida Library Directory with Statistics, 2001, pp. 153–202). The average annual total expenditure for each study respondent was $3,760,913.58 with the state average being $514,278.57. The average expenditure per capita for each study respondent was $24.19, which is 21.4% higher than the State of Florida average expenditure per capita of $19.93 (Florida Library Directory with Statistics, 2001, pp. 153–202).

The 40 study respondents were analyzed using the number of years experience as an HLA (the only demographic question asked of respondents). Approximately 32.5% (13) of the respondents had less than five years experience; approximately 30% (12) of the respondents had between six and ten years of experience; and approximately 37.5% (15) of the respondents had over 11 years of experience as an HLA in Florida public libraries (White, 2002, p. 384). The average years of service for survey respondents was 10.1 years, with a range of 1–27 (White, 2002, p. 126).

The study respondents were analyzed using the six PLA's categories of population served. These categories were:

Less than 49,999 (SP1), between 50,000 and 99,999 (SP2), between 100,000 and 249,999 (SP3), between 250,000 and 499,999 (SP4), between 500,000 and 999,999 (SP5), and over one million (SP6). An analysis of the study respondents' SPs is depicted in Table 3. With the exception of the SP5 category of respondents, the study population was equally distributed and

Table 3. Service Population Comparisons of Respondents.

Service Population Ranges	Total Number of LAU in the Range in Florida	Total Number of Respondents in the Range	Percentage of Total (%)
0–49,999 (SP1)	29	15	51.7
50,000–99,999 (SP2)	10	5	50.0
100,000–249,999 (SP3)	20	14	70.2
250,000–499,999 (SP4)	9	4	44.4
500,000–999,999 (SP5)	5	1	20.0
Over one million (SP6)	2	1	50.0
Total	75	40	53.3

reflective of the whole population of LAU in Florida when considering the demographic breakouts and the geographical coverage of the study respondents.

GENERAL FINDINGS

The general survey findings from the study indicated that, on average, LAUs used 2.6 different PM systems, with a range of nine (1, 10). A majority of respondents (over 75%) indicated their reliance on performance measures implemented before 1990 to provide their LAU with PM information, i.e. OM, quality management measures, and performance-based budgeting.

The study results indicated that a majority of respondents primarily used quantitative performance measures, i.e. OM. Respondents stated their LAU used OM, "because they were standard and easy to come by," and "the data that served us best is what we could count" (White, 2002, pp. 188–191). Results indicated that electronic output measures (EOM) were the most frequently implemented performance measure that had been developed since 1991 among all respondents for reporting efficiency/effectiveness or service impact.

The majority of respondents perceived customer satisfaction as the performance measure they would use to effectively demonstrate accountability or effectiveness in all of the quality or service criteria examined. This is contradicted, however, by the respondents, as most LAU did not make a formal attempt to collect such customer satisfaction data on a regular basis. Respondents reported perceived customer satisfaction was not what a majority of stakeholders or the library requested in terms of PM information to effectively report service quality. Customer satisfaction was also not a PM information source that respondent's perceived as positively impacting service quality in their LAU.

The results indicated respondents did not consistently use the same types of performance measures to determine the effectiveness of similar quality criteria except within service criterion. These indications may illustrate the need for improved understanding of the use of PM by survey respondents and an improved understanding of the organizational culture in which HLA operate.

The majority of respondents indicated they collected customer satisfaction feedback annually or "as required." Results indicated a majority of respondents collected, used, and maintained outdated or erroneous customer feedback and technology evaluation PM information to base critical strategic, administrative, resource allocation, and service provision decisions.

Approximately 54.0% of respondents did not include library customers in the PM process in their LAU (White, 2002, p. 254). One respondent stated, "It is risky for administrators that work as 'at will' employees to invite evaluation and measurements by those who are not library professionals" (White, 2002, p. 386). PM information is reported intensively, but inconsistently, within the library organization, and decreased in the frequency of recipients as recipients became further removed from the library organization itself.

The majority of the respondents perceived that patrons primarily requested no type of PM information from libraries to demonstrate service effectiveness. The majority of the respondents also perceived that the LAU requested no type of PM information from partners and program collaborators to demonstrate service effectiveness. These results may demonstrate a lack of communication or understanding existing between the governing body, customers, partners, and program collaborators, and the LAU regarding the type of PM information required to provide evidence to demonstrate service effectiveness. The results also indicate that a majority of LAU were collecting and reporting evidence to demonstrate service effectiveness than was different from the evidence required by their stakeholders.

Survey respondents also reported their perceptions on the effectiveness of PM within their LAU. The majority of respondents indicated the PM process in their LAU was not a valuable process and did not allow them to make more effective decisions. Respondents generally perceived the time required to conduct PM within their LAU would have been better spent providing direct customer service than collecting data that no one appreciated.

As a result of the combination of these findings, the researcher perceived that a majority of LAU were expending resources to collect, maintain, and use PM information that they perceived to be unnecessary and devalued.

ANALYSIS OF RESOURCE USAGE QUESTIONS

Question 3 of the study asked respondents, "What resources are being allocated for performance measurement in Florida public libraries?" Three sub-questions were designed to collect data to address the overarching question. Sub-question 3.1 asked, "What is the total amount of staff time dedicated solely to performance measurement in an average year?" and Question 16 in the attitudinal survey collected data to address this question.

The data analysis of Question 16 determined that 75% of all respondents allocated no more than 5% of the total annual staff time available in their LAU to conduct PM. Based on survey responses, an estimated range of 174.098–317.07 FTE of the 2,991.0 total FTE (Florida Library Directory with Statistics, 2001, p. 153) working in the 40 respondent LAU's were reported as being allocated for some portion of their work time to implement or conduct PM. A respondent estimate of 334.73–609.75 FTE in staff time was allocated to implement or conduct PM in Florida public libraries was calculated based on the survey responses (White, 2002, p. 163). From the survey data, the researcher estimated 6.0–11.0% of the statewide library workforce of 6,016 FTE (Florida Library Directory with Statistics, 2001, pp. 153–202) reported working in the 75 LAU in Florida are involved in conducting PM. This translated to 14,438.4–26,470.4 staff hours expended in 2002 on PM in Florida public libraries. "By way of comparison, if the minimum estimate of 334.73 FTE allocated statewide to conducting PM in Florida public libraries in FY 2000 were the staff of one LAU:

• This LAU would have more FTE staff than all but one of the respondents in this study.
• This LAU would have enough staff to operate 23 of the 40 responding LAUs at FY 2000 staffing levels" (White, 2002, p. 163).

Sub-question 3.2 asked, "What is the total overall percentage of the budget dedicated to conducting performance measurement last year?" Question 17 in the attitudinal survey collected data to address this question.

The data analysis of Question 17 determined 89.7% of all respondents allocated 5% or less of the overall LAU budget to conduct PM. An estimated range of $4,121,858.92–$8,376,302.36 (Florida Library Directory with Statistics, 2001, pp. 153–202) of the $150, 436,534.00 (Florida Library Directory with Statistics, 2001, pp. 153–202) of total expenditure reported by respondents was allocated to conducting PM in FY 2000. A statewide estimate of $7,926,651.77–$16,108,273.77 (Florida Library Directory with Statistics, 2001, pp. 153–202) was allocated to conducting PM in Florida public libraries in FY 2000. The statewide estimate range did not appear to include the value of staff time allocated to PM in Florida libraries. Approximately, 2.5–5.1% of the $318,570,893.00 (Florida Library Directory with Statistics, 2001, pp. 153–202) reported total expenditure of the 75 LAU in Florida to provide public library service was allocated to conduct PM in FY 2000. A statewide estimate of $7,926,651.77–$16,108,273.77 was calculated from the study to be allocated to conducting PM in Florida public libraries in FY 2000 (White, 2002, p. 166). By way of comparison, if the minimum estimate of $7,926,651.77 allocated to conducting PM in Florida public libraries in FY 2000 was one funding account:

- It would be "equal to approximately 24.1–49.0% of the total State Aid Funds received by Florida's public libraries in FY 2000" (White, 2002, p. 166).
- It would be "two to four times more than the statewide total expenditure for electronic information collection acquisition" (White, 2002, p. 166).

Sub-question 3.3 asked, "What is the total training time provided to staff members in the past year dealing specifically with using performance measurement?" Question 18 in the attitudinal survey collected data to address this question.

The data analysis of Question 18 determined that 95% of all respondents allocate less than 5% of all training time to training staff to conduct PM (White, 2002, p. 167). "Research in librarianship and other related professions/industries has yet to determine a baseline range of staff training for PM in public libraries. Statistics were not available detailing the total amount of training time provided to library staff in Florida public libraries. Therefore, the researcher was not able to infer a statewide total of PM staff training time and was unable to determine whether this level of staff training for PM is appropriate for public libraries in Florida" (White, 2002, p. 168).

In order to assess the overall responses of the attitudinal questions regarding HLA's perceptions of the use and effectiveness of PM in Florida public libraries, the researcher created Fig. 2, which shows the Likert Category Response Frequencies for Questions 1–15.

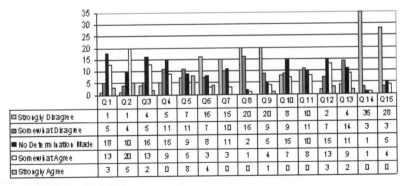

	Q1	Q2	Q3	Q4	Q5	Q6	Q7	Q8	Q9	Q10	Q11	Q12	Q13	Q14	Q15
Strongly Disagree	1	1	4	5	7	16	15	20	20	8	10	2	4	35	28
Somewhat Disagree	5	4	5	11	11	7	10	16	9	9	11	7	14	3	3
No Determination Made	18	10	16	15	9	8	11	2	5	15	10	15	11	1	5
Somewhat Agree	13	20	13	9	5	3	3	1	4	7	8	13	9	1	4
Strongly Agree	3	5	2	0	8	4	0	0	1	0	0	3	2	0	0

Fig. 2. Questions 1–15 Likert Category Response Frequencies.

Figure 2 illustrates that six of fifteen questions garnered a majority positive response. Three of fifteen questions garnered a majority no determination made response, while six of fifteen questions garnered a majority negative response.

Five of the six majority positive response questions were Questions 6–9 and 11 which were all stated in a negative manner. The negatively stated questions evaluated respondent's perceptions to the converse information sought by the researcher. The negatively stated questions had the lowest response rates; however, they did not yield the lowest perceived mean response value of the 15 questions. Question 14, regarding the Legislature's role in distributing PM, yielded a mean response value 56.9% lower than any of the negatively stated questions. Overall, HLA perceptions of the use and effectiveness of PM in Florida public libraries was neutral at best, with respondents being equally distributed between the extremes of perception (i.e. effective, not effective).

When combined with the findings regarding resource expenditure and staff time commitments to conducting and implementing PM in Florida public libraries, the study findings seemed to suggest that substantial resources were used annually to conduct a process (PM) that was not perceived to be effective by at least half of those who conducted the process and utilized its results.

CORRELATION FINDINGS

A correlational analysis was conducted "between responding HLA (Head Library Administrator) experience as a HLA in Florida Public libraries and the scores from the attitudinal survey questions 1–20, and 25–28. The correlation coefficients were calculated in order to determine the existence and strength of any statistical relationships that may exist…" (White, 2002, p. 244). Table 4 illustrates the correlation coefficients between HLA experience and various PM aspects.

Table 5 illustrates the correlations coefficients between responding HLA experience as a HLA in Florida public libraries and the scores from attitudinal survey questions.

None of the correlation coefficients determined a significant relationship, defined as a correlation coefficient lower than −0.50 and higher than +0.50, existed between HLA experience and the attitudinal survey scores for Questions 1–20 and 25–27. The correlation coefficients for HLA experience and Questions 4, 16, and 18 were the highest-ranking positive correlation

Table 4. Correlation Analyses of HLA Experience and Various
PM Aspects.

Question Number	Correlation Value for HLA Experience	Question Number	Correlation Value for HLA Experience
1	(0.03)	13	0.06
2	(0.03)	14	(0.07)
3	0.00	15	0.11
4	0.25	16	0.27
5	0.00	17	0.13
6	(0.06)	18	0.29
7	(0.04)	19	(0.22)
8	0.18	20	(0.13)
9	0.20	25	(0.02)
10	(0.18)	26	0.07
11	(0.04)	27	(0.08)
12	0.17		

Values within parentheses denote negative numbers.

Table 5. Correlation Analysis of SP level, SA status, and Various PM
Aspects.

Question Number	Correlation of SP Level	Correlation of SA Status	Question Number	Correlation of SP Level	Correlation of SA Status
1	0.28	0.23	13	0.28	(0.12)
2	0.31	0.36	14	(0.02)	0.00
3	0.03	0.28	15	0.16	0.17
4	0.20	0.31	16	0.57	(0.02)
5	0.46	0.11	17	0.33	(0.02)
6	0.08	(0.16)	18	0.24	(0.30)
7	(0.18)	(0.04)	19	(0.10)	(0.19)
8	(0.33)	(0.06)	20	(0.28)	0.03
9	0.02	(0.03)	25	(0.22	(0.06)
10	0.01	0.06	26	(0.19)	(0.01)
11	0.18	0.21	27	(0.10)	(0.01)
12	0.30	0.16			

Values within parentheses denote negative numbers.

coefficients. Question 4 dealt with the effectiveness of PM results to report
the total organizational impact of the library. Questions 16 and 18 dealt
with staff time in the PM process and the amount of training time provided
to staff regarding PM.

The results of the correlation analysis indicated 11 of the 23 correlation coefficients were negative. The correlation coefficients for HLA experience and Questions 10, 19, and 20 had the lowest-ranking negative correlation coefficients. Question 10 dealt with respondent's perceptions of the degree of consensus between HLA regarding the types of performance measures used to report service quality. Questions 19 and 20 dealt with the frequency of PM in regard to determining customer satisfaction and technology evaluation.

A correlation coefficient was calculated for the total number of reported performance measures being used by each respondent, obtained in Question 21 of the attitudinal survey, and the amount of HLA experience of each respondent in order to address sub-question 1 of overarching Question 4. The correlation coefficient was calculated to be –0.18, which indicated that the relationship between the number of performance measures used by re-spondents and the HLA experience of the respondent was not significant.

Table 5 illustrates only one of the correlation coefficients determined a significant relationship, defined as a correlation coefficient lower than –0.50 and higher than +0.50, existed between SP level or SA receiving status and the attitudinal survey scores for Questions 1–20 and 25–27. The correlation between scores from Question 16 and SP level resulted in a correlation coefficient of 0.57. Therefore, there was a positive correlation between the size of the SP of the LAU and the amount of resources allocated to conduct PM within the survey respondents. This relationship could be explained by the overall size of the budget for a larger LAU as opposed to that of a smaller LAU and the higher PM and administrative experience levels of the HLA in larger SP LAU.

The correlation coefficients for SP level and Questions 5, 16, and 17 were the highest-ranking positive correlation coefficients for SP-level calcula-tions. Question 5 dealt with the priority of PM in respondent's LAU. Questions 16 and 17 dealt with staff time in the PM process and the budget amounts allocated to conducting PM. The correlation coefficients for SA status and Questions 2, 3, and 4 were the highest-ranking positive corre-lation coefficients for SP-level calculations. Question 2 dealt with the re-spondent's perception of the results of PM in their LAU. Question 3 dealt with the results of the PM process providing stakeholders with an accurate account of the overall quality of library service. Question 4 dealt with the results of the PM process effectively reporting the total organizational im-pact of the library.

The results of the correlation analysis indicated that 8 of the 23 corre-lation coefficients calculated with SP level were negative and that 12 of the 23 correlation coefficients calculated with SA receiving LAU status were negative. The correlation coefficients for SP level and Questions 8, 20, and 25 had the lowest-ranking negative correlation coefficients for SP-level calculations. Question 8 dealt with respondent's perceptions of PM undermining the library's ability to provide effective service. Question 20 dealt with the frequency of technology evaluation. Question 25 dealt with what types of PM information did the respondent's governing body require in order for the library to demonstrate effective service. The correlation coefficients for SA status and Questions 6, 18, and 19 had the lowest-ranking negative correlation coefficients for SA status calculations. Question 6 dealt with the respondent's perceptions of whether PM would be used if not required by governing bodies or funding agencies. Question 18 dealt with the amount of time allocated to training staff in PM. Question 19 dealt with the frequency of customer service measurement in respondent's LAU.

The data analysis for several of the survey questions were designed to answer Question 4, which asked, "Are there any correlations between the amount of experience of head library administrators and the usage and perceptions of impact of performance measurement in Florida's public libraries?" Six sub-questions were designed to collect data to address this question.

Sub-question 4.1 asked, "Is there a correlation between the amount of experience as head library administrator to the number of performance measurements used?" Question 21 and the "Years of Head Library Administrator Experience" demographic question on the attitudinal survey were used to address this question. The correlation coefficient was calculated to be –0.18, indicating that no significant relationship exists between the amount of HLA experience and the number of performance measures used in respondent's LAU.

Sub-question 4.2 asked, "Is there a correlation between the amount of experience as head library administrator to the perception of the impact of performance measures?" Questions 8 and 13, and the "Years of Head Library Administrator Experience" demographic question on the attitudinal survey were used to address this question.

The correlation coefficients calculated were as follows: HLA experience and Question 8 yielded a 0.18 coefficient and HLA experience and Question 13 yielded a 0.06 coefficient. Therefore, a significant relationship, defined, as a correlation coefficient lower than −0.50 and higher than +0.50, does not exist between HLA experience and the attitudinal survey scores from Questions 8 and 13.

Sub-question 4.3 asked, "Is there a correlation between the amounts of experience as head library administrator to library administrators' perceptions of the accuracy of performance measures?" Questions 3, 7, 10, and 11 and the

"Years of Head Library Administrator Experience" demographic question in the attitudinal survey were used to address this question.

The correlation coefficients calculated using HLA experience were as follows: HLA experience and Question 3 yielded a 0.00 coefficient; HLA experience and Question 7 yielded a −0.04 coefficient; HLA experience and Question 10 yielded a −0.18 coefficient; and HLA experience and Question 11 yielded a −0.04 coefficient. Therefore, a significant relationship, defined, as a correlation coefficient lower than −0.50 and higher than + 0.50, did not exist between HLA experience and the attitudinal survey scores from Questions 3, 7, 10, and 11.

Sub-question 4.4 asked, "Is there a correlation between the amounts of experience as head library administrator to library administrators' perceptions of the effectiveness of performance measures?" Question 4 and the "Years of Head Library Administrator Experience" demographic question in the attitudinal survey were used to address this question. The correlation coefficient was calculated to be 0.20, indicating that no significant relationship exists between the amount of HLA experience and the respondent's perception of how PM results effectively report the total organizational impact of the library.

Sub-question 4.5 asked, "Is there a correlation between the amount of experience as head library administrator to library administrators' perceptions of the necessity of performance measures?" Questions 5, 6, 9, and 15 and the "Years of Head Library Administrator Experience" demographic question in the attitudinal survey were used to address this question.

The correlation coefficients calculated using HLA experience were as follows: HLA experience and Question 5 yielded a 0.00 coefficient; HLA experience and Question 6 yielded a −0.06 coefficient; HLA experience and Question 9 yielded a 0.20 coefficient; and HLA experience and Question 11 yielded a 0.18 coefficient. Therefore, a significant relationship, defined, does not exist between HLA experience and the attitudinal survey scores from Questions 5, 6, 9, and 15.

Sub-question 4.6 asked, "Is there a correlation between the amounts of experience as head library administrator to library administrators' perceptions of the current benefit of performance measurement in their organizations?" Questions 1, 3, 4, 12, and 13 and the "Years of Head Library Administrator Experience" demographic question in the attitudinal survey were designed to address this question.

The correlation coefficients calculated using HLA experience were as follows: HLA experience and Question 1 yielded a −0.03 coefficient; HLA experience and Question 3 yielded a 0.00 coefficient; HLA experience and

Question 4 yielded a 0.25 coefficient; HLA experience and Question 12 yielded a 0.17 coefficient; and HLA experience and Question 13 yielded a 0.06 coefficient, indicating that no significant relationship existed between HLA experience and the attitudinal survey scores from Questions 1, 3, 4, 12, and 13.

The data analysis for some survey questions were designed to answer overarching Question 5, which asked, "Are there any correlations between the amount of experience as head library administrator to the resources allocated to performance measurement?" Three sub-questions were designed to address this question.

Sub-question 5.1 asked, "Is there a correlation between the amount of experience as head library administrator to the total amount of staff time dedicated to conducting performance measurement?" Question 16 and the "Years of Head Library Administrator Experience" demographic question in the attitudinal survey were used to address this question. The correlation coefficient was calculated to be 0.27, thus no significant relationship existed between the amount of HLA experience and the amount of staff time allocated to conducting PM.

Sub-question 5.2 asked, "Is there a correlation between the amount of experience as head library administrator to the overall percentage of the budget dedicated to conducting performance measurement?" Question 17 and the "Years of Head Library Administrator Experience" demographic question in the attitudinal survey were used to address this question. The correlation coefficient was calculated to be 0.13, indicating that no significant relationship existed between the amount of HLA experience and the amount of budget allocated to conducting PM.

Sub-question 5.3 asked, "Is there a correlation between the amount of experience as head library administrator to the total training time provided to staff members dealing specifically with using performance measurement?" Question 18 and the "Years of Head Library Administrator Experience" demographic question in the attitudinal survey were used to address this question. The correlation coefficient was calculated to be 0.29, so, no significant relationship was established between the amount of HLA experience and the amount of staff training time dedicated to PM.

CORRELATION OF DEMOGRAPHIC FACTORS

The data analysis for some survey questions was designed to answer Question 6, which is, "Do demographic factors such as the service population size or whether libraries receive State Aid affect the use and perceived impact of performance measurement in Florida's public libraries?" Demographic analyses for Questions 1–20 and 25–27 were used to address this question. Correlation coefficients calculated using SP levels and SA status are displayed in Table 4.26 (White, 2002).

Sub-questions 6.1 asked, "Does the service population size affect the use and perceived impact of performance measurement in Florida's public libraries?" Correlation coefficients showed only Question 16 of the 23 attitudinal questions, with a correlation coefficient of 0.57, showed a significant relationship. Question 16 dealt with the amount of staff time allocated to PM.

Sub-question 6.2 asked, "Does whether or not libraries receive State Aid affect the use and perceived impact of performance measurement in Florida's public libraries?" None of the 23 attitudinal questions demonstrated a significant relationship between SA status and respondent's perceptions of the use and impacts of PM. In Questions 1–29, responses were analyzed demographically to determine if there were any discernable relationships between the study's demographic factors, i.e. amount of HLA experience, SP level and SA status, and the responses provided using the mean response values of each demographic category. Correlation analysis found only one instance of a significant relationship, i.e. defined in the study to be a correlation ratio over 0.50, though in many cases some degree of relationship between the demographic factors and the responses was demonstrated.

The general finding of the analysis of the mean response values suggests that each of the three demographic factors affect the perceived mean value of the responses for Questions 1–29 regarding the use of PM and its perceived impact to some degree. Generally, as amounts of HLA experience and SP levels increase, the perceived use of PM and the degree of impact decline. Also, SA receiving LAU generally had significantly higher mean response values than did LAU not receiving SA.

CONCLUSIONS

As previously stated, the study's primary purpose was to determine the current usage and perceived impact of PM in Florida public libraries through studying the "Evaluation" and "Information" components of the researcher's PM theoretical model.

Theoretically, as an organization proceeds through the PM process, the results of each component's activities are used to initiate the next component's activities. When the "Information" component is completed, the resulting data and information is then used by library administrators to provide corrective feedback to each step of the process and to address accountability, service quality, or other stakeholder concerns, i.e. the two purposes of PM in this study. The feedback from library administrators into the PM process should be directed to each component of the process in order to improve the overall effectiveness of the process and to ensure that all of the strategic value of the information produced is used to the greatest benefit by the organization. The theoretical operation of the PM process model, especially the "Evaluation" and "Information" components of the model, is the focus of the conclusions.

A major conclusion related to the study is that a majority of respondents indicated in spite of using many different types of PM, up to 11 different types of PMs in one LAU alone, the use of PM has made little perceived positive impact on Florida public libraries and the services they provide. Respondents, especially noted evaluating technology and staff-related issues, i.e. time required to learn and conduct PM process, lack of understanding of PM, and resistance, as being areas where little impact had been made by existing performance measures. Respondents also indicated increasing the implementation of technology in the PM process would be a key requirement to effectively conduct PM in the future.

A majority of respondents perceived the PM process as inaccurate and imprecise and not a top priority in their LAU. A majority of respondents did not perceive that PM use had greatly enhanced their ability to effectively demonstrate or report organizational impact or service quality, though many respondents reported limited positive impacts in the areas of reporting resource use and improving public relations with the communities they serve. The limited amount of perceived positive impact was further diminished when the amount of resources allocated to conduct PM in FY 2000 was considered.

An estimated $7.9–$16.1 million was allocated to conduct PM in FY 2000. The total budgetary amount allocated to conducting PM in Florida public libraries was equivalent to 24.1–49.0% of the SA distributed to Florida's public libraries in FY 2000, two to four times the total amount spent statewide on electronic information resources, or 2.0–5.0% of statewide public library income. Additionally, an estimated 335–609 staff FTE was used to conduct PM in FY 2000.

During the PM process in Florida public libraries, a majority of respondents indicated performance data and information regarding customer satisfaction and technology evaluation were collected annually or "as required." While annual reporting of PM information to stakeholders was a standard practice in governmental and nonprofit organizations, it was probable that the collected PM information was out of date or erroneous when analyzed and used by the LAU to report their performance. Once the PM information was analyzed, the resulting data and knowledge was not widely or consistently disseminated to individuals within or agencies outside of the library organization in a majority of respondents. For example, LAU staff members were not always included in the PM process, nor did they always receive the resulting data and knowledge created from the PM process.

The resulting data, information, and knowledge of the PM process were not effectively cycled into the PM process itself. Respondents did not indicate PM information was used to evaluate the "Evaluation" or "Information" components of the process model, the effectiveness of the process as a whole, nor did a majority of respondents indicate PM information being extensively cycled into the "Planning" and "Acquisition" components of the PM process model.

A significant number of respondents indicated that their governing bodies and customers did not require any type of PM information from the LAU, nor did LAU require PM information from their partners and program collaborators. Even when the type of PM information required by governing bodies and customers to demonstrate quality and effectiveness is known by LAU, a majority of LAU did not collect the same type of PM information perceived as required by their governing bodies and customers. Thus, many respondents were collecting, maintaining, and reporting outdated, erroneous, or unnecessary PM information to the LAU's governing body, stakeholders, and partners or program collaborators.

RECOMMENDATIONS

The first recommendation to come from this study was that LAUs need to review their PM processes in order to ascertain whether needed or required PM information is effectively collected and reported to all appropriate recipients. The review should include stakeholders, customers, partners or program collaborators, and individuals or organizations with PM expertise and be performed regularly to allow for timely corrective feedback of the effectiveness of the PM process. The review should ensure that the PM process is connected to all other aspects of the organization and its processes.

After the PM process review, HLA and LAU staff should be provided an increased knowledge and understanding of PM use through the provision of training and practicums specifically designed to meet the requirements of the revised PM process in their LAU. Appropriate technologies should be implemented, with appropriate training, to minimize resource consumption, while maximizing potential strategic and community impact value of the PM process. The results of the HLA PM process review will provide governing bodies, stakeholders, partners, and program collaborators with an increased knowledge and understanding of the PM process through improved direct communication and reporting of required PM information between all PM process participants. Appropriate technologies should be implemented to maximize stakeholder and community awareness of the strategic needs, accomplishments, and value of the LAU.

The second recommendation was to review existing PM information management processes within the LAU, including the communication and reporting of PM information, participants and roles in the PM information management processes, and selecting and aligning PM needs among participants. Identify areas of improvement and initiate regular reviews of the process to allow for corrective feedback.

To reduce the amount of incorrect or unnecessary data collected, the LAU should integrate existing and future information management systems with PM information management processes and resources.

The researcher revised the initial PM model using the study findings and Purpose I conclusions. The revised PM model is illustrated in Fig. 3.

In the revised PM process model, the information flows (red lines) were adjusted to account for the study findings of the use of PM information. The empty triangles in the revised model indicate an inconsistent or diminished flow of PM information to the "Planning and Acquisition" and "Outputs" components of the model. The "Evaluation" component of the model receives no PM information, while the "Resources" and "Activities" components of the model receive the majority of the PM information produced in the process.

In the literature review of this study, four theoretical factors were identified as sources of problems in the PM process in libraries: a lack of consensus as to the types and value of PM, a lack of understanding of how to use and interpret PM information, organizational structures and cultures impeding the PM process, and a lack of precision in the PM process. Evidence was found to indicate that all four theoretical problem factors currently exist in the PM process of Florida public libraries. All of these problem factors impede the creation and operation of a PM in Florida public libraries.

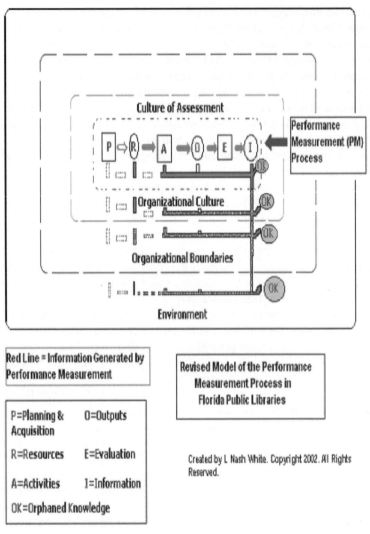

Fig. 3.   Revised Performance Measurement (PM) Process Model.

A majority of respondents perceived little change would occur in their PM use and impact over the next three years, though several respondents identified social and political changes in their community as affecting their PM process in the future. The majority of respondents perceived output-oriented measures used in their LAU would continue to be more effective to use than newer performance measures over the next three years. The study findings indicated that a significant number of respondents lacked an understanding of or commitment to the use of PM and the management of the resulting PM information. Because of this lack of understanding or commitment, a majority of respondents did not support a library culture, which values the PM process or the resulting information or value. The lack of a culture that supports the PM process may be responsible for an apparent lack of understanding or communication of PM information needs of stakeholders and partners, the lack of process and value alignment in the overall PM process, the negative perceptions of impact from using PM, the lack of priority in conducting PM, and the allotment of resources allocated to conducting PM.

The third recommendation was that statewide and regional library agencies, i.e. the State Library, Florida Library Association, and multitype library cooperatives, and leaders should undertake to improve their understanding of the PM process, the management of the resulting PM information, and their combined strategic and community impact value. Positively conveying and demonstrating the importance and value of a culture of assessment in all organizational activities could achieve this understanding. The results would formulate the foundation required to develop a culture of assessment that fits Florida public libraries' needs. HLA should then exemplify the values of the culture of assessment as described by Lakos, i.e. "walk the walk, and talk the talk." By providing support and leadership for the PM process and its use in their LAU, the HLA's commitment, perceptions, and values will lead the drive toward the implementation and adoption of the culture of assessment in their LAU.

To ensure that PM training and education are provided to all Florida library staff, the regional and state agencies libraries should provide continuing education opportunities in the area of PM to library practioners and their stakeholders. The PM process and results will more closely align with desired organizational outcomes and their reporting as the understanding of the PM process and the potential derived value becomes better appreciated by both practioners and stakeholders. Corresponding to the educational opportunities for practioners, students and prospective practioners in library and information studies programs entering the profession need an improved understanding of the practical application of evaluation theories, measures, developments, and the PM process. Many graduates of library and information studies programs immediately become HLA or are required to perform administrative functions, such as performance evaluation upon entry into the profession. Ensuring their understanding of current practices and future developments will allow new professionals to acclimate more readily into a culture of assessment, and/or to initiate or support a culture of assessment in their workplace.

Researchers in the profession should provide direction and guidance to practioners in investigating and improving the understanding and operation of the PM process and the culture of assessment. Research efforts and results should support the development of future PM processes and the culture of assessment. Expanding the research into PM would provide needed resources for practioners and students to better understand the practical application of PM and the dynamics of a culture of assessment.

IMPLICATIONS FOR PRACTICE

The study's implications for practice include research evidence and recommendations designed to increase the understanding and appreciation of the PM process and the culture of assessment in Florida public libraries. The findings of this study can provide immediate utility to the profession by serving as the basis for LAU to examine their PM processes and begin developing enhanced understandings and abilities to use PM more effectively.

The results of the studies, including the revised models of the PM process and the culture of assessment, serve as a guide to practioners for evaluating existing PM processes and developing new PM and PM processes. The study's results serve as a practical resource for the training of professionals in the field and students who will become library professionals in the PM process and the culture of assessment.

The study provides library stakeholders with a resource they can use to examine their existing communication methods, PM information management, and roles of participation in the PM process of their public library. As stakeholders become more aware of the PM process and how it operates in their public libraries, stakeholders will better appreciate the value and the efforts required to obtain the PM information. Redundant and erroneous work collecting and managing PM information could be reduced or eliminated in the PM process, thus saving valued resources for addressing other pressing needs. Stakeholders would derive better services while reducing resource expenditure, thus improving the perceived community impact of the library on the communities they serve.

IMPLICATIONS FOR RESEARCH

The study's implications for research are a baseline dataset of information, data, and participant perceptions for immediate future research in the area of PM use and impact in Florida public libraries and in other possible settings. The study's findings benefit researchers in the fields of librarianship, public administration, information and knowledge management, and organizational informatics, which is the study of how technology affects the social and cultural aspects of organizations and how the social and cultural aspects of organizations affect technology use.

This study was the first study of the PM processes of Florida public libraries. Other incentives for research was the delivery of a detailed body of evidence and the need for an understanding of the existing PM process, its participants, and the social and cultural affects on the PM process. In addition, an understanding of the management and communication of PM information within the library organization and between the library organization and its stakeholders was made available to researchers.

The results of the study serve as a guide for future research. The study's findings concerning the perceptions of the current use and impact of PM and the lack of a culture of assessment identify the challenges and successes of PM in the field. The identified challenges and successes, as well as the revised models of the PM process and the culture of assessment, serve as points of embarkation for future research into the PM process and other organizational research interests.

RECOMMENDATIONS FOR FUTURE RESEARCH

Recommendations for future research in the area of PM, the PM process, and the culture of assessment in Florida public libraries based on the findings of the study are listed below. The recommendations are listed in order according to the researcher's perceptions of the priority or necessity of the research to establish future improvements and refinements in the PM process.

1. Replicate the study to determine the reliability of results. Determine the scope and application of the study findings to other public library settings.
2. Describe in detail the micro and macro PM information utilization processes and behaviors in LAU, especially by HLAs.

3. Determine the organizational, cultural, and technological factors affecting the communication and reporting of PM information between stakeholders, governing bodies, and public libraries.
4. Model and research the orphaned data and knowledge process to understand its creation, while identifying methods to reduce its production and costs or to regain the value of the orphaned data and knowledge.
5. Identify methods to increase the use of technology in the PM process and reduce the resources required in conducting PM.
6. Develop new PM measures that address the study findings, such as technology evaluation measures and community impact of library service.

CONCLUSION

This study of the use and perceptions of PM by Florida public LAUs demonstrate a less than effective utilization of PM processes and resources. While the public is increasing their demand for accountability and responsiveness from Florida public libraries, HLAs have difficulty in responding to the request due to mixed perceptions of the types of measurement to utilize and the perceptions of the effectiveness of PM in public libraries. HLAs showed little consensus for how to improve the PM process or the direction that improvement should pursue. The results demonstrated a need for increased education and understanding of PM processes among HLAs in Florida public libraries.

REFERENCES

Ammons, D. N. (2000). *Municipal benchmarks: Assessing local performance and establishing community standards*. Thousand Oaks, CA: Sage Publications.

Creswell, J. W. (1994). *Research design: Qualitative and quantitative approaches*. Thousand Oaks, CA: Sage.

DeProspo, E. R., Altman, E., & Beasley, K. E. (1973). *Performance measures for public libraries*. Chicago, IL: PLA.

Hatry, H. P., Blair, L., Fisk, D. M., Greiner, J. H., Hall, J. R., & Schaenman, P. S. (1979). *Efficiency measurement for local government services – some initial suggestions*. Washington, DC: Urban Institute.

Hernon, P., & Altman, E. (1996). *Service quality in academic libraries*. Chicago: American Library Association.

Himmel, E. I., & Wilson, W. J. (1998). *Planning for results: A public library transformation process*. Chicago: American Library Association.

Institute for Museum and Library Services (IMLS). (2000). *Perspectives on outcome based evaluation for libraries and museums.* Washington, DC: Institute for Museum and Library Services (IMLS).

Kraft, D. H., & Boyce, B. R. (1991). *Operations research for libraries and information agencies: Techniques for the evaluation of management decision alternatives.* San Diego, CA: Academic Press, Inc.

Risher, H., & Fay, C. (Eds) (1995). *The performance imperative: Strategies for enhancing workforce effectiveness.* San Francisco, CA: Jossey-Bass.

Scriven, M. (1991). *Evaluation thesaurus* (4th ed.). Newbury Park: Sage Publications.

Shafritz, J. M., & Ott, J. S. (Eds) (1997). *Classics of public administration* (4th ed.). Fort Worth, TX: Harcourt Brace College Publishers.

Suchman, E. A. (1967). *Evaluation research: Principles and practice in public service and social action programs.* New York: Sage Foundation.

United Way of America's Outcome Measurement Resource Network. (1995–2002). Available online: http://www/unitedway.org/outcomes/.

Van House, N. A., Lynch, M. J., McClure, C. R., Zweizig, D. L., & Rodger, E. J. (1987). *Output measures for public libraries: A manual of standardized procedures* (2nd ed.). Chicago: American Library Association.

White, L. N. (2002). *Does counting count: An evaluative study of performance assessment in Florida public libraries.* Published doctoral dissertation thesis. Tallahassee, FL: Florida State University.

Withers, F. N. (1974). *Standards for library service: An international survey.* Paris: UNESCO.

FURTHER READING

Altman, E. (1990). Reflections on performance measures fifteen years later. In: C. C. Curran & F. William Summers (Eds), *Library performance, accountability, and responsiveness: Essays in honor of Ernest R. DeProspo* (pp. 9–16). Norwood, NJ: Ablex Publishing Corporation.

American Library Association. (1980). *Library effectiveness: A state of the art.* New York: American Library Association.

Babbie, E. (1998). *The practice of social research* (8th ed.). Belmont, CA: Wadsworth Publishing.

Bassett, G. (1993). *The evolution and future of high performance management systems.* Westport, CT: Quorum Books.

Belasen, A. T. (1999). *Leading the learning organization: Communication and competencies for managing change.* Albany, NY: State University of New York Press.

Bell, C. R. (1994). *Customers as partners: Building relationships that last.* San Francisco, CA: Berrett-Koehler Publishers.

Benton Foundation. (1996). *Americans chart a future for public libraries.* Washington, DC: W.W. Kellogg Foundation.

Bertot, J. C., McClure, C. R., & Ryan, J. (2001). *Statistics and performance measures for public library networked services.* Chicago: American Library Association.

Best, D. P. (Ed.) (1996). *The fourth resource: Information and its management.* Hampshire, England: ASLIB Gower.

Bjornlund, L. (1999). *Beyond data: Current uses of comparative performance measurement in local government*. Washington, DC: International City/County Management Association.

Black, S. A., & Porter, L. (1996). Identification of the critical factors of TQM. *Decision Sciences, 27*(1), 1–21.

Blagden, J., & Harrington, J. (1990). *How good is your library? A review of approaches to the evaluation of library and information services*. London: ASLIB.

Blank, J. L. T. (Ed.) (2000). *Public provision and performance: Contributions from efficiency and productivity measurement*. Amsterdam: Elsevier.

Boekhorst, P. te. (1995). Measuring quality: The IFLA guidelines for performance measurement in academic libraries. *IFLA Journal, 21*(4), 278–281.

Bogan, C., & English, M. J. (1994). *Benchmarking for best practices: Winning through innovative adoption*. New York: McGraw-Hill.

Boisse, J. A. (1996). Adjusting the horizontal hold: Flattening the organization. *Library Administrative & Management, 10*(2), 77–81.

Bourn, J. (1995). Public sector management. International library of management (Vol. 2). Vermont: Dartmouth Publishing.

Boyce, B. R., Meadow, C. T., & Craft, D. H. (1994). *Measurement in information science*. San Diego, CA: Academic Press.

Brewer, J. (1995). Service management: How to plan for it rather than hope for it. *Library Administration and Management, 9*(4), 207–210.

Brimson, J. A. (1994). *Activity based management: For service industries, government entities, and nonprofit organization*. New York: Wiley.

Brocka, B., & Brocka, M. S. (1992). *Quality management: Implementing the best ideas of the masters*. Homewood, IL: Business One Irwin.

Brockman, J. R. (1992). Just another management fad? The implications of TQM for library and information services. *ASLIB Proceedings, 44*(7/8), 283–288.

Brockman, J. (Ed.) (1997). *Quality management and benchmarking in the information sector*. London: Bowker-Saur.

Brooking, A. (1999). *Corporate memory: Strategies for knowledge management*. London: International Thomson Business Press.

Brooks, T. A. (1981). *An analysis of library-output statistics*. Austin, TX: University of Texas.

Brophy, P., & Coulling, K. (1996). *Quality management for information and library managers*. London: ASLIB Gower.

Brown, M. G. (1996). *Keeping score: Using the right metrics to drive world-class performance*. New York: Quality Resources.

Brusha, C. H., & Harter, S. (1980). *Research methods in librarianship*. New York: Academic Press.

Campbell, J. D. (1996). Building an effectiveness pyramid for leading successful organizational transformation. *Library Administration & Management, 10*(2), 82–86.

Carr, D. K., & Johansson, H. J. (1995). *Best practices in reengineering: What works and what doesn't in the reengineering process*. New York: McGraw-Hill.

Chen, C. (1978). *Quantitative measurement and dynamic library service*. Phoenix, AZ: Oryx Press.

Childers, T., & Van House, N. A. (1989). *The public library effectiveness study: Final report*. Washington, DC: U.S. Dept. of Education.

Childers, T., & Van House, N. A. (1993). *What's good? Describing your public library's effectiveness*. Chicago: American Library Association.

Ciborra, C. U., Braa, K. C., Cordella, A., Dahlbom, B., Failla, A., Hanseth, O., Hepso, V., Ljungberg, J., Monteiro, E., & Simon, K. A. (2000). *From control to drift: The dynamics of corporate information infrastructures.* Oxford, England: Oxford University Press.

Clark, A., & Dawson, R. (1999). *Evaluation research: An introduction to principles, methods, and practice.* London: Sage.

Collier, D. A. (1993). *The service/quality solution: Using service management to gain competitive advantage.* Milwaukee, WI: ASQC Quality Press.

Curran, C., & Clark, P. M. (1989). Implications of tying state aid to performance measures. *Public Libraries, 28*(6), 348–354.

Davis, F. W., & Manrodt, K. B. (1996). *Customer-responsive management: The flexible advantage.* Cambridge, MA: Blackwell.

Dillman, D. A. (1978). *Mail and telephone surveys: The total design method.* New York: Wiley.

Dixon, N. M. (1999). *Common knowledge: How companies thrive by sharing what they know.* Boston, MA: Harvard Business School Press.

Drucker, P. F. (1980). *Managing in turbulent times.* New York: Harper and Row.

Earl, M. J. (Ed.) (1995). *Information management: The organizational dimension.* New York, NY: Oxford University Press Inc.

Edosomwan, J. A. (Ed.) (1987). Integrating productivity and quality management. In: *Industrial engineering* (Vol. 14). New York: Marcel Dekker, Inc.

Evans, J., Anderson, D. R., Sweeney, D. J., & Williams, T. A. (1990). *Applied production and operations management.* St. Paul, MN: West Publishing Company.

Finch, B. J., & Luebbe, R. L. (1995). *Operations management: Competing in a changing environment.* Orlando, FL: Dryden Press, Inc.

Fisher, W. (1995). Does TQM really help anyone? *Library Acquisitions: Practice and Theory, 19*(1), 49–52.

Florida Department of Library and Information Services. (1997). *Access for all: Libraries in Florida's future.* Tallahassee, FL: Florida Department of Library and Information Services.

Florida Department of Library and Information Services. (2000). *Florida library directory with statistics.* Tallahassee, FL: Florida Department of Library and Information Services.

Florida Department of Library and Information Services. (2001). *Florida library directory with statistics.* Tallahassee, FL: Florida Department of Library and Information Services.

Florida Library Association Public Library Standards Working Committee, Berger, L., & Weaver, B. (1995). *Standards for Florida public libraries: A vision for the 21st century.* Princeton, NJ: Library Development Solutions.

Gale, B. T. (1993). *Managing customer value: Creating quality and service that customers can see.* New York: Free Press.

Garrod, P., & Kinnell, M. (1996). Performance measurement, benchmarking, and the UK Library and information services sector. *Libri, 46*(3), 141–148.

Gill, J., & Johnson, P. (1997). *Research methods for managers* (2nd ed.). London: Paul Chapman Publishing Ltd.

Glass, G. V., & Hopkins, K. D. (1995). *Statistical methods in education and psychology* (3rd ed.). Boston, MA: Allyn and Bacon.

Glazier, J. D., & Powell, R. R. (Eds) (1992). *Qualitative research in information management.* Englewood, CO: Libraries Unlimited, Inc.

Goleski, E. (1995). Learning to say, "Yes": A customer service program for library staff. *Library Administration and Management, 9*(4), 211–215.

Gray, S. T. (1997). *Evaluation with power: A new approach to organizational effectiveness, empowerment, and excellence.* San Francisco: Jossey-Bass Publishers.

Haavind, R. (1991). *The road to the Baldridge award: Quest for total quality.* Stoneham, MA: Butterworth-Heinemann.

Halachmi, A., & Bouckaert, G. (Eds) (1996). *Organizational performance and measurement in the public sector: Toward service, effort, and accomplishment reporting.* Westport, CT: Quorum Books.

Hall, P. D. (1994). Historical perspectives on non-profit organizations. *In the Jossey-Bass handbook of nonprofit leadership and management* (pp. 3–43). San Francisco, CA: Jossey-Bass Publishers.

Harris, M. (1991). The customer survey in performance measurement. *British Journal of Academic Librarianship, 6*(1), 1–27.

Hays, R. D. (1996). *Internal service excellence: A manager's guide to building world class internal service unit performance.* Sarasota, FL: Summit Executive Press.

Hernon, P. (1992). Library and information science research: Not an island unto itself. *LISR, 14*(1–3), 1–3.

Hernon, P. (1996). Service quality in libraries and treating customers as customers and non-customers as lost or never-gained customers. *Journal of Academic Librarianship, 22*(3), 171–172.

Hernon, P., & Altman, E. (1998). *Assessing service quality: Satisfying the expectations of library customers.* Chicago: American Library Association.

Hernon, P., & McClure, C. R. (1990). *Evaluation and decision making.* Norwood, NJ: Ablex Publishing Corporation.

Hernon, P., & Whitman, J. R. (2001). *Delivering satisfaction and service quality: A customer-based approach for libraries.* Chicago: American Library Association.

Hershfield, A. F., & Boone, M. D. (1972). *Approaches to measuring library effectiveness: A symposium.* Syracuse, NY: Syracuse University Press.

Heskett, J. L. (1990). *Service breakthroughs: Changing the rules of the game.* New York: Free Press.

Hunt, V. D. (1993). *Managing for quality: Integrating quality and business strategy.* Homewood, IL: Business One Irwin.

Jensen, B. (2000). *Simplicity: The new competitive advantage in a world of more, better, faster.* New York, NY: Perseus Publishing.

Johnson, R. S. (1993). *TQM: Leadership for the quality transformation.* Milwaukee, WI: ASQC.

Kaplan, A. (1964). *The conduct of inquiry; methodology for behavioral science.* San Francisco: Chandler Publishing Company.

Kaplan, R. S. (2001). Strategic performance measurement and management in nonprofit organizations. *Nonprofit Management and Leadership, 11*(3), 353–370.

Kaplan, R. S., & Norton, D. P. (1996). *The balanced scorecard: Translating strategy into action.* Boston, MA: Harvard Business School Press.

Kearney, R. C., & Berman, E. M. (1999). *Public sector performance: Management, motivation, and measurement.* Boulder, CO: Westview Press.

Kemp, R. L. (1995). The Creative management of library services. *Public Libraries, 34*(4), 212–215.

Keyes, J. (1992). *Infotrends: The competitive use of information.* New York: McGraw-Hill, Inc.

Kling, R. (2001). *What is social informatics?* [Online]. Available: http://www.slis.indiana.edu/si/concepts.html

Lakos, A. (1998). Building a culture of assessment in academic libraries. Paper presented at a panel discussion at *Living the Future II conference* (pp. 3–7). University of Arizona, Tucson, AZ, April 12.

Lakos, A. (1999). The missing ingredient – culture of assessment in libraries. *Performance Measurement and Metrics, 3.*

Lancaster, F. W. (1988). *If you want to evaluate your library* .... Champaign, IL: University of Illinois.

Lancaster, F. W. (1977). *The Measurement and evaluation of library services.* Washington, DC: Information Resources Press.

Lawes, A. (1993). The benefits of quality management to the library and information profession. *Special Libraries, 84,* 142–146.

Lawler, E. E., II. (1980). *Organizational assessment: Perspectives on the measurement of organizational behavior and the quality of work life.* New York: Wiley.

Lee, S., & Clack, M. E. (1996). Continued organizational transformation: The Harvard college library's experience. *Library Administration & Management, 10*(2), 98–104.

Leedy, P. D. (1993). *Practical research: Planning and design.* New York, NY: Macmillan Publishing Company.

Leimkuhler, F. F. (1977). Operations research and systems analysis. In: F. W. Lancaster (Ed.), *Evaluation and scientific management of libraries and information centers* (pp. 131–164). Bristol: Noordhoff International.

Letts, C., Ryan, W., & Grossman, A. (1999). *High performance nonprofit organizations: Managing upstream for greater impact.* New York, NY: Wiley.

Liu, K., Clarke, R. J., Andersen, P. B., & Stamper, R. K. (Eds) (2000). *Information, organization, and technology: Studies in organizational semiotics.* Norwell, MA: Kluwer Academic Publishers.

Locke, L. F., Spirduso, W. W., & Silverman, S. J. (1993). *Proposals that work: A guide for planning dissertations and grant proposals* (3rd ed.). Newbury Park, CA: Sage Publications.

Losee, R. M., & Worley, K. A. (1993). *Research and evaluation for information professionals.* San Diego, CA: Academic Press, Inc.

Lubans, J. J., & Chapman, E. A. (Eds) (1975). Reader in library systems analysis. Reader series in library and information science (Vol. 1975). Englewood, CO: Microcard Edition Books.

Lynch, B. P. (1985). *Management strategies for libraries: A basic reader.* New York: Neal-Schuman Publishers.

Lynch, M. J. (1990). Measurement of library output: How is it related to research. In: C. C. Curran & F. W. Summers (Eds), *Library performance, accountability, and responsiveness: Essays in honor of Ernest R. DeProspo* (pp. 1–8). Norwood, NJ: Ablex Publishing Corporation.

McClelland, S. B. (1995). *Organizational needs assessments: Design, facilitation, and analysis.* Westport, CT: Quorum Books.

McClure, C. R. (1990). Integrating performance measures into the planning process: Moving toward decision support systems. In: C. C. Curran & F. W. Summers (Eds), *Library performance, accountability, and responsiveness: Essays in honor of Ernest R. DeProspo* (pp. 17–32). Norwood, NJ: Ablex Publishing Corporation.

McClure, C. R., & Hernon, P. (Eds) (1990). *Library and information science research: Perspectives and strategies for improvement.* Norwood, NJ: Ablex Publishing Corporation.

130   LARRY NASH WHITE

McGee, J. V., Prusak, L., & Pyburn, P. J. (1993). *Managing information strategically.* New York, NY: Wiley.

Miles, M. B., & Huberman, A. M. (1984). *Qualitative data analysis: A sourcebook of new methods.* Beverly Hills, CA: Sage Publications.

Miller, W. C. (1993). *Quantum quality: Quality improvement through innovation, learning, and creativity.* White Plains, NY: Quality Resources.

Milner, E. M. (2000). *Managing information and knowledge in the public sector.* London: Routledge.

Moore, N. (1989). *Measuring the performance of public libraries.* New York: UNESCO.

Moorman, J. A. (1997). Standards for public libraries: A study in quantitative measures of library performance as found in state public library documents. *Public Libraries,* (Jan/Feb), 32–39.

Mullis, R., Mullis, A., Cornille, T., Handy, D., Handy, A., & Huber, J. (2000). *Born to read program evaluation.* Tallahassee, FL: Florida State University.

Murray, V., & Tassie, B. (1994). Evaluating the effectiveness of non-profit organizations. *In the Jossey-Bass handbook of nonprofit leadership and management* (pp. 302–324). San Francisco, CA: Jossey-Bass Publishers.

Noble, P., & Ward, P. L. (1976). *Performance measures and criteria for libraries.* Public Library Occasional Papers (Vol. 3). England: Orchard & Ind.

Obloj, K., Cushman, D. P., & Kozminskis, A. (1994). *Winning: Continuous improvement theory in high-performance organizations.* Albany, NY: State University of New York.

Oldham, C. (1977). An Examination of cost/benefit approaches to the evaluation of library and information services. In: F. W. Lancaster (Ed.), *Evaluation and scientific management of libraries and information centers* (pp. 165–184). England: Noordhoff.

O'Neil, R. M., & Osif, B. A. (1993). A total look at TQM: A TQM perspective from the literature of business, industry, higher education, and librarianship. *Library Administration and Management, 7*(4), 244–254.

Ormes, S. (1996). Access is limited in quantity and quality. *Library Association Record, 98*(1), 68.

Park, M. W. (1998). *InfoThink: Practical strategies for using information in business.* Lanham, MD: Scarecrow Press, Inc.

Patton, M. Q. (1980). *Qualitative evaluation methods.* Beverly Hills, CA: Sage Publications.

Peters, B. G., & Pierre, J. (2001). *Politicians, bureaucrats, and administrative reform.* London: Routledge.

Pfeffer, J., & Sutton, R. L. (1999). *The knowing-doing gap: How smart companies turn knowledge into action.* Boston, MA: Harvard Business School Press.

Poll, R. (1991). Problems of performance evaluation in academic libraries. *INSPEL, 25*(1), 25–36.

Pritchard, R. D. (1990). *Measuring and improving organizational productivity: A practical guide.* New York: Preager.

Pritchard, R. D. (1995). *Productivity measurement and improvement: Organizational case studies.* Westport, CT: Preager.

Prusak, L. (Ed.) (1997). *Knowledge in organizations.* Boston, MA: Butterworth-Heinemann.

Robbins, J. (Ed.) (1988). *Rethinking the library in the information age.* Washington, DC: United States Department of Education.

Robbins, J., & Zweizig, D. (1988). *Are we there yet? Evaluating library collections, reference services, programs, and personnel.* Madison, WI: University of Wisconsin–Madison.

Rust, R. T., & Oliver, R. L. (Eds) (1994). *Service quality: New directions in theory and practice.* Thousand Oaks, CA: Sage Publications.

St. Clair, G. (Ed.) (1996). Total quality management in information services. In: *Information Services Management* (Vol. 6). London: Bowker-Saur.

Schement, J. R. (1996). A 21st century strategy for librarians. *Library Journal,* 34–36.

Shaffer, K. R. (1972). *The experience of management.* Metuchen, NJ: Scarecrow Press.

Smith, M. (1996). *Collecting and using public library statistics.* New York: Neal-Schuman Publishers.

Snyder, H. (1997). Protecting our assets: Internal control principles in libraries. *Library Administration and Management, 11*(1), 42–46.

Special Libraries Association. (1998). *Knowledge management: A new competitive asset.* Washington, DC: Special Libraries Association.

Stephens, N. D. (1985). *Archives of library research from the Molesworth institute.* New York: Haworth Press.

Tague-Sutcliffe, J. (1996). *Measuring information: An information services perspective.* San Diego, CA: Academic Press.

Thompson, A. A., & Strickland, A. J., III. (1984). *Strategic management: Concepts and cases.* Plano, TX: Business Publications.

Thompson, J. (1991). *Redirection in academic library management.* London: Library Association Publishing.

Thomas, J. C. (1994). Program evaluation and program development. *In the Jossey-Bass handbook of nonprofit leadership and management* (pp. 342–366). San Francisco, CA: Jossey-Bass Publishers.

Tiefel, V. (1989). Output or performance measures: the making of a manual. *C&RL News, 50,* 475–478.

Travica, B. (1998). *New organizational designs: Information aspects.* Stamford, CT: Ablex Publishing Corporation.

Tushman, M. L., & Anderson, P. (1997). *Managing strategic innovation and change.* Oxford, England: Oxford University Press.

United State Census Bureau. (2001). *State and county quick facts for Florida.* (September). Available online: http://www.quickfacts.census.gov/qfd/states/ 12000.html

Van House, N. A., Lynch, M. J., McClure, C. R., Zweizig, D. L., & Altman, E. (1977). *Output measures for public libraries: A manual of standardized procedures* (1st ed.). Chicago: American Library Association.

Wallace, D. P., & Van Fleet, C. (2001). *Library evaluation: A casebook and can-do guide.* Englewood, CO: Libraries Unlimited.

Wilson, P. F., & Pearson, R. D. (1995). *Performance-based assessments: External, internal, and self-assessment tools for total quality management.* Milwaukee, WI: ASQC Quality Press.

Wedgeworth, R. (Ed.) (1993). *World encyclopedia of library and information science* (3rd ed.). Chicago, IL: ALA.

Zweizig, D., Johnson, D. W., Robbins, J., & Besant, M. (1994). *Tell it! Evaluation sourcebook and training manual.* Madison, WI: University of Wisconsin.

Zweizig, D., & Rodgers, E. Jo. (1982). *Output measures for public libraries: A manual of standardized procedures.* Chicago: American Library Association.

APPENDIX: FLORIDA PUBLIC LIBRARY
PERFORMANCE MEASUREMENT STUDY

Introduction
Thank you for your participation. This 33 question survey should take
approximately 25 minutes or less to complete. If you have any questions or
experience difficulties in completing the survey, please contact Larry Nash
White at **E-mail:** white_l@firn.edu **Telephone 850-567-3627** or
cinfo@orgdoctors.com

Instructions
Instructions for completing each section of the survey are provided at the
beginning of each of the five (5) sections. Reminder! The survey needs to be
completed and returned to Larry White on/**before October 10, 2001.**
Participants are encouraged to return the survey (via e-mail when possible)
using the addresses below: **E-mail:** white_l@firn.edu **Standard Mailing: Attn:
Larry White** or cinfo@orgdoctors.com **6284 Crestwood Drive Tallahassee,
FL 32311.**

Online Assistance
Online assistance (in terms of examples and definitions) is available to you.
To access the online assistance, click on the **Help!** Link wherever you see it.
The **Help!** Link will take you to a Web site that provides answers to
potential problems and further explains the instructions for the survey with
examples. The Help! Link will be located at the top and bottom of each page
of the survey.

Section # 1
Please insert the Participant Identification Number (PIN) that was provided
to you in the accompanying **PIN #** e-mail in the response box to the right.

How many years experience as a Florida public library head administrator
do you have? Please round up to the next whole number. Number of years
⇒

Section # 2
Perceptions of Performance Measurement (15 Questions)
Please read each statement below and select the rating between 1–10 that
best describes your level of agreement with the statement in relation to your
public library administrative unit using the scale below.

Please record your selection in the response box at the end of each question.
Agreement Level Lowest Agreement < - - - - - - - - - > **Highest Agreement**
Help!!

Score 1 2 3 4 5 6 7 8 9 10
(1) The results obtained from using performance measurement are worth more than the resources expended to obtain the performance measurements.
Response ⇒
(2) I have a positive view of the results generated from the use of performance measurement in my library administrative unit. **Response** ⇒
(3) The results obtained from the use of performance measurement system(s) provide stakeholders with an accurate account of the overall quality of library service. **Response** ⇒
(4) The results from using performance measurement system(s) effectively report the total organizational impact of the library. **Response** ⇒
(5) Performance measurement is one of the top five priorities for my library administrative unit. **Response** ⇒
(6) The library administrative unit would no longer use performance measurement if it were no longer required by government agencies to receive financial resources. **Response** ⇒
(7) In the reality of my library administrative unit, the focus of performance measurement is to just complete it; not to focus on how well it gets completed or how the results will be used. **Response** ⇒
(8) In my library administrative unit, conducting effective performance measurement undermines the library's ability to provide effective service.
Response ⇒
(9) The overall "community good" that the library administrative unit provides out weighs any need of Help!! accounting for resources.
Response ⇒

Section # 2 Contd.
Help!!

Agreement Level Lowest Agreement < - - - - - - - - > **Highest Agreement**
Score 1 2 3 4 5 6 7 8 9 10
(10) Most library administrators agree on the type of performance measures to be used to report service quality. **Response** ⇒
(11) Most library administrators lack an understanding of how to interpret performance measurement results. **Response** ⇒
(12) The precision of performance measurement in our library administrative unit lends credibility to library administrators' decision making. **Response** ⇒
(13) Performance measurement has greatly improved the library's abilities to provide quality service. **Response** ⇒
(14) Florida's State Aid to libraries should be dispersed to library systems based solely on a competitive comparison of performance measurements to be determined by the Legislature. **Response** ⇒

(15) An annual weeklong workshop on performance measurement should be required of all Florida public library administrators. **Response** ⇒

Section # 3
Performance Measurement Resources (Three Questions)
This section of the study will collect data on the resources allocated to performance measurement within the library administrative unit. Help!!

(16) Please estimate the overall percentage of the total paid staff time in the administrative unit dedicated solely to performance measurement in an average year. Please round to the nearest whole number. Please select one option and record the option number in the box below.

Option 1	Option 2	Option 3	Option 4	
Less than 1%	1–5%	6–10%	More than 10%	**Response** ⇒

(17) What was the total overall percentage of the budget dedicated to conducting performance measurement last year in the library administrative unit? Please select one option and record the option number in the response box below.

Option 1	Option 2	Option 3	Option 4	
Less than 1%	1–5%	6–10%	More than 10%	**Response** ⇒

(18) What percentage of total training time provided to staff members in the past year dealt specifically with using performance measurement? Please select one option and record the response in the box below.

Option 1	Option 2	Option 3	Option 4	Option #
Less than 1%	1–5%	6–10%	More than 10%	**Response** ⇒

Section # 4
Performance Measures Usage Nine Questions
This section will obtain information on how and what performance measures are used for in your library administrative unit.

(19) Performance measurements collected for evaluating customer service are conducted how often?
Please select one option and record the response in the box below.

Option 1	Option 2	Option 3	Option 4	Option 5
Daily	Weekly	Yearly	As required only	Never

Response ⇒

(20) Performance measurements collected for evaluating technology are conducted how often? Please select one option and record the response in the box below.

Option 1	Option 2	Option 3	Option 4	Option 5
Daily	Weekly	Yearly	As required only	Never

Response ⇒

(21) What types of performance measurement are currently being used in your library administrative unit? Please record an "X" in each response box that applies. For each type of measurement used, please indicate the year the measurement was first implemented. If the implementation date is not known, please leave blank.

Used Date

____NonElectronic Output Measures

____Electronic Output Measures

____United Way Outcomes Measurements

____Quality Management Measurements (i.e. TQM) for definitions

____Sterling Measurements or examples, click

____Six Sigma the online

____Performance-Based Budgeting Measurements assistance link

____Balanced Score Card (BSC) below.

____Other Methods

If you use performance measures other than those listed above, please describe them in the boxes below. If you do not use any other performance measurement methods, skip to the **Question 22.**

Type of Measurement(s):

(1)

(2)

(3)

How are measurements used?

(1)

(2)

(3)

When was this type of measurement implemented?

(1)

(2)

(3)

Question 21 Contd.

Why were these types of measurement implemented?

(1)

(2)

(3)

(22) Excluding the State Library of Florida, who receives performance measurement data from your library administrative unit at least annually? Please record an "X" in each response box that applies.

Department of Education (State or Federal) **Response** ⇒ ____
Friends/Trustees/Volunteers of the library **Response** ⇒ ____
Library Associations (State or National) for definitions **Response** ⇒ ____
Library Multitype Cooperatives or examples, **Response** ⇒ ____
Local Community Groups click the **Response** ⇒ ____
Local Government Officials online **Response** ⇒ ____
Local Media assistance **Response** ⇒ ____
Local School Officials below. **Response** ⇒ ____
Program Collaborators/Partners **Response** ⇒ ____
Staff (Library) **Response** ⇒ ____
Suppliers/Vendors **Response** ⇒ ____
Others (If used, name of Others) > **Response** ⇒ ____

(23) Who regularly participates in the actual performance measurement process in your library? Place an "X" in the Participates Column Box for each type of person/group who participates in performance measurement in your library administrative unit. Select all that apply.

Participates in Performance Measurement
Director/Assistant Director ____
Head of Information Sys/Technology ____
Branch Manager/Department Head ____
Front Line Staff ____
Library Users ____
Friends Groups/Volunteers/Trustees ____
Library Advisory Board ____
Local Government Officials ____
Local Media/Community Groups ____
Outside Consultants ____
Public Relations (PR) Staff Member ____
(Specially trained and dedicated to PR only)
Performance Measurement (PM) Staff Member ____
(Specially trained and dedicated to PM only)
Other (Please specify): ____

Reporting Performance Results
(24) Do you use performance measures to perform the following evaluation actions in your library administrative unit? If the type of performance measurement is used, select the evaluative action that it is primarily used for listed below. Select only one for each evaluative action. If the type of

performance measurement is not used, place an "**X**" in the "Not Applicable" box for each type of performance measurement.
Reporting Efficiency/Effectiveness ____
Reporting Service Impacts ____
Not Applicable ____
NonElectronic Output Measures ____
Electronic Output Measures ____
United Way Outcomes ____
Quality/Process Management Measurements ____

Reporting Efficiency/Effectiveness ____
Reporting Service Impacts ____
Not Applicable ____
Sterling Measurements ____
Six Sigma ____
Pay for Performance ____
Balanced Score Card (BSC) ____
Other Methods ____

(25) The governing body of the library administrative unit primarily requests what type of evidence to demonstrate service effectiveness? Circle the appropriate response.

Option # Response
(1) Cost-benefit analysis (2) Efficiency scores (3) Process review
(4) Outcomes/Impact (5) Other (6) None

(26) The patrons of the library administrative unit primarily request what type of evidence to demonstrate service effectiveness? Circle the appropriate response.
Option # Response
(1) Cost-benefit analysis (2) Efficiency scores (3) Process review
(4) Outcomes/Impact (5) Other (6) None

(27) The library administrative unit primarily requests what type of evidence from service partners to demonstrate service effectiveness?
Option # Response
(1) Cost-benefit analysis (2) Efficiency scores (3) Process review
(4) Outcomes/Impact (5) Other (6) None

Section 5
Performance Measurement Impact Five Questions
This section will obtain information on the impact of performance measures usage in your library administrative unit.

(28) Making a Difference with Performance Measurement
In theory, performance measures are utilized in order to improve the library administrators' ability to improve and report the quality of service in their administrative unit. In order to determine whether this is true, please indicate below how each type of performance measurement has impacted the quality of service provided by your library administrative unit. If your library administrative unit does not use a particular type of performance measurement, select the choice "N/A" (Not Applicable). Place an "X" in the appropriate box below.

N/A	Very negative	Somewhat negative	No difference made	Somewhat positive	Very positive
Non-Electronic Output Measures					
Electronic Output Measures					
United Way Outcomes Measurements					
Quality Management Measurements					
Sterling Measurements					
Six Sigma					
Performance-Based Budgeting Measurements					
Balanced Score Card (BSC)					
Other Methods					

(29) What type of performance measurement would you use to respond most effectively to requests from your governing body to demonstrate accountability or effectiveness for each of the following quality or service criteria? Please select one option (from the list below) for each quality or service criteria and record the option number in the appropriate response box to the right of each question.

Option 1	**Option 2**	**Option 3**	**Option 4**	**Option 5**
Outputs	Cost-effectiveness	Customer Satisfaction	Outcomes Assessment	New measure Needed

Option #
(a) Overall Service Quality **Response** _____
(b) Overall Customer Service Rating **Response**_____
(c) Availability of Information **Response**_____
(d) Effective Resource Usage **Response**_____
(e) Access to Information **Response**_____
(f) Effectiveness of Technology **Response**_____
(g) Community Impact **Response**_____
(h) Human Resource Development **Response**_____
(i) Quality of Information Provided **Response**_____

(30) What type(s) of performance measurements will your library administrative unit be using in three years? **Why?** Reply below.

(31) Please describe any negative impacts from the use of performance measurement on your library administrative unit in the box below. Please list all of the negative impacts that apply in your library administrative unit. If there are no negative impacts, please state this.

(32) Please describe any positive impacts from the use of performance measurement on your library administrative unit in the box below. Please list all of the positive impacts that apply in your library administrative unit. If there are no positive impacts, please state this.

(33) How would you respond to the following statement:
"Everyone knows that libraries are a good thing for the community. We also know that the total operating budget of the library administrative unit is a small percentage of the overall governing body operating budget. So, why should anyone really care about performance measurement in public libraries?" **Do you agree with these statements? Please explain your response**.

Thank you for completing this survey. Your effort is appreciated

The survey needs to be completed and returned to Larry White on/before October 10, 2001. Participants are encouraged to return the survey (via e-mail when possible) using the addresses below: **E-mail**: white_l@firn.edu **Standard Mailing: Attn: Larry White** or cinfo@orgdoctors.com **6284 Crestwood Drive Tallahassee, FL 32311**.

CONTRACTING PUBLIC LIBRARY MANAGEMENT TO PRIVATE VENDORS: THE NEW PUBLIC MANAGEMENT MODEL

Robert C. Ward and Michael Carpenter

INTRODUCTION

An international management movement known as New Public Management (NPM) emerged during the 1970s and 1980s. It relies on the normative use of economic market models, transaction cost theory, and public choice theories to deliver public services. While the manifestations of this new approach have taken many different avenues across the world, in the United States the primary manifestations have been found in the "Reinventing Government" movement (Gore, 1993), and the "Competitive Sourcing" plan of the Bush Administration (Office Management and Budget, 2002, 2003). A central component of NPM practices in the United States is the use of "outsourcing" of government service delivery to private or non-profit organizations.

Fueling the development of NPM in the United States have been the fiscal problems faced by local, state, and federal governments since the 1970s. Governments in the United States are faced with conflicting pressures to increase the levels of service delivery, but to do so in a climate of reducing taxes. Advocates of NPM claim that reliance on NPM principles will

Advances in Library Administration and Organization, Volume 23, 141–172
Copyright © 2006 by Elsevier Ltd.
All rights of reproduction in any form reserved
ISSN: 0732-0671/doi:10.1016/S0732-0671(05)23004-3

promote efficiency and cost savings in government, thus allowing service levels to rise while limiting cost and tax increases (Rondinelli, 2003; Savas, 1987). On the other hand, critics of NPM claim that outsourcing cases in this country often result in either failures to deliver services or outright corruption. The end result, according to the critics of NPM, is that government capacity is hollowed-out, and, ultimately, democratic accountability to the citizen is lost (deLeon & Denhardt, 2000; Milward, 1996).

The library profession has also been influenced by the emergence of NPM. During the past 30 years, outsourcing has been adopted by the library profession, especially in terms of internal operations. The extensive development of outsourcing in the library profession eventually led to a study being conducted by the American Library Association on this area of service delivery (Martin, 2000). The section of the Martin study related to the outsourcing of public library management generated controversy in the library profession and reflected the broader debate occurring in the public management field over the use of NPM principles for the delivery of government services. We restrict the current study to public libraries (local government libraries of general scope intended for public use); other types of libraries such as Federal governmental departmental libraries and military libraries will form the subject of another study.

In essence, NPM makes little or no distinction between the role of government in society and free market principles. To NPM advocates, government should not be run like a business, but rather business should run government (Lane, 2000). To these advocates of NPM, substitution of public goods theories with concepts such as decentralization, market competition, deregulation, load shedding, privatization, user fees, and enterprise management leads to a more responsive government service (Arnold, 1998; Ferlie, 1996). In public administration, opposition to NPM reflects a more traditional view of the public sector which emphasizes a positive role for public service in our society (Frederickson, 1996). The public administration critics of NPM charge that NPM undermines representative democracy, and circumvents constitutional systems developed to sustain democracy by removing public accountability from government (Goodsell, 1993; Moe, 1994; Terry, 1998).

A similar level of debate has emerged in the library profession. NPM advocates in the library profession claim that only the use of outsourcing will save public libraries from fiscal extinction (Dubberly, 1998). Opponents of NPM in the library field, on the other hand, believe that the use of outsourcing, especially in public library management, will result in the loss of democratic accountability, and the eventual privatization of public libraries (Schuman, 1998). The end result of this debate is that NPM advocates in the library profession call for embracing the movement, and opponents call for active opposition to the movement.

The Use of Outsourcing for Public Library Management

While the debate over the application of NPM principles in the library profession reflects the broader debate raging in public management, often the debate is based more on emotions than fact. In an attempt to sort emotions from fact, we have assumed the task of examining actual cases involving the application of NPM principles to public library management. We seek to discover if the application of such principles have led to the proposed increases in services claimed by the advocates of NPM, or if it has resulted in the reduction in public accountability postulated by the NPM critics. Of the thousands of public libraries in the United States, at the time of this research project, we have found only eight cases in which outsourcing of the management of a public library has occurred. Of the eight cases, only seven cases have data available for examining this phenomenon. The seven cases are:

Calabasas, California
Hemet, California
Riverside County, California
Jersey City, New Jersey
Linden, New Jersey
Fargo, North Dakota
Lancaster, Texas

The outsourcing of the management of a public library as opposed to the outsourcing of particular functions such as cataloging, binding, and building maintenance, is not a common practice in the United States. To this day, the vast majority of public libraries continue to operate as either public board systems or as in-line agencies of local governments. An examination of these seven cases shows that the reasons for such a decision to outsource the management often reflect the emergence of unusual conditions not normally associated with the operation of a public library.

While each of the cases has specific issues related to the decision to outsource, generally the decision originated from one of three reasons.

1. Dispute over a local intergovernmental contract for library service delivery, and specifically the levels of services delivered and the costs for such services: Calabasas and Riverside County.

2. Inability to attract qualified candidates for the director position: Hemet and Lancaster.
3. Dissatisfaction with the current or past director's performance and professional knowledge: Fargo, Jersey City, and Linden.

While specific justifications to outsource vary from case to case, generally they all relate to a single overriding issue, namely the perceived failure of administrative accountability within the specific public library program.

The Concept of Administrative Accountability in Public Administration

Administrative accountability is a cornerstone of the system of representative democracy found in the United States. Broadly stated, administrative accountability is measured by the level of control exercised by elected officials, the representatives of the citizenry, over appointed officials. Both legally and economically, this control is often described as the principal/agent relationship, with the elected official defined as the principal and the appointed official defined as the agent. Often this relationship is seen as a simple linear relationship between an order giver and an order taker. However, administrative accountability in a representative democracy is anything but simple, and involves multiple layers of relationships composed of law, philosophy, and professional ethics (Chang, de Figueiredo, & Weingast, 2001).

Romzek and Dubnick (1994) have sought to classify these varying levels of administrative accountability. The first level of administrative accountability relates to the internal rules, regulations, and legal mandates that form the basis for the creation of a public agency. Administrators, at this level of accountability, adhere to the established requirements necessary to deliver the appropriate government services. The second level of accountability relates to the professional standards and training needed to actually perform the designated work of the agency and maintain the professional processes related to their area of work. The third level of administrative accountability refers to the legal relationship between the elected official and the appointed official within a democracy. This is the traditional level of principal/agent relationship and is grounded within the constitutional system that establishes the government itself. The final level of administrative accountability relates directly to the citizen and applies to both the elected principal and the appointed agent. In essence, both the principal and agent are legally and morally bound to perform their duties within the political wishes of the citizen/customer.

The advocates of NPM argue that traditional public management has focused on the first two levels of accountability, namely organizational and professional accountability, and ignored the other levels of legal and political accountability. According to NPM advocates, such as Niskanen (1971), public bureaucrats have used their expertise and position to engage in an unethical game of information monopoly to advance their agency and professional interests. NPM theorists believe that bureaucrats have a distinct advantage in terms of information and expertise over the elected officials. The elected official lacks specific technical knowledge in terms of public policy arenas. Due to this lack of technical knowledge, elected officials are reluctant to intervene or object to the bureaucrat's advice. Bureaucrats use their technical information position to manipulate the decision-making process, seeking to maximize agency budget gains while minimizing program effects, thus shirking their primary legal and political responsibilities for personal and professional gain.

Shirking of legal and political accountability on the part of bureaucrats in a democracy is one of the major reasons proponents of NPM advocate that government should adopt a broad-based program of outsourcing government services. In the minds of NPM proponents, government bureaucrats have failed because they have emphasized accountability to the first two levels, hierarchy and professional, while ignoring accountability to the last two levels, legal (principal/agent) and political (customer/citizen). Consequently, administrative focus on the hierarchical and professional levels of accountability leads to inefficient operations, unnecessary red tape, and irresponsible behavior.

The argument presented in favor of NPM is that only by emphasizing the legal (principal/agent) and political (customer/citizen) levels of accountability can we return government to a responsive system that fulfills citizen wants. Since, in a representative democracy, elected officials have the sole legitimate authority for defining public wants, their stated preferences should always have priority over any hierarchical or professional accountability. Thus, by focusing on the specific legal and political ends of accountability, managers are able to obtain specific outcome measures, and achieve designated public service demands (Savas, 1994). The end result of such an approach returns administrative accountability to its rightful focus, namely the legal and political levels of accountability.

Outsourcing facilitates this type of administrative accountability by clearly identifying and separating the purchaser of government services from the provider of government services. By separating providers from purchasers, a process is unleashed which negates the shirking behavior of bureaucrats, namely the unleashing of economic self-interest. Under this approach, both the separate purchaser and provider have a vested self-interest in finding and implementing the optimal way in which to deliver the government service. The self-interest factor is at work because both parties have an interest in dividing the gain achieved and mutually reaping the benefits of this new exchange. Thus, by separating government administration from hierarchical and professional accountability we create a clear contractual relationship between a service seller and a service buyer. This separation allows for the introduction of competitive market principles into a non-competitive arena and assures economic efficiency by introducing pricing and profit incentives (Lane, 1997a, b, 2000). Thus, NPM advocates claim that three critical outcomes will accrue to government if it adopts these new public/private principles. The first claim is that administrative accountability will return to its proper focus on legal (principal/agent) and political (customer/citizen) accountability. The second claim is that government will experience an economic and efficiency gain by introducing a profit incentive into public service delivery. The third claim is that this economic efficiency gain leads to a greater citizen use and satisfaction with services and products delivered, thus, ultimately, strengthening the political accountability level of democracy.

In terms of the outsourcing of public library management, we need to examine the extent to which the separation of administration from government actually led to the achievement of these stated claims of NPM. Such an examination will require an in-depth look at the cases.

Methodology

In terms of the outsourcing of public library management, we need to examine the extent to which the separation of administration from government actually leads to the achievement of the stated benefits claimed by NPM advocates. If the NPM advocates are correct, an examination of the use of outsourcing should reveal gains in three areas: an increased level of direct accountability to elected or appointed officials by contractors versus public employees; an increase in the economic efficiency of the use of public funds; and an increase in public use or satisfaction with the public goods that are provided by the agency. If the basic premises of NPM are correct, we should see gains in all three areas: accountability, efficiency, and use/satisfaction.

In order to measure gains in the areas of accountability, efficiency, and use/satisfaction, a researcher must locate three separate, but related, units of data. In terms of accountability, one must obtain information related to the previous system of governance of the agency plus the new contract developed between the local government and the private service provider. At the time of this research, a search of the various reports on public library management outsourcing discovered that there were eight reported cases in the United States. Of the eight cases, the researchers were able to obtain information related to the previous systems of operation and contracted systems of operation for seven of the eight.

In terms of efficiency, the researcher must obtain the previous operating expenses for the agency during the time of direct local government control, and the new operating expenses in effect during the new contract period. In the seven cases under study, the various state laws related to the operation of public libraries in these states require that each of the public libraries shall report to their state libraries full financial information related to the operation of their libraries, including both revenue and expenditure information by line item and staffing. This information is subsequently provided by the state libraries to the National Center for Educational Statistics (NCES), and is available in public records from both sources.

To measure use/satisfaction, the researcher must locate the previous annual performance measures of the agency during the local government control period, and the new annual performance measures in effect during the private contract regime. Once again, by state law this type of information, containing uses by categories of services, hours of operation, staffing levels, and units of collection inventory, must be reported annually to the various state libraries. Additionally, this type of information is also reported to the NCES, and is public record available through their data services.

Thus, for seven of the eight reported cases, the necessary information required to examine the impact that outsourcing had on accountability, efficiency, and use/satisfaction was available. Additionally, each of those seven cases was reported on widely in their local press, the professional trade journals, and even, in certain cases, national newspapers. Thus, supplemental sources of contextual information are available to expand the analysis of the various data sets for each one of the seven cases.

In order to foster this examination, we will group the cases according to their areas of administrative failure as previously specified.

WHY LIBRARIES HAVE OUTSOURCED THEIR MANAGEMENT

Intergovernmental Library Service Contract Dispute

The first level of case analysis involves disputes over local intergovernmental contracts for library service delivery, and specifically the levels of services delivered and the costs of such services. The two examples of this type of problem involve the city of Calabasas and Riverside County, both in California.

In the first example, Calabasas, we see an issue arise over administrative accountability in terms of the fiduciary relationship. Calabasas did not exist as a city until 1991. Before 1991, it was part of the unincorporated area of Los Angeles County. As part of the unincorporated area of the county, the residents of the area received library service through the County of Los Angeles Public Library system, paid for by a library tax applied to property within the County. In 1991, Calabasas incorporated as a city, and became independent of the Los Angeles County government. Since the county was no longer able to assess the property within Calabasas for library services, Calabasas had to contract with the Los Angeles County Public Library. The library contract funding came through a property tax within the City of Calabasas, which paid for County Library services. At this time, 1991, Calabasas was one of 50 cities within Los Angeles County that contracted with the county library system for library services.

The primary issue concerning fiduciary accountability revolved around the perception of the citizens of Calabasas that the city was not receiving a full measure of services in relation to the contract charge from the County Library. An internal study done by the City of Calabasas found that, in 1997, Calabasas paid Los Angeles County Library $530,000 in property taxes for library services, but only received $250,000 worth of services.

While Calabasas was claiming that it was not receiving full return on its contract payment, the County Library argued that the city was receiving a full return based on the costs incurred by the County Library. The dispute simmered without mutual reconciliation. Finally, in April 1998, Calabasas decided that it could maximize its resources by seeking an alternative method of library services delivery, and voted to withdraw from the contract with the County Library.

Since all the materials, staff, and a majority of the equipment belonged to the Los Angeles County Library, Calabasas needed to create a complete library from scratch. The city contracted the entire library operation out to a private company, which in turn oversaw the development of library services and collections, the hiring of staff, and the daily operation of the library (DiMattia, Lifer, & Rogers, 1998).

The issue of fiduciary accountability also emerges in the Riverside County, California library contract. From 1911 to 1997, Riverside *County* contracted with the *City* of Riverside to provide library service to county residents. Under the terms of the contract, the city-appointed Board of

Library Trustees served as both the city and county's policy-making body, and the city library director served as the county library director. Additionally, all library employees were employees of the City of Riverside, not the county. While the City of Riverside maintained control over all matters related to library policy and library employment, the County of Riverside retained exclusive ownership of all capital assets purchased with county funds such as the collections and buildings.

In 1993, a state-mandated change in property taxes used to support the county's library service resulted in a major reduction in county property tax revenues. Because of the reduction in tax revenues, the City Library reduced library service levels by reductions in service hours, staff layoffs, and reductions in materials purchased. County residents complained that the City of Riverside refused to reduce administrative costs rather than service costs, while levying a 10 percent overhead charge for the county contract. Additionally, the county government charged that the City was providing less service than paid for by the contract, and was refusing to involve the County government in the decision making process. The issue of fiduciary accountability to contracting governments became the central point of contention.

To respond to citizen demands for improved library services, the County government decided to withdraw from the Riverside City contract, effective July 1, 1997, and establish an independent County Library. In order to accomplish the transition without the loss of library service, the County contracted with a private company to manage the library operations and employ all staff working in the library. The contract for library service was overseen by a newly established County Librarian position, who served primarily as the Contract Administrator, and a newly established County Library Board of Trustees, who oversaw and approved all library policies (Baker, 1998).

Fiduciary accountability in public library management. As stated previously, NPM advocates claim that outsourcing facilitates administrative accountability by advancing two critical elements within a principal/agent relationship. The first element is the clear identification and separation of the purchaser of government services (principal) from the provider of government services (agent). The second element is the creation in both the separate purchaser and provider of a vested self-interest in finding and implementing the optimal way in which to deliver the government service. The second element leads to efficiency since both parties are interested in dividing the gain achieved and mutually reaping the benefits of this new exchange. By advancing these two elements, NPM advocates claim that we create a clear contractual relationship between a service seller and a service buyer (principal/agent). Such a separation allows for the introduction of competitive market principles into a non-competitive arena and assures economic efficiency by introducing pricing and profit incentives. Increased economic efficiency leads to greater user/customer satisfaction with services and products (Lane, 1997a, b, 2000).

Both the Calabasas and Riverside County incidents exhibit failure to fulfill fiduciary accountability because of information asymmetry and goal conflict. Principals (elected officials) are at a disadvantage because agents (bureaucrats) possess a greater level of technical information and expertise allowing agents the opportunity to manipulate information in a manner advantageous to the agent, and detrimental to the principal. Agents are motivated to manipulate the information in this manner because their goals are different from the principal's goals. While principals and agents are rational utility maximizers, they seek to maximize different things. The principal (elected official) seeks to maximize constituent interests, while the agent (bureaucrat) seeks to maximize budgets. Since agents are in the stronger position in terms of information, they are able to manipulate the information to maximize their budget interests, but at the expense of minimizing the principal's constituent interests (Niskanen, 1971).

Underlying both the Calabasas and Riverside cases is the above assumption related to information asymmetry and goal conflict. Both the Calabasas City government and the Riverside County government claimed that the contracting libraries, Los Angeles County Public Library and Riverside City Library, were somehow manipulating information in order to maximize their budgets while minimizing the level of services delivered. Since the agents, Los Angeles County and Riverside City, had failed in their fiduciary accountability of advancing the interests of the principals over the interests of the agents, they no longer could be considered reliable agents. In such a situation, the principal is left with no other alternative but to seek another, more reliable, agent. Both Calabasas and Riverside County could have established their own local government agency, but they rejected that option based on the claim advanced by NPM advocates that outsourcing to the private sector would lead to both greater fiduciary accountability and a greater gain in the service/cost delivery ratio. If NPM advocates of outsourcing are correct, then we should see these claims confirmed in the fiduciary and service/cost measures that emerged in Calabasas and Riverside County since the contracts were implemented.

Both the Calabasas and Riverside contracts are forms of *service contracts*. In general, service contracts are between governments and private sector firms to deliver predefined services for a specified time periods. Usually such contracts involve the private firm not only delivering the service, but also having exclusive control over the management of the service, and the employment of all workers involved in the service delivery. In the United States, service contracts are common tools for local government service delivery, and account for over 25 percent of municipal services (Rondinelli, 2003). Common examples of such service contracts are waste collection, hospital management, emergency medical services, and bus operations.

The first point to examine in terms of NPM principles is whether there is a clear identification and separation of the purchaser of government services from the provider of government services. In the case of both Calabasas and Riverside County, there is only a limited separation between purchaser and provider.

Calabasas contracts with a private firm to hire and supervise all staff. The contract also allows the company to have control over the automation of the library, purchase of supplies and book collections, and day-to-day operation and management of the library. On the other hand, the city created an advisory Library Commission that oversees, with the consent of the City Council, all library policies, overall budget allocations, hours of operation, public programs, and any major cost items. The City Clerk is the contract manager, who reports directly to the City Council on contract performance and issues related to non-compliance. In addition, under the terms of the contract, the City retains ownership of all buildings, equipment, furniture, and collections purchased for the Library (City of Calabasas, 2001).

The Riverside contract contains requirements relating to the hours of operation in the library branches, staffing levels at all branches, and levels of book purchases for each regional service zone covered by the library. As in the case of Calabasas, there is an advisory Library Commission which oversees all policies related to the library and its operations. The contract administrator for Riverside County is the County Librarian who is a county employee. The County Librarian supervises the private firm, and must approve all operational policies and material purchases. While the employees of the library are employees of the private firm, the County Librarian must approve the hiring of all managerial and supervising staff. As in Calabasas, all buildings, equipment, and collections remain the property of the County government (County of Riverside, 1997).

Thus, the contracts in Calabasas and Riverside County marginally meet the first requirement of NPM. Although there is a clear identification and separation between purchaser and provider, that separation is severely limited. The major functions one would associate with service contracts such as budgetary control and procedure setting remain under the control of the local governments. The only clear separation appears at the level of employment, and here one sees that both the operational staff and the management staff are removed from the local government's employment roles, and placed in a private sector employment status.

Overall, one can conclude that a major gain occurred in terms of the agent's accountability to the principal. While the limitations within the contracts hamper the concept of complete and clear separation from principal and agent, the additional restrictions ensure that elected officials in both communities have a greater level of oversight and control of the agency than was previously in existence with either Los Angeles County or the City of Riverside. Thus, the introduction of outsourcing, in these two cases, did lead to a stronger level of legal accountability.

The second level of accountability that NPM claims will be strengthened by outsourcing is the political or citizen/customer level. Supposedly, a strengthening of legal accountability will be translated into better public services reflecting the true wants and wishes of the citizen/customer (political accountability). Thus, to measure a return to political accountability, we need to examine the service measures. These service measures also reflect the second element of the NPM philosophy, namely that, by creating both a separate purchaser and provider, we create a vested self-interest in finding and implementing the optimal way in which to deliver the government service. In the case of both Calabasas and Riverside County, we find some measures suggesting that the second element did have some positive, but qualified, effect.

While Calabasas saw an increase in staffing from 6.5 FTEs in FY 1998–1999 to 7.7 FTEs in FY 2001–2002 and, since the hours of operation between FY 1998–1999 and FY 2001–2002 remained constant, there was a positive impact in the level of staff to public service hours. Additionally, the materials held by the library also increased in the same period, rising from 16,025 items to 25,465 items, a 58 percent increase. The increase in items held also was reflected in an increase in items checked-out, rising from 78,511 in FY 1998–1999 to 113,687 in FY 2001–2002. During this same time period, reference services also increased by an impressive 222 percent, and visits to the library went up by 79 percent. Overall, total service units increased by 61 percent (National Center for Educational Statistics (NCES), 1999, 2002).

On the cost side of the service/cost ratio, the results are not as positive. Budget figures for Calabasas show a very different picture of the gains achieved at the service levels. Initially, Calabasas saw an initial efficiency gain by contracting with a private firm rather than the Los Angeles County Library. The last year of contract with Los Angeles County, FY 1997–1998, saw a contract figure of $530,000. The first year of contract with the private firm, FY 1998–1999, saw a total operating expense of $446,385, a net decrease of $83,615. However, the operating expense decrease did not stabilize, and by FY 2001–2002 the operating expenses for the library rose to $767,330. Additionally, the unit costs for service delivery rose by six percent (NCES, 1998, 2002). In the end, we can conclude that any gains in services were the result of increases in the budget for the library and not the result of changes in the operational efficiency of the overall system.

Riverside County also experienced some positive service results. FTEs rose from 62.97 in FY 1996–1997, the last year of the contract with Riverside City, to 111.6 in FY 2001–2002. Hours of operation also increased from 507 h/week in FY 1996–1997 to 971 h/week in FY 2001–2002. Materials purchases also increased, with collection holdings rising from 917,348 items in FY 1997–1998 to 975,278 items in FY 2001–2002, a six percent increase in holdings. However, actual public use of the library declined. Comparing FY 1997–1998 to FY 2001–2002 circulation dropped from 2,704,794 to 2,033,578 (−25 percent), reference services from 794,231 to 584,993 (−25 percent), and library visits from 1,979,429 to 1,463,860 (−26 percent). Overall, total service units delivered declined by 25 percent. The drop in public use of the system is all the more disappointing since the expenditures for the system rose from $6,785,671 in FY 1997–1998 to $8,010,278 in FY 2001–2002, an 18 percent increase. The combination of an increase in the budget and a decline in use resulted in the unit costs for service and product delivery rising from one dollar and 24 cents in FY 1997–1998 to one dollar and 96 cents in FY 2001–2002, an increase of 58 percent (NCES, 1998, 2002). While the results in Calabasas might be attributable to an increase in the budget, in the case of Riverside County there is a clear measure of the outsourcing contract's failure to improve service, and actually an increase in costs with a corresponding decrease in public use – just the opposite result than that predicted by the NPM advocates.

From the available data, it would appear that the second and third premises of NPM, namely locating the optimal way to deliver government services and increased public satisfaction, was not manifested in either case. In the case of Calabasas, we see an increase in public use units, but with a corresponding increase in operational costs. In Riverside, we see major decreases in service delivery units with major increases in operational costs, a clear sign of both service and productivity failures.

One last element to examine in both cases is a premise within NPM philosophy that outsourcing will lead to better performance by the introduction of self-interest due to an ability to mutually share the economic gain that is achieved. Under the terms of the initial contract entered into by Calabasas, the private firm, in addition to its annual contract, was to receive a 7.5 percent handling fee on all collection resources purchased or licensed for the library. In contrast to Calabasas, Riverside County was more cautious in its approach to handling charges. From FY 1997–1998 to FY 1999–2000, the county provided no handling charges, and strictly limited the contract to a fixed amount. After the firm successfully performed under the initial contract for three years, the county modified the contract. Under the new contract, the firm received a 2 percent handling fee on all material purchases.

This handling charge was never specifically defined as a performance bonus, but it does provide an incentive for the firm to increase the number of items owned by the Library and is indirectly evident in both the eight percent increase in holdings in Riverside and the 58 percent increase in holdings in Calabasas. When one compares the performance of the two libraries and takes into account that high performance only occurs in the library with the generous handling charge, one might conclude that the NPM premise related to the division of gain might have some validity.

The evidence suggests that NPM principles in the area of fiduciary accountability have a positive impact. However, we see that an improvement in legal/fiduciary accountability does not, by itself, lead to either an improvement in political (citizen/customer) accountability or to efficiency within the agency or service.

Although both Riverside County and Calabasas exemplify a perceived failure at the fiduciary level of legal accountability, two of our other cases, namely the public libraries of Hemet and Lancaster, also deal with a failure of legal (principal) accountability, but this time in relation to the provision of necessary professional knowledge.

Inability to Attract Qualified Candidates for the Director Position

Although both the Riverside County and Calabasas cases represent classic information asymmetry and goal conflict in the principal/agent relationship, two of the other cases, namely Hemet and Lancaster, exhibit a problem in terms of information asymmetry, but not goal conflict. In both cases, the agents' goals were not in conflict with the principal since the agents had already left their positions of authority. However, in the vacuum that was created by the agents' departures, the issue of lack of information arose. In such an environment, proponents of NPM suggest that principals should design organizational structures in such a way that they can facilitate their control over the situation (McCubbins, Noll, & Weingast, 1987; Potoski, 2002; Whitford, 2002; Lewis, 2003).

The Hemet Public Library was in the process of developing plans for a new 47,000 square foot city library when the library director resigned. (Although Hemet is in Riverside County, its library has never been part of the Riverside County system). The library's Board of Trustees immediately started a recruitment process for a new library director, specifically someone who had had previous experience with library capital projects. While the recruitment process was extensive, the Board was unable to locate candidates who possessed previous experience handling such a large capital project.

In consultation with the city manager, the Library Board of Trustees decided that the Library was at a critical point in its development, and the success of the capital project was crucial for the future of the Library. Rather than take the risk on hiring someone without capital project experience and professional knowledge, the Library Board and the Hemet city government decided to seek a "temporary" solution. In December, 1999, Hemet contracted with a private firm that possessed the necessary background in library capital projects to assume the administration of the library and oversight of the library building project. The contract called for the firm to complete the new library-building project within a two-year period and to provide management of the library during that two-year period. The understanding between the city and the firm was that, at the end of the capital project, the Board of Trustees and the City Manager would examine the performance of the firm. After review of the performance of the private firm, Hemet and its Library Board of Trustees could exercise their option to hire a new full-time library director, and the contract with the private firm could end. In December, 2001, the Hemet city government renewed the contract with the private firm for an additional two years and elected not to hire a permanent library director (Trovillion, 2002).

The Lancaster (Texas) Veterans Memorial Library faced a problem similar to that confronting Hemet. Like Hemet, Lancaster had a major capital project approved for an expanded city library. Unlike Hemet, though, the director of the library completed the building project and then resigned. While the physical building was completed, the building still needed additional interior work to complete the project and bring the library online. None of the remaining library staff possessed professional training or experience in managing a library.

In order to deal with the immediate crisis, the Library Board and the city elected to hire a private firm to take over both the completion of the capital project and to provide ongoing professional management to the library. In the case of Lancaster, though, the city elected to offer the firm a five-year contract, renewable on an annual basis, to continue operation of the library. The contract with the private firm went into effect on July 1, 2001, and will remain in force until September 30, 2006 (Trovillion, 2002).

Both Hemet and Lancaster experienced a failure of legal (principal) accountability in terms of technical information. In the case of Hemet, the proposed capital project required a level of professional expertise that was not forthcoming. In the case of Lancaster, the decision by their professional director to leave in the middle of the project created a professional vacuum at a critical time. No matter the reasons for the problem, both cities experienced a failure at the level of professional accountability and turned to the private rather than the public sector to resolve their crisis.

Both Hemet and Lancaster used variations on a form of outsourcing contract known as the *Build-Operate-Transfer agreement*. Under normal conditions, such agreements between private and public sectors involve a process whereby the private firm agrees to finance the building of a public service infrastructure and then is given a limited amount of time to run the service in order to recover its initial financing and profit. At the end of the predetermined time frame, the firm relinquishes ownership of the infrastructure to the public sector, which then has the option of either operating the service directly, or engaging the vendor in a service contract (Rondinelli, 2003). Generally, these agreements provide for turnkey systems, and are commonly used in Africa, Asia, and South America to build toll roads, port expansions, public hospitals, and power facilities. These agreements are also used in the United States for building toll roads and water/waste treatment facilities.

The hiring of an outside firm to consult with a local public library undertaking a major capital building project is a common practice in the United States. This is especially the case in small- to medium-size public libraries where, although the administrative staff members may have professional training, they have not encountered large capital projects during their career. This practice, hiring outside expertise for such projects, is also encouraged in the professional literature of the library field, and supported by the professional national associations.

While both Hemet and Lancaster did not use a private firm to finance the capital project, they did utilize a private firm to oversee the capital project and also agreed to have the firm provide the operational function for the facility for a limited time period. In this sense, the agreements in Hemet and Lancaster approximate the Build-Operate-Transfer Agreement model, although limiting the level of private firm investment in the project.

As in the cases of Riverside County and Calabasas, we again see mixed results in terms of attaining the gains proposed in the NPM model. Hemet retains a limited managerial role for the private firm in terms of operations of the library. Staff members, other than managers, remain employees of the city government and are subject to evaluation by the city manager. Policy and reporting functions remain with the city, and are under the control of the city manager and the library's board of trustees. The city manager LAO retains control over all materials and service purchases. Thus, there is only a slight amount of separation between purchaser and provider, with the private firm providing only managerial direction of the operation, and limited day-to-day oversight (City of Hemet, 1999).

In terms of optimizing resources in order to achieve a greater gain in service delivery, the results seem to support the decision to utilize a private firm. While hours of operation and staffing levels remain flat, overall service delivery measures show a gain of 20 percent from FY 1998–1999 to FY 2001–2002. Circulation experienced a 15 percent increase during this period, an 18 percent gain in library visits, and an impressive 80 percent gain in reference services. The increases in services were also matched by an increase in funding for the operation, which rose by six percent during the same time period. More impressive though, is the fact that the large increase in services, with a minimal increase operating expenses, resulted in a 12 percent reduction in the unit costs (NCES, 1999, 2002). It would seem that Hemet clearly achieved an efficiency gain.

Interestingly, the findings from Hemet seem to contradict portions of the NPM theory, especially compared to the performance of Riverside. Like Riverside, Hemet restricted the contract with the vendor to the provision of management services. No handling charge clause appears in the contract to encourage the firm to greater effort. Yet, in the case of Hemet, we see performance gain and efficiency gain, while in Riverside we see just the opposite. In these two cases, it would seem that the lack of gain-sharing does not necessarily lead to a lack of performance, thus bringing into question the validity of the gain-sharing premise within NPM theory.

While the results from Hemet are somewhat confusing in terms of gain-sharing, the results from Lancaster are, on the surface, more promising. From FY 2000–2001 to FY 2001–2002, the library's collection was increased by 13 percent. During this same time, circulation use increased by 175 percent, library visits rose by 211 percent, and reference services experienced a 124 percent increase. Even more impressive than the increase in use was the gain in efficiency. While the library's operating expenses were only increased by four percent, there was a 62 percent decrease in the unit cost for service delivery (NCES, 2001, 2002).

While initially the results from Lancaster seem to support the basic theory of NPM, one must qualify this finding by noting that the two years of data are not necessarily comparable. During FY 2000–2001, the library was operating in a smaller facility with a limited collection. Also, during this same time period, the library was involved in constructing a newer and larger facility. The first year of the private firm's contract, FY 2001–2002, coincides with the opening of the new and larger library with a larger and newer collection of materials. It is highly likely that the opening of the new library played a major role in the increased use of the library, and the subsequent reduction in the unit cost figure. Nonetheless, one has to recognize that handling a 177 percent increase in business with only a four percent increase in the operating budget is an impressive feat.

In order to explore the results from Lancaster further, we examined the figures for the library in the year previous to the beginning of the building project (FY 1998–1999) and compared those figures with the results from FY 2001–2002. Again, performance improvement is clear, with circulation increasing by 124 percent, reference services up by 53 percent, and visits increasing by 30 percent. While the performance results are still very good, an examination of the operating expense figures show that from FY 1998–1999 to FY 2001–2002 the budget rose by 70–70 percent (NCES, 1998, 2002). It would be reasonable to assume that the opening of a new and larger facility combined with an increase in the budget could explain the service increases. Still, the gains in service are impressive, especially when one looks at the unit cost figures, which fell by three percent.

In exploring the differences between performances by Hemet and Lancaster, an examination of the contract structure points to major differences between the two agencies. Unlike Hemet, Lancaster sought to create a clear separation between purchaser and provider. In terms of employees, Lancaster established a phase-in program that brought all library employees under the hiring and firing authority of the private firm over a 12-month period. By the end of 2001, all employees, both management and staff, had become employees of the private firm and were no longer covered by the city's civil service system. Thus, in terms of employment, the contract clearly separated purchaser from provider (City of Lancaster, 2001).

In terms of materials purchased, while the City of Lancaster retained ownership of materials, the private firm had exclusive control over all materials selected and purchased for the library and of any supporting materials utilized in the operation. While other purchases, such as equipment, are subject to approval by the city manager and city council, materials purchases are under the control of the firm. Again, we see an attempt to separate purchaser from the provider.

In terms of policies and operational regulations, Lancaster's Library Board of Trustees is advisory, and all authority within these areas is subject to the control and authority of the city council. While the council establishes broad operating policy for the library, the firm retains authority in terms of day-to-day operational policies, especially as it relates to staff and procedures. Contract management is under the authority of the city manager.

The final area of difference between Hemet and Lancaster relates to the handling charge. As stated previously, Hemet provided for no additional handling charge to encourage the firm. On the other hand, Lancaster provided an additional five-percent handling charge on all materials purchased, and on all accounting and payment functions performed by the firm.

Lancaster is closer to the ideal NPM model in the sense that purchaser and provider are separate, the provider has freedom to operate, and there is mutual gain shared between the parties. However, when we examine the performance of Lancaster versus Calabasas, where separation is limited but performance reaches the same high levels, the only common element both libraries share is the handling charge. Yet this finding is offset by the fact that another high performing library, Hemet, contained no handling charge. Once again, we have some evidence that the division of gain may or may not have some validity.

A final area of consideration relates to accountability, and these two cases, again, show that the use of outsourcing contracts did have a major impact on *legal* accountability. Prior to the decisions to outsource the Hemet and Lancaster libraries, the local library boards of trustees had major responsibility in terms of approving operating policies and budget expenditures. After the implementation of outsourcing both policy and budget authority were removed from the control of the boards, and placed directly into the hands of the city managers and councils. The end result in terms of the claimed benefits achieved by NPM was that in both the Hemet and Lancaster cases we see increases in *political* accountability.

Dissatisfaction with the Director's Performance and Professional Knowledge

The Hemet and Lancaster examples show the use of NPM as a means of dealing with a failure of professional accountability related to a lack of technical information within the library's principal/agent relationship. While serious, the failure to acquire technical expertise in the performance of one's duties is not an unusual phenomenon in either the public or private sector. However, failure of professional accountability as it relates to advancing personal or professional values over the lawful orders of elected or appointed officials is a far more serious issue. The advancement of professional norms or opinions in direct contradiction of elected officials wishes challenges the very basis of the principal/agent relation, and closely approximates the criticisms leveled by NPM advocates. There are three cases of such failures, and the subsequent use of management outsourcing. They are Fargo, North Dakota, Jersey City, New Jersey, and Linden, New Jersey.

As Romzek and Dubnick (1994) state, the second level of administrative accountability exhibits itself through professional norms and ethics. This level of accountability is a form of self-imposed accountability that assures the agency that the persons working within the agency possesses the necessary expertise and values to fulfill the agency charges. However, this second level may conflict with their third level of administrative accountability, namely legal, or the principal/agent relationship. This third level is the classic definition of administrative accountability, and spells out the specific relationship that exists between the administrator and the citizen's representative, namely the elected or appointed official.

The issue of which level of accountability, professional versus legal, has the higher moral and ethical demand has filled volumes of professional literature. In public administration, the issue came to the forefront of ethical consideration during the famous Friedrich/Finer debate of the 1940s. Further consideration of the issue became central in the field of public administration when the Nuremberg Trials held that compliance with lawful orders provided no defense when viewed in light of immoral and criminal actions. Yet, academic discussions on this matter often devolve to the arena of personal and professional work decisions not carrying the moral weight of the issues faced at Nuremberg or advanced in the Friedrich/Finer debate.

The result of the minimization of the accountability issue, at least as NPM advocates view matters, is that the professional bureaucrats of our government agencies place a greater loyalty to their professional norms and peers than to the agencies that employ them. Consequently, this focus on professional norms undermines the position of the elected representative of the people and leads to excessive and unwarranted professional restrictions. The result of such a focus is that government agencies and services fail to comply with the wishes of elected officials, and this, in turn, leads to dysfunctional programs. NPM advocates claim that only by forcing the professionals to comply with the wishes of elected officials through outsourcing, can we hope to turn government back to its proper focus, namely the citizen's wants. All three of the following cases (Fargo, Jersey City, and Linden) exhibit elements related to these claims.

The Fargo Public Library Board of Trustees was unable to hire a library director with whom it, and the staff, felt comfortable. In five years, the Board had hired three separate directors, all of whom failed to meet the Board's management expectations. When the Board of Trustees bought out the last library director's contract, it mounted a national recruitment process for a new director. Unfortunately, the Board of Trustees' preceding actions made it difficult to attract any candidates who were qualified for the position. In January 2001, after six months without a director, the Board of Trustees and the City of Fargo finalized a contract with a private firm to manage the library. The two-year agreement specifically stated that the contract was for daily operational management, library reorganization, and recruitment of a qualified library director (Trovillion, 2002).

The private firm recruited a new library director, under contract to the firm, who was able, over the two-year period, to reorganize the library, resolve staff issues, and rebuild the credibility of the library. While the Board of Trustees was pleased with the private firm's work, the City Council became dissatisfied when the firm proposed an operating budget that exceeded the Council's budget expectations. Shortly after the budget request, the Board of Trustees voted to end the contract, effective November 1, 2003, citing late payment of bills. The Board of Trustees then negotiated the release of the Library Director from the firm's contract in order to offer that person the same position, but as a local government employee ("Fargo Public," 2003).

In the case of Jersey City, the Board of Trustees was dissatisfied with the library management's ability to automate the library. The Board's frustrations were further exacerbated by the fact that all library employees, including the director, were covered by the local civil service system, and could not be removed from their positions without following extensive due process procedures (Trovillion, 2002).

In order to end-run the civil service procedures, the Board sought to create a separate work force using a private firm to manage the library. Under the agreement, the private firm would hire new employees as positions became vacant who were private employees not covered by civil service. A state court blocked the move to create a separate workforce, forcing the development of a new contract that specifically prohibited creation of a library workforce outside the civil service system (Rogers & Oder, 1998).

In spite of the thwarting of the original intent of the trustees, the Board of Trustees engaged the private firm to develop a "management restoration plan," and approved the service contract on July 14, 1998. The firm's contract called for the development of a library automation plan, provision of management services, development of a detailed reorganization proposal, and a plan for eventually moving away from outsourcing and back to a full in-line government agency status (Flagg, 1998).

The Library Board of Trustees and firm attempted to reorganize the library, but staff and community resistance and resentment led to a rancorous and hostile work environment. Eventually, the Board of Trustees canceled the contract with the private firm, effective January 1, 2002, and promoted a longtime library employee to head of library operations ("Jersey City," 2001).

The Library Director of the Linden Library had held the position for many years, and was near retirement. The Board of Trustees became disenchanted with the Library Director's job performance, and specifically felt that the Director was unwilling to update and change the library's operation, causing the library to stagnate and fall into disarray. For over a year the Board of Trustees proceeded to micromanage the Library, further straining an already fragile Board of Trustees/Director relationship.

After a year of micro-management and without the knowledge of the Director, the Board of Trustees opened discussions with a private company to manage the library after the Director's retirement. Upon learning of these discussions, the Director went on an extended sick leave, further aggravating the management problem. The Board of Trustees, with the consent of the City Council, immediately contracted with a private firm to manage the Library and to provide an interim Director. The contract became effective on September 2, 2000 (Trovillion, 2002).

The final two-year contract signed by the library covered both the management and operation of the Library, and designated a specific individual to serve as the interim director. Under the terms of the contract, the Linden city government provided funds to cover all expenses associated with managing the library, including salaries and benefits, maintaining and expanding the library's collection, and community programing. The unionized library staff reported to the private company, but remained employees of the Library, not the private company. The Board of Trustees established and controlled all library policies, and the city retained ownership of all facilities, furnishings, and materials while continuing to provide building maintenance. After the initial two-year contract was completed, the Library signed a two-year renewal, and retained the private company – no "permanent" library director replaced the retired library director (City of Linden, 2000).

However, the relationship between the Linden Library's Board of Trustees and the private firm began to erode over the course of the contract. As in the case of Fargo, late payment of outstanding bills created concern about the quality of management. Eventually, on February 29, 2004, the Library and the private firm issued a public statement praising the work of the private firm in completing the requirements of the contract. Like Fargo, the private firm's Library Director's contract was ended, and the private firm's Director was hired as a permanent city employee (Oder, 2004).

The operations of the Fargo, Jersey City, and Linden public libraries are all governed by an outsourcing method called *management contracts*. Under a management contract, the government retains ownership of all operational elements and infrastructure, while the private firm provides the management expertise and oversight required for operating the service. Under this approach, government retains both policy and legal control, but the firm exercises authority in terms of routine management decisions. In countries other than the United States, this type of contract is often used to manage government owned resorts and hotels, agricultural industries, and mining operations. In the United States, such contracts appear in the operation of public hospitals, correctional facilities, and public utilities (Rondinelli, 2003).

Both New Zealand and Australia have used management contracts to replace permanent public employment with short-term contracts. The underlying assumption for the use of these types of contracts is that their use will lead to a focus, by management, on the primary principal/agent relationship, namely the elected official and citizen consumer. The dominant view in this area is that professional public administration is a closed career system that undermines accountability due to its professional focus rather than its legal/ political focus. The broadest use of this type of approach was the State Sector Act of 1988 in New Zealand which ended the "tenure-until-retirement" arrangement for senior public managers (Yeatman, 1998).

Of the two schools of thought about the utility of this type of contract, the first believes that such an approach will lead to management taking over the political policy arena since they will have an unfettered hand in the daily operation of the agencies (Clarke & Newman, 1997; Pollitt, 1993). The second school of thought holds that such an approach will lead to just the opposite result, namely, that political officials will take over the management of public agencies (Halligan, 1997; Pierre, 1995). The research data on the results tends to support the second school of thought (Hojnacki, 1996; Talbot, 1996). Generally, the data seem to suggest that while such an approach undermines merit principles, political control is strengthened through both recruitment and the enforcement of a return to direct responsibility back to elected officials (Boston, 1991). In cases of Fargo, Jersey City, and Linden, we find data that would seem to support the findings from previous research, namely a strengthening of legal accountability at the expense of public employment principles.

The data from the three libraries, Fargo, Jersey City, and Linden, once again show mixed results. From FY 2000–2001 to FY 2001–2002, the Fargo Public Library performance improved under the direction of the private firm. With only a five percent increase in the collection size, the library experienced a 14 percent increase in circulation and a 16 percent increase in library visits. Reference services also increased by 36 percent. Overall, total service units increased by 16 percent. However, during the same time period, the expenditures for the library also increased by 18 percent, and unit costs increased by two percent. When one looks at the percent of rise in service units compared to the percent of rise in expenditures coupled to the fact that the unit costs remained reasonably stable, we can assume that increases in service and budget were linked (NCES, 2001, 2002). We can interpret that the increase in use was attributable to the increase in expenditures and not to efficiency gains.

Jersey City increased library funding from FY 1997–1998 to FY 2000–2001 by only one percent. While the Jersey City Library achieved a nine percent gain in circulation, its library collection declined by seven percent, visits fell by 23 percent, and reference service decreased by 47 percent. In the end, total units of services declined by 22 percent while unit costs rose by 29 percent (NCES, 1998, 2001).

The results from Linden are similar to the performance at Jersey City. From FY 1998–1999 to FY 2001–2002, library budget figures decreased by six percent, but circulation declined by 18 percent, materials holdings fell by 28 percent, library visits decreased by 12 percent, and reference service suffered a 68 percent decrease. Overall, total units of service declined by 21 percent, and unit costs rose by 18 percent (NCES, 1999, 2002).

When examining the performance of the three libraries, and the differences achieved, one is struck by the different approach taken by Fargo versus that taken by Jersey City and Linden. In the case of Jersey City and Linden, the boards of trustees and the private firms invested time in developing staff training programs. However, in the case of Fargo we see the emphasis placed on employee relations. Under the program established by the Fargo board of trustees and its vendor, employees not only received an extensive retraining program delivered in-house, they also were engaged in discussion groups with the library management, and employee relations programs. Previous employee issues were dealt with directly by the new management, and an employee representative was appointed as an ex-officio member of the Board of Trustees. The end result for Fargo was the stabilizing of the employer/employee relationship. On the other hand, in both Jersey City and Linden the focus on a training program did not resolve the issues creating a tense and unproductive work environment.

The interesting thing about these performance results is the fact that although the majority of the NPM literature stresses profit incentives as a major motivator for employee performance, the data from Fargo would suggest that human relations factors play a greater role in employee improvement than profit incentives. While we are unable to claim a direct link between employee satisfaction and agency performance, the results from Fargo suggest that such a linkage may exist and should be researched further by NPM advocates.

As for incentives to the firm in terms of dividing the projected gain in productivity, we also see mixed results. While Fargo had the most significant gain in use, the contract with the firm offered the least gain-sharing incentive. The Fargo contract allowed for a five percent handling charge on all materials purchased for the library, but no other incentive was provided. The Linden contract also contained a handling charge fee, but it was a set figure of $208,500 annually. The Jersey City contract offered extensive bonus payments for a wide variety of services. An additional $25,000 bonus was offered for establishing a library foundation. Another $25,000 bonus was set for developing a marketing plan. Bonus schedules were also developed for the number of hours of staff training provided and for staff evaluations, and an additional $25,000 bonus was provided for developing a management restoration plan. In spite of the provision of bonus payments, only Fargo showed a significant increase in citizen use for overall services, bringing into question, in these three cases, the validity of the NPM concept of division of gain as an incentive for service improvement.

In terms of legal (principal) accountability, however, we can see an increase in the direct authority of the Board of Trustees over the management of the libraries. However, this increase, while significant on paper, has underlying issues needing in-depth exploration.

The establishment of credibility and trust between a principal and agent (Board of Trustees and a Library Director) is critical for successful management of a public library. The basis for such a working relationship exhibits itself in the actual performance on the part of both parties. Directors must be able to show by actual results that they have the abilities necessary to handle problems and issues on an on-going basis. Trustees, on the other hand, must show that they are able to establish working policies that assist the agency in the completion of its mission, while respecting the competencies of the director and staff to implement such policies. When suspicions arise on the part of either party, in terms of the above qualities, the working relationship begins to deteriorate. If the parties fail to address the problem, the situation may result in a full-blown rift between the two parties and a failure of the agency to complete its mission.

All three of the above cases show a failure of management and trustees to establish such a working, and mutually supporting, principal/agent relationship. While the underlying issues creating the rift between management and trustees vary in each case, fundamentally, they are experiencing the inability to establish this balance between the two conflicting demands for technical expertise and democratic accountability. In this sense, the cases exhibit a basic issue faced in any type of principal/agent relationship within a democratic form of government. However, the ground for the conflicts vary for each case, as does the decision to outsource management.

Excessive turnover in upper management within an agency usually signals a problem in the selection and hiring process. Fargo's Board of Trustees hired three directors over a five-year period. None of the Directors seemed able to establish a solid working relationship with either the Board of Trustees or the library staff. Staff complaints about the management's abilities further undermined confidence between the Board of Trustees and the three Directors. In each case, the Board concluded that a mistake had occurred in the selection process and that they needed to seek new leadership for the agency. However, the continuing personnel actions by the Board of Trustees led to a perception within the professional library community that the Board of Trustees was unwilling to address the true underlying issues, and Fargo was a "no-win" situation for any candidate seeking the position of Director. This resulted in a lack of viable and experienced candidates applying for the position and the necessity to seek a private firm to manage the library.

The Library Director hired by the private company was able to establish a working relationship between management and staff. While credit goes to the individual hired in the position to see and deal with the underlying staff problems, an additional factor was the length of the contract. The two-year contract created an environment where the firm was given the necessary time to establish both a working staff relationship and a process of problem resolution. In previous conflicts, the Board had elected to take the easy solution to staff complaints and removed the Director. The new contract period, however, forced the Board of Trustees to deal directly with staff problems. Eventually, after a successful two-year probationary period, the Board of Trustees and staff felt a renewed confidence in the individual hired as Director, and retained the Director as their employee. The resolution of staff issues created an atmosphere which allowed the agency to return to its public mission. It would appear that the approach used by the firm to resolve staff issues rejected the profit incentive position advanced by NPM advocates, and instead returned to the human relations school's position that public employees are motivated by factors beyond just financial gain.

The Jersey City case also shares common problems with Fargo, but the approach selected by the Board of Trustees further aggravated an already strained employer/employee relationship. While Boards of Trustees may reasonably question the technical expertise of management in areas such as organizational computing not normally associated with their professional training, the common response to this problem is to seek outside assistance. Often libraries facing a problem of lack of technical expertise elect to hire outside consulting and contracting firms to provide the necessary knowledge. However, in the case of Jersey City, the Board of Trustees sought to use outsourcing not only to resolve this problem, but also as a means to attack a cornerstone of public employment in the United States, namely civil service system coverage.

Under the rationale of needing assistance with library automation, the Board of Trustees attempted to advance a strategy of undermining civil service coverage for its employees by creating a separate private workforce within the library. Using attrition as a means of worker replacement, the Board sought to create, over time, a private sector workforce for the library who could be hired or fired at will by the library's management and Board of Trustees. The library employees rightly perceived this as an attempt by the Board of Trustees to remove them from the protections of civil service coverage and led to a community and system wide staff response against the private firm and the Board.

The example of Jersey City reinforces one of the arguments against out-sourcing of public services, namely that the use of outsourcing advances an unstated anti-government employment philosophy and agenda. The failure of the principal/agent relationship, in this case, lies squarely at the feet of the principal. This failure runs counter to the perceived problem as defined by NPM advocates, namely public employees, and instead focuses the failure in the principal/agent relationship on the actions of the principal.

Linden's case also exhibits some problems in terms of the principal/agent relationship, but, in this case, failures appear on both sides of the relationship. The Linden Board of Trustees lost confidence in the director because the Director did not exhibit the type of assertive behavior the Trustees felt was appropriate. By implication, the Board of Trustees perception of failure was due to a lack of willingness on the part of the Director to adopt current professional practices. On the other hand, the Director felt personally affronted by the lack of confidence exhibited by the Board of Trustees. In such an environment of mutual lack of confidence, the probability of agency mission failure is high.

The Board of Trustees in Linden apparently felt uncomfortable directly confronting these matters with the Director and sought to compensate by micromanaging the daily operations. While the actions by the Board are humanly understandable, they further undermined its relationship with the Director. The Board also failed in maintaining the principal/agent relationship by electing to open discussions with the private firm in a secretive manner. When the director learned of the secret discussions, the director also failed in maintaining the principal/agent relationship by using extended sick time, thus leaving the library with a management vacuum. Once both parties in the relationship had failed to maintain their respective role, the only resolution left to the crisis was to seek new leadership for the library. Contrary to NPM claims, in this case, the failure of the principal/agent relationship was due to the actions of both parties, not solely the agent.

In terms of the first claimed benefit for the use of outsourcing, namely a return to the proper legal accountability status of principal and agent, one of the cases exhibits such a result, another case has mixed results, and the final case fails to achieve the goal. Both Fargo and Linden successfully reasserted the dominant position of the Board of Trustees in terms of library operations. Fargo's method of employee problem resolution strengthened the Board's legal accountability position. However, Linden's method of micromanagement, while strengthening their legal accountability, achieved this end at the cost of undermining the principal/agent relationship. The third case, Jersey City, however, failed in its efforts to reassert its position of authority over its agents. The hostility of both the employees and the community to the board's efforts eventually resulted in an ending of the contract with the vendor, and thus a weakening of the board's prestige. Thus, one would have to conclude that the claim by NPM advocates of a return to a focus on legal accountability on the part of the agents may not occur in all cases.

From an ethical standpoint, the actions by principals in all three of the above cases undermined the basic foundations for any type of principal/ agent relationship. Specifically, the principals in these cases operated as if there were no reciprocal obligations on their part in terms of the agent. In terms of the basic concept of "agency" there is always a responsibility placed on the agent to put the welfare of the principal before the agent's welfare. However, in any principal/agent relationship the principal may not ask the agent to act in ways that are professionally or morally unethical or, in the case of the public sector, result in harm to the public interest. In essence, principals are required to respect the organizational agent's professional, moral, personal, and physical integrity, and to make no requests that would result in such harm to either the organizational agent's personal standing or the public interest. The actions by the principals in all three of these cases show some degree of disregard for the agent's professional, moral or ethical standing as it relates to the public interest.

CONCLUSION

Examination of the preceding seven cases shows that NPM claims related to returning government to its proper principal/agent focus, and thus achieving gains in performance, are somewhat questionable. All seven cases show some increase in the level of legal accountability within the principal/agent relationship, the first claimed benefit of NPM. These findings also support previous research findings that the introduction of NPM theories into the provision of government-funded services leads to political officials increasing their influence over the management of public agencies (Hojnacki, 1996; Talbot, 1996; Boston, 1991). However, the majority of the cases exhibit a failure in the claimed second benefit, namely an increase in the political stakeholder/citizen satisfaction level. In all seven cases, we see either a decline in political stakeholder/citizen use of the agency after the introduction of NPM theory or an increase in operational costs with only varying levels of impact on stakeholder/citizen use of the agency. Additionally, the cases show that, even where there is clear separation between purchaser and provider with a prescribed division of gain, the theory does not always live up to its claimed second benefit.

   In addition to the above findings, this research shows that underlying assumptions within NPM theory related to information asymmetry and goal conflict require further refinement. Several of the above cases show that conflict within the principal/agent relationship does not necessarily originate within the proposed budget-maximizing behavior of the agent. Rather, these cases show that conflict within the principal/agent relationship may occur within the political maximizing behavior of the principal, and have nothing to do with the agent's information advantage. Furthermore, rather than conflict arising between the principal and agent due to goal conflict over constituent wants versus budget maximization, we find several cases which seemed fueled by the principal's ideological agenda, not constituent wants. The predisposition by certain principals toward a specific political agenda would support the claim that NPM, in certain cases, provides a new political tool rather than an economic or managerial tool.

As for criticisms that NPM hollows out government and undermines democratic principles, the data from the case studies can neither directly affirm nor directly disprove. However, if one accepts citizen use as a shadow measure of citizen's preferences, then the decline in public use would tend to support a critic's view of NPM impacts on government. Additionally, if one accepts the underlying argument that public libraries are an agency founded to support the Jeffersonian ideal of development of an informed and enlightened citizenry, decline in use could signal the emergence of a serious problem. Public libraries, in the United States, are the only publicly funded agencies chartered with providing authoritative general information and reading materials, without charge, to the general citizenry. These libraries, along with publicly funded schools, are the primary mechanisms our society has developed to create and maintain the Jeffersonian ideal of an informed citizenry. The maintenance and strengthening of an informed citizenry is critical for the sustenance of our democracy. If the citizenry turns away from the use of such agencies due to the misuse of NPM theories, then we will have fatally wounded democracy.

REFERENCES

Arnold, P. E. (1998). *Making the managerial presidency* (2nd ed.). Lawrence, KS: University Press of Kansas.

Baker, R. L. (1998). Outsourcing in Riverside County: Anomaly, not prophecy. *Library Journal, 123*(5), 34–37.

Boston, J. (1991). The theoretical underpinnings of public sector restructuring in New Zealand. In: J. Boston, J. Martin, J. Pallot & P. Walsh (Eds), *Reshaping the state: New Zealand's bureaucratic revolution.* Auckland, New Zealand: Oxford University Press.

Chang, K. H., deFigueiredo, R. J. P., Jr., & Weingast, B. R. (2001). Rational choice theories of bureaucratic control and performance. In: W. F. Shugart II & L. Razzolini (Eds), *Elgar companion to public choice* (pp. 271–292). Cheltenham, UK: Edward Elgar.

City of Calabasas. (2001). *Library services agreement.* Calabasas, CA.

City of Hemet. (1999). *Special services agreement.* Hemet, CA.

City of Lancaster. (2001). *Contract for library management services of the Lancaster Veterans Memorial Library.* Lancaster, TX.

City of Linden. (2000). *Contract for library management and operations.* Linden, NJ.

Clarke, J., & Newman, J. (1997). *The managerial state.* London: Sage.

County of Riverside, Board of Supervisors. (1997). *Agreement with library systems and services, LLC, for provision of library services [and annual renewals],* Riverside, CA.

DeLeon, L., & Denhardt, R. A. (2000). The political theory of reinvention. *Public Administration Review, 60*(2), 89–97.

DiMattia, S., Lifer, E., & Rogers, M. (1998). Calabasas secedes from LA County PL. *Library Journal, 123*(9), 13.

Dubberly, R. A. (1998). Why outsourcing is our friend. *American Libraries, 29*(1), 72–74.

Ferlie, E. (1996). *The new public management in action.* Oxford: Oxford University Press.

Flagg, G. (1998). Jersey city board ignores protests, votes to privatize. *American Libraries, 29*(7), 14–15.

Frederickson, H. G. (1996). Comparing the reinventing government movement with the new public administration. *Public Administration Review, 56*(3), 263–270.

Goodsell, C. (1993). Reinventing government or rediscovering it. *Public Administration Review, 53*(1), 85–86.

Gore, A. (1993). *From red tape to results: Creating a government that works better and costs less. Report of the national performance review.* Washington, DC: United States Government Printing Office.

Halligan, J. (1997). New public sector models: Reform in Australia and New Zealand. In: J. E. Lane (Ed.), *Public sector reform: Rationale, trends and problems* (pp. 17–46). London: Sage.

Hojnacki, W. (1996). Politicization as a civil service dilemma. In: H. Bekke, J. Perry & T. Toonen (Eds), *Civil service systems in a comparative perspective* (pp. 137–164). Bloomington, IN: Indiana University Press.

Jersey City Free Public Library, Board of Trustees. (2001). *Renewal contract for management consultant services to the Jersey City free public library,* Jersey City, NJ.

Lane, J.-E. (1997a). Incorporation as public sector reform. In: J.-E. Lane (Ed.), *Public sector reform: Rationale, trends and problems* (pp. 283–300). London: Sage.

Lane, J.-E. (1997b). Conclusion. In: J.-E. Lane (Ed.), *Public sector reform: Rationale, trends and problems* (pp. 301–307). London: Sage.

Lane, J.-E. (2000). *New public management.* London: Routledge.

Lewis, D. E. (2003). *Presidents and the politics of agency design: Political insulation in the United States bureaucracy, 1946–1997.* Palo Alto, CA: Stanford University Press.

Martin, R. S. (Ed.) (2000). *The impact of outsourcing and privatization on library services and management.* Chicago: American Library Association.

McCubbins, M. D., Noll, R., & Weingast, B. (1987). Administrative procedures as instruments of political control. *Journal of Law, Economics, and Organization, 3,* 243–277.

Milward, H. B. (1996). Symposium on the hollow state: Capacity, control and performance in interorganizational settings. *Journal of Public Administration Research and Theory, 6*(2), 193–195.

Moe, R. C. (1994). The "reinventing government" exercise: Misinterpreting the problem, misjudging the consequences. *Public Administration Review, 54*(2), 111–122.

National Center for Educational Statistics. (1998). *Data file, public use: Public libraries survey: Fiscal year 1998.* Washington, DC: United States Department of Education.

National Center for Educational Statistics. (1999). *Data file, public use: Public libraries survey: Fiscal year 1999.* Washington, DC: United States Department of Education.

National Center for Educational Statistics. (2001). *Data file, public use: Public libraries survey: Fiscal year 2001*. Washington, DC: United States Department of Education.

National Center for Educational Statistics. (2002). *Data file, public use: Public libraries survey: Fiscal year 2002*. Washington, DC: United States Department of Education.

Niskanen, W. (1971). *Bureaucracy and representative government*. Chicago: Aldine.

Oder, N. (2004). One contract ends, efforts continue. *American Libraries, 129*(8), 16–17.

Office of Management and Budget. (2002). *The President's management agenda*. Washington, DC: Superintendent of Documents, Government Printing Office.

Office of Management and Budget. (2003). Performance of commercial activities. *Federal Register, 68*, 32134–32142.

Pierre, J. (Ed.) (1995). *Bureaucracy in the modern state: An introduction to comparative public administration*. Aldershot: Edward Elgar.

Pollitt, C. (1993). *Managerialism and the public services* (2nd ed.). Oxford: Blackwell.

Potoski, M. (2002). Designing bureaucratic responsiveness: Administrative procedures and agency choice in state environmental policy. *State Politics and Policy Quarterly, 2*, 1–23.

Rogers, M., & Norman, O. (1998). NJ Judge Nixes Jersey City outsourcing contract. *Library Journal, 123*(19), 12.

Romzek, B. S., & Dubnick, M. (1994). Issues of accountability in flexible personnel systems. In: P. W. Ingraham & B. S. Romzek (Eds), *New paradigms for government: Issues for the changing public service* (pp. 263–294). San Francisco: Jossey-Bass.

Rondinelli, D. A. (2003). Partnering for development: Government-private sector cooperation in service provision. In: D. A. Rondinelli & G. S. Cheema (Eds), *Reinventing government for the twenty-first century: State capacity in a globalizing society* (pp. 219–239). Bloomfield, CT: Kumarian Press.

Savas, E. S. (1987). *Privatization: The key to better government*. Chatham, NJ: Chatham House.

Savas, E. S. (1994). On privatization. In: F. S. Lane (Ed.), *Current issues in public administration* (5th ed., pp. 404–413). New York: St. Martin's Press.

Schuman, P. G. (1998). The selling of the public library: It's not just "outsourcing," it's "privatization". *Library Journal, 123*(13), 50–52.

Talbot, C. (1996). *Ministers and agencies: Control, performance and accountability*. London: CIPFA.

Terry, L. D. (1998). Administrative leadership: Neo-managerialism and the public management movement. *Public Administration Review, 58*(3), 194–200.

Trovillion, A. (2002). *Report on privatization of public libraries – pro and con*. Tallahassee, FL: Florida House of Representatives, Committee on Tourism.

Whitford, A. B. (2002). Bureaucratic discretion, agency structure, and democratic responsiveness: The case of the United States attorneys. *Journal of Public Administration Research and Theory, 12*, 3–27.

Yeatman, A. (1998). Trends and opportunities in the public sector: A critical assessment. *Australian Journal of Public Administration, 57*(4), 138–147.

CAREER DEVELOPMENT DIRECTIONS FOR THE PUBLIC LIBRARY MIDDLE LEVEL MANAGER

Janine Golden

INTRODUCTION

Leadership development is a significant issue in public libraries and library administrators debate, among other topics, how to achieve it for the middle-level manager. At the present time, library organizations use leadership and management workshops, seminars, and institutes to assist with managers' organizational learning processes. Current literature indicates that additional strategies such as career planning, mentoring, networking, acquiring adequate qualifications and experience, professional involvement, and continuing education are used not only to facilitate middle-level managers' career development, but also to help organizations fill the leadership gaps within their ranks.

The Problem Statement

Which combination of career development strategies creates the best pathway for these public library middle-level managers aspiring to become public library directors is not known. The need for the profession to explore

Advances in Library Administration and Organization, Volume 23, 173–244
ISSN: 0732-0671/doi:10.1016/S0732-0671(05)23005-5

this path has become critical because the significant number of leaders who are graying and who plan to retire is creating a "potential erosion of leadership stability in the information community over the next 5 to 10 years" (Katz & Salaway, 2003, p. 8). With the departure of the older baby boomers, "a serious collective loss is imminent in terms of experience and expertise. There are few experienced, trained, middle-level managers, supervisors, and administrators within the middle age group of librarians who could ensure appropriate succession in the libraries following such a massive retirement exodus" (Curran, 2003, p. 134).

Although graduate schools of business are now emphasizing leadership skills, schools teaching library and information science were and are largely neglecting those same skills. "Many in the mainstream profession of library and information science education believe that such a topic has little place and importance for the LIS student and thus there is no room in or outside the curriculum" (Sheldon, 1991, p. 69). Formal library education courses have attempted to provide skills needed to manage libraries; however, the leadership factor has been understood primarily as an *innate personality characteristic* and, as such, not generally incorporated into the LIS curriculum. Instead, librarians have been viewed as gateways to sources of information for other career fields studying the leadership concept (Sheldon, 1991).

In order to help strengthen and expand the future leadership pool, three components are needed: (1) the establishment of stronger methods of effective training and development; (2) programs built to identify potential leadership candidates, since not all individuals may choose to move into more senior leadership positions; and (3) indicators to assist these potential leaders in determining which methods are necessary to pursue a successful career developmental path (Katz & Salaway, 2003). In all cases, libraries recognize a need for career professional development strategies.

The library and information science profession specifically is concerned about the issue of leadership. Elements involved with the existence of a call for leadership renewal exist: the erosion of leadership stability, perceptions of leadership, and the identification of potential managerial leadership candidates.

Erosion of Leadership Stability

Two issues have contributed to the erosion of leadership stability. The first is the graying of the workforce. The demographics of the baby-boom generation point to a future in which there will be a much older workforce but "one that may be far too small to meet America's organizational needs" (Goldberg, 2000, p. 15). According to Goldberg the problem is twofold. First, there are too few people to replace the previous generation. Second, more people are leaving the workforce earlier than ever before. The average age of retirement has declined steadily, dropping from 67 in 1950 to 62.7 in 1995. The Employee Benefit Research Institute's 1997 Retirement Confidence Survey indicates that the trend toward early retirement in all probability will continue.

The American Library Association (ALA) engaged Decision Demographics of Arlington, Virginia to calculate how many librarians would reach age 65 in each of the next 30 years. They found using 1990 census data that 87,409 people said they were librarians and had a Master's degree or above. They then used the age of those 87,409 people in 1990 to project when each of them would reach age 65. The highest number (18,469) will be 65 during the years 2010–2014. Logically, then, what may be surmised is that, with this reduction in the number of librarians will come a corresponding reduction in the size of the leadership pool. However, along with the graying and retiring of the current workforce comes a second issue: the resultant shift in organizational memory and experience. Research literature shows that there has been a lack of growth in succession management systems over the past 15 years. In 1984, 68 percent of organizations reported having formal succession plans in place, but in 1999 this had dropped to 61 percent (Bernthal, Rioux, & Wellins, 2004).

Perceptions of Leadership
As Bernthal noted in a 2004 Development Dimensions International (DDI) study, there exists a real leadership shortage. The library field is certainly no different. Riggs (1997) reported that, although leadership had become a common word in the business profession and in everyday use by the late 1980s, the existence of books and journal articles on library leadership at that time were scarce.

Ten years later, Moran examined the topic of leadership and found that, although there was an outpouring of literature about it, leadership within the context of libraries is still "characterized by ambiguity and inconsistency" (Moran, 1992, p. 377). The body of literature expresses concern with the leadership, or lack thereof, in today's library managers (Evans, Ward, & Rugaas, 2000). According to Sayles "Jobs get done and functions get performed with managers who are leaders, but they don't add up to organizational effectiveness without leadership" (Sayles, 1993, p. 82).

Identification of Potential Managerial Leadership Candidates
In the DDI study, Bernthal et al. found that three-quarters of businesses have difficulty finding qualified leaders. Programs built to identify potential

managerial leadership candidates and establish stronger programs for their effective training and development would help to strengthen the numbers of potential future managerial leaders (Bernthal et al., 2004). The need is to establish individuals interested in moving into more senior leadership positions since not all may choose to do so.

Herb White found that the profession is challenged to locate and preserve the "wild ducks," those who stand on principle, ask difficult questions, and are not afraid to buck the system (White, 1987, p. 69). Mech's study noted that existent leaders agree that it is the responsibility of the library director to identify and help transform talented individuals into efficient managers (Mech, 1989). In agreement are Haycock and McCallum, "If libraries are to craft bold mission statements, reconceptualize services and embrace marketing, then the profession needs visionaries, entrepreneurs and leaders as never before" (Haycock & McCallum, 1997, p. 34).

In his work, Sayles identified the necessity of a combination of leader/ manager. Applying the title *working leader*, he noted that "jobs get done and functions get performed with managers who are not leaders, but they don't add up to organizational effectiveness without leadership" (Sayles, 1993, p. 83). Concurring with Mintzberg, Sayles found that *action-oriented manager* seeks to do something, to change something, and to make tomorrow different from today; thus the action-oriented manager is indispensable.

It is the middle-level leader/managers of today who are faced with two major challenges: the changing nature of their leadership roles and the need to restructure their career plans if they intend to advance. The first challenge is that the leadership role is actually changing; leader/managers have greater responsibilities in operating with fewer staff members but a wider scope of duties. Giesecke found that "the traditional hierarchical bureaucracy is no longer correct so that even ... the tried and true rules of management don't work anymore. Middle-level (leader) managers are expected to be a manager of professional librarians who themselves are a form of manager, and to negotiate with – rather than order staff to complete tasks in order to accomplish organizational goals" (Giesecke, 2001, p. 7).

The demands of this changing workplace include (a) a working environment that is faced with the downsizing and flattening of many organizations, (b) an organizational culture in which rapid technological change creates a shift of responsibility for decisions, and (c) external conditions and trends, including an increased focus on the consumer, that involve demands for improved efficiency.

The second challenge presenting itself to the middle-level leader/manager is the need for them to restructure their own career progression paths if they are intent on advancement. Many managers expect rewards in the form of career progression, but organizations are significantly downsizing and de-layering. Thus, as hierarchical layers are stripped away, so are thoughts of traditional career progression, particularly in a governmental, or civil service infrastructure (Thomas & Dunkerley, 1999). As such, traditional career models have been superceded. Leader/managers now have to find new methods of professional advancement through self-development by diversifying skills and/or adding professional qualifications thereby increasing their own marketability.

Purpose and Significance of the Study

This study relied on three types of strategies that are similar to those identified in Farmer and Campbell's work: (1) professional strategies which include involvement with professional groups at various levels; (2) organizational strategies which are carried out by or within organizations; and (3) educational strategies which relate to more formal learning and training (Farmer & Campbell, 1998). The fact remains that there is little agreement about which set or combination of career development strategies creates the best pathway for the middle-level leader/manager aspiring to become a public library director. This study set out to:

1. Determine the career paths of directors of major public libraries relative to educational background, experience, and years of service.
2. Focus on selected career development *strategies* to identify which were most useful and most closely associated with achievement of success by public library directors by
   (a) investigating a selected group of strategies researched in the current literature: professional involvement, recognizing/taking opportunities, qualifications, mentorship, experience, networking, career planning, training and development, and continuing education;
   (b) determining the public library directors' use of the strategies chosen and the level of significance of these strategies to their career success; and
   (c) analyzing the relevance of these strategies to the successful career development for middle-level managers. Since selected strategies are perceived by the directors to be major contributors in their own career trajectory, they are then to be considered as useful elements for middle-level managers to apply to their own career advancement.
3. Investigate the role and value of selected *factors* that contributed to the successful career paths of public library directors by

(a) examining a selected group of *external* factors relative to public library directors' perceptions of the extent that these factors affected their career success: luck/serendipity, gender, age, and geographic mobility and

(b) investigating the correlation of these *external* factors to determine if a relationship exists among the individual factors and strategies.

4. Collect base-line data from the directors for future study of a selected group of *internal* factors (innate or developed) chosen: ability, flexibility, communication, determination, proactivity, hard work, personality, intelligence, and enjoyment. The expectation is that since certain factors play a significant role in career development, the acknowledgement of their existence and effect need to be known.

Limitations of the Study

There are two major limitations to this study. The first concerns the treatment of the internal factors in this research: only base-line data was gathered in order to recognize the existence of these *internal* factors owned and acknowledged by public library directors. They are viewed by this study as either innate or developed characteristics. Measurement of the correlation between these factors and career advancement is beyond the scope of this study; however, the correlation of these factors among themselves is included. Statistics are gathered only for future reference.

The second limitation concerns the selected grouping of *external* factors chosen for this study. In the literature, numerous external factors are identified as potentially influential in career success. Luck or serendipity, gender, age, and geographic mobility are chosen because they were specifically mentioned in research on the career success of public library directors. This selection allows for future comparison studies.

Research Questions

This study was designed to investigate selected factors and strategies that perceptibly contribute to the leadership and successful career development of current public library directors so that they may then be considered as useful elements for middle-level managers to apply to their own career advancement. To achieve this objective, five primary research questions were investigated:

1. What were the career paths taken by directors of major public libraries?
2. How do library directors rate the importance of individual external factors on their career success?

a. What are the relationships among the importance ratings of individual external factors?
3. How do library directors rate the influence of individual internal factors on their career success?
4. To what extent do library directors report using selected career development strategies to achieve career success?
   a. How do library directors rate the influence of individual strategies on their career success?
   b. What are the relationships among the importance ratings of individual strategies?
   c. What are the relationships between importance ratings of individual external factors and the importance ratings of individual strategies?
5. Which career development strategies are recommended by library directors to assist middle-level managers in the successful pursuit of their careers as future library directors?

LITERATURE REVIEW

Considering that a currently graying workforce is ready to retire, this study may assist organizations in achieving their goals of filling the leadership gap within their ranks by focusing on strategies and factors helpful to the middle-level manager. By determining what factors and strategies are used by the public library directors, those that they perceived to be of significance, and those that they recommend to assist the middle- level leader/manager, pathways can be established offering direction for the career development of current middle-level leaders/managers.

The reviewed literature points out that the library and information science profession specifically is concerned about the issue of leadership, in general, ways in which leaders can be identified, and approaches to leadership (Ward, 2000). To assist with this study, three major areas based on the study's research questions were used to address the issues and help formulate a framework for the review of pertinent research and publications: the involvement of strategies and factors in successful career paths of library directors, career strategies impacting career success, and relevance of strategies to the middle-level public library leader/manager.

This study not only includes the required relevant research studies but also the work of credible and well-known practitioners and leading consultants in the leadership and management fields. This was done in order to provide context for the middle-level public library leader/manager for whom the study hopes to be most beneficial. The review of the literature was organized into three main areas: career paths of major library directors, strategies impacting career success, and context for middle-level public library managers.

Career Paths of Major Library Directors

Throughout the literature many elements are considered to be possible influences on career development. Farmer and Campbell (1998) classified these into internal factors, external factors, and strategies. They proposed that internal factors such as ability, flexibility, communication, determination, proactivity, hard work, personality, intelligence, and enjoyment are the aspects, innate or developed, that might affect career success. Farmer and Campbell also examined external factors that they describe as influencing career success but over which people have little or no control. The factors they focused on are luck, serendipity, gender, family support, age, and geographic mobility.

They categorized professional involvement, recognizing/taking opportunities, mentoring, experience, qualifications, and networking as external factors over which people do have a greater or lesser degree of control. It is the latter set of external factors that, for purposes of this study, are known as strategies and are related to additional selected studies as discussed in the literature.

Factors and Strategies found in Relevant Library and Information Sciences Studies

Two primary and six secondary studies are particularly applicable to this study and have provided a model for the extended set of library director career development factors and strategies that appears in this study. The two primary studies modeled and extended for this research are those conducted by Farmer and Campbell (1998) and Greiner (1985).

In their research, Farmer and Campbell examined the relationship between continuing professional development (CPD) and additional factors influencing career success. They conducted interviews with people they perceived to be successful within the information, human resources, and accounting professions. Those within the information professional category fell into two major groups: the directors and senior managers, and the middle-ranking managers.

Given the factors/strategies of personality, networking, geographic mobility, presentation, gender, age, and accent, 55 information professionals (92 percent) perceived both personality and networking as being the most significant factors contributing to career success in general. Participants ranked determination, hard work, personality, ability, and experience as the top five influencing factors on career success. The information professionals then chose the four most important factors affecting their *own* career success with hard work, networking, ability, and experience topping the list. Finally, Farmer and Campbell asked these professionals about achieving career success. Their top three perceptions for success were: (1) recognize and take opportunities, (2) have a clear definition of success and what it means to you, (3) update and develop your skills, (4) plan your career, (5) be flexible, and (6) move to different posts/places.

The second primary study, used as a model and expanded for this study, was conducted by Greiner in 1985. As part of her research, Greiner conducted a nationwide survey of male and female public library directors serving areas of 100,000 people or more. With an initial population of 420 directors (256 males, 163 females, and 1 unidentified gender) she gathered personal, educational, and professional data about each director, and statistical data about his or her library/library system. Her research focused on (1) the existing conditions in the profession relating to salaries and library support and (2) the career development process with regard to steps in the advancement from the beginning of a professional career to achievement of the position of library director.

Based on a response of 321 or 76.43 percent (189 males, 132 females), Greiner's research on the directors' career development process explored both strategies and factors. She reviewed steps in the advancement from the beginning of a professional career to achievement of the directors' current position.

The strategies reported in Greiner's study are qualifications, professional membership, directorship aspirations (career planning), mentoring, and career breaks. Factors indicated in Greiner's survey included timing/luck, age, gender, and mobility.

Secondary studies found to contain elements useful to this study have been conducted by Pergander (2003), Haycock and McCallum (1997), Chatman (1992), Harris and Tague (1989), McNeer (1988), and Ferriero (1982). These particular works have been reviewed because their characteristics are relative to library directors enabling comparisons and contrasts relevant to this study.

Career Strategies Impacting Career Success

A review of the literature recognizes the possible need for career professional development strategies. Because of the constant rate of change in organizations, leadership positions in the future will likely require different competencies. Bernthal at DDI found that organizations are "gearing up for the projected leadership gap by increasing their budgets for training and development" (Bernthal et al., 2004, p. 3).

What are suggested by the current literature are actions that will ensure a supply of high-quality leading managers. By assuming that individuals can be taught the characteristics of leadership, libraries can raise the caliber of managers through the teaching and encouraged use of career leadership development strategies. The library profession should formulate, agree upon and adopt a plan designed to develop leaders that the library organizations must possess if they are to survive (Hendry, 1996). Exposing the middle-level manager to issues and solution-finding at the higher level in addition to using these career development strategies will enable libraries to offer potential leaders this guidance.

The literature mentions nine predominant career professional development strategies: (1) career planning, (2) training and development, (3) continuing education, (4) networking, (5) mentorship, (6) qualifications, (7) experience, (8) professional involvement, and (9) recognizing/taking opportunities.

Context to Middle Level Public Library Managers

According to Mintzberg there is no job more vital to our society than that of the leader/manager. "It is the manager who determines whether our institutions serve us well or whether they squander our talents and resources" (Mintzberg, 1975, p. 61).

Throughout the 1980s and up to the present, library management is established as an important area of study in the major indexes and databases and as something distinct from the traditional concerns of librarianship (Barter, 1994). Bailey describes it as "an area of a professional librarian's career that cannot be ignored .... a creative activity of motivating people to work together to implement the libraries' missions and objectives" (Bailey, 1982, p. 7).

The role of the public library manager today needs to incorporate individuals who "can operate cost-effective and cost-efficient services, are receptive to new ideas and are familiar with the legal and ethical issues surrounding information provision. They are sensitive to the political environment surrounding inside and around the organization, can adapt their service to the changing needs of the organization, and can continually demonstrate the value of the information service to the achievement of the organization's goals" (Johnson, 1999, p. 323).

Because of the recognized resurgence of leadership renewal, middle-level public library managers aspiring to become directors are involved in acknowledging changes. These changes are major elements that have and are occurring in the career development process beginning with their own current roles.

McAnally and Downs (1973) offered a list of the pressures which alter the role of the library leader/manager: the information explosion, the expansion of technology, the high rate of inflation, the new theories of management, the growing atmosphere of conflict present in many organizations, and the increasing stress placed on the directors.

Many of the interpersonal and organizational skills that made leaders/ managers successful in the past remain important for modern ones to emulate. However, those leaders/managers in the twenty-first-century organizations require a broadening of skills and talents to lead new types of organizations (Stueart & Moran, 2000).

There are two factors that have a major impact on creating changes in the practice of leadership/management by the public library middle-level manager. The first is the demands of the changing workplace and the second is a restructured career progression path.

Prominently indicated in the survey of current research literature are changes that are driven by (1) the working environment, (2) the organizational culture, (3) external conditions/trends, and (4) the changing role itself for the middle-level leader/manager.

Within the working environment, there are two elements that are major considerations for the leader/manager. In today's employment environment downsizing or "rightsizing" has become commonplace and has occurred so frequently in the last 10 years that it has become acknowledged as an organizational necessity (Sicker, 2002). The current buzzword *restructuring* is often a euphemism for layoffs (Wessel, 1993). Unlike past trends where mostly blue-collar jobs were cut, the American Management Association Survey on Downsizing reports that 54.6 percent of the jobs cut are supervisory, middle management, and professional/technical positions (American Management Association, 1993). As a result, "there is a greater degree of job insecurity in the current employment environment, regardless of position or status with an organization than at any time in the post-World War II era" (Wessel, 1993, p. A1).

The second consideration relating to the working environment is the flattening of the organization. The removal of layers and flattening of organizational structures raise a number of challenges for the middle-level manager. Thomas and Dunkerley (1999) illustrate this in concluding that middle-level managers are working harder, longer, with wider roles and greater responsibilities. Many leaders/managers expect rewards in the form of career progression, yet organizations are significantly downsizing and delayering their organizations. Thus, as hierarchical layers are stripped away, so are the thoughts of traditional career progressions, particularly in a governmental (civil service) infrastructure.

Not only has the existence of new technology altered the culture of the organization, but the rapidity of technological change created the shift of responsibility for decisions. The reality is that managers spend most of their working lives in interdisciplinary and interfunctional teams interacting with people who may have totally different working styles (i.e., LIS and IT). And the effectiveness of a team depends on how well these different managerial preferences are accepted and integrated in the group decision-making processes. Because organizations today are restructuring and having to respond to new environmental challenges, one team member can no longer have all of the answers. "The careers of both professionals and managers are inextricably bound with those of others" (Davies, 1995, p. 3) thus making team management a viable tool for assisting with career development.

The third factor creating change in the practice of management is a direct result of external conditions and trends. Pressures such as the drive for improved efficiency, the new consumerism (i.e., quality and quantity of services, value for money (Griffiths & King, 1994)), the changing market, reorganizations and restructuring, legislative changes, and new technology require further examination of the management techniques applied by the middle-level manager. In addition, public libraries face challenges and are asking employees to do more with less without the ability to promise long-term employment as compensation. "The issue has become how an organization gets passion without promise, and devotion without dividends" (Bell, 1998, p. 27).

Currently, because staffing and budgeting concerns have reduced the number of tiers in organizational structures, directors need to be more involved with day-to-day issues, which in turn create additional pressures for these managing leaders. Today, the role of the public library manager needs to incorporate individuals who "can operate cost-effective and cost-efficient services, are receptive to new ideas, are familiar with the legal and ethical issues surrounding information provision, are sensitive to the political environment with the organization, can adapt their service to the changing needs of the organization, and can continually demonstrate the value of the information service to the achievement of the organization's goals" (Johnson, 1999, p. 323).

Even assuming that a leader/manager does want to progress up the administrative ladder, there are roadblocks in the way. Stueart and Moran

(2002) listed two of these roadblocks: libraries being and having been in a non-growth stage for a number of years, and management plateauing which may be due to a lack of openings in the positions directly above the manager level. If there are positions that exist directly above the manager's level, these positions may be held by individuals who are only slightly older than the employee seeking the advancement and thus, not ready to retire. To the middle-level manager seeking advancement, the traditional career models appear to be superceded.

And once again, because of organizational decentralization and delayering, few organizations can predict with any confidence the extent of services they will be providing 5–10 years down the road and what the service level requirements will be (Sicker, 2002). The message is that the career as it has been known, "a series of upward moves with steadily increasing income, power, status, and security," is a thing of the past (Hall, 1996, p. 1).

Because of this, the burden of career planning/management is being shifted from the organizational resource department to the manager. As stated by Sicker (2002), the word *career* within an organization has now become a *job to be done* that meets customers' needs and brings a return on investment to the shareholders.

McNeer (1988) found three predominant areas of suggested professional activity in her study: apprenticeships, professional/scholarly activity (experiences and contacts made in professional organizations), and personal initiative. What the current literature suggests is that the managerial leader is finding additional new methods of professional advancement. By developing a diversification of skills and interests and adding professional qualifications the managers are increasing their own marketability. The DDI study suggested that leadership development is a joint venture where leaders "take responsibility for their own development and organizations support them through the process" (Bernthal et al., 2004, p. 2). In their survey, almost three-quarters of the leaders/managers polled indicated that they pursue development activities to make themselves more marketable for other jobs.

Leonard Sayles (1993) identified the type of change in management:

- Everything has changed.
- Customers are much more demanding, and are increasingly demanding customization.
- Customer needs are in flux.
- The market is more turbulent.
- The new manager's role is one of completely rethinking the past.
- All the things that you have been told about managing are totally wrong.

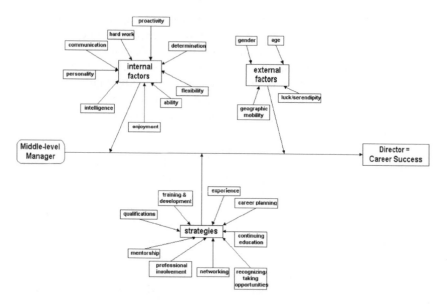

Fig. 1. Career Development Model (Golden, 2005).

With this in mind, this study's intent was to explore the best path for the middle-level manager/leader aspiring to become a public library director in light of the above challenges. The career paths of current public library directors along with external factors and the strategies they used to advance their careers are explored and their suggested best practices indicated. Fig. 1 illustrates a career development model created for this research (Golden, 2005).

RESEARCH DESIGN AND METHODOLOGY

This study used elements of the quantitative approach to research by describing current conditions (survey research) and investigating relationships between and among the career development factors and strategies (correlational). However, elements of the qualitative approach are used specifically in the data collection and analysis of the open structured questions.

Development of this survey/investigative research design began with the construction of a data collection instrument (the questionnaire) appropriate to five formulated research questions.

- What were the career paths of major library directors?
- How do library directors rate the importance of individual external factors on their career success? What are the relationships among the importance ratings of individual external factors?
- How do library directors rate the influence of individual internal factors on their career success?
- To what extent do library directors report using selected career development strategies to achieve career success? How do library directors rate the influence of individual strategies on their success? What are the relationships among the importance ratings of individual strategies? What are the relationships between importance ratings of individual external factors and the importance ratings of individual strategies?
- Which career development strategies are recommended by library directors to assist middle-level managers in the successful pursuit of their careers as future library directors?

The design of this study was instrumental in the investigation, examination and analysis of career paths of major library directors; their perceptions of the effect of internal and external factors on their career success; strategies which assisted in achieving career success and could contribute to a developmental tool for aspiring middle-level managers; the relationships among the importance ratings of the individual external factors; and the relationships among the importance ratings of individual strategies.

The study design was also loosely modeled upon the work of Jane Farmer and Fiona Campbell (1998). Replicating their concept of the relationship of internal and external factors a new study was constructed with selected factors and potential influential strategies as acknowledged by public library directors as contributory to their successful career attainment.

Instrumentation

A self-developed questionnaire was constructed taking into account various questions from those presented by Farmer and Campbell (1998), Chatman (1992), and Greiner (1985). Questions from those studies were combined with self-constructed questions formulated in response to the five research questions specific to this study. With each question corresponding to one of the research questions presented, a pilot study was performed to test whether the survey questions measured the identified career development strategies and factors indicated in the proposed research. With the use of the pilot study, both validity and reliability were established.

Rather than using all open-ended queries, the survey includes structured questions with a group of fixed responses as well as an unstructured format to enhance reliability (see survey located in the appendix). The open-ended questions used are found to be an added benefit for the exploratory component of the investigative research process.

The survey instrument was designed to gather personal, educational, and professional data about the library directors. The intent was to use a simple web-based questionnaire containing structured groupings of questions and answers resulting in the production of enough information to examine not only the career development strategies used and recommended by the directors, but also the relationships among those selected variables as they relate to director career achievement.

Population of the Study

The letter announcing the survey with an invitation to participate was sent to public library directors in the United States whose service area encompasses a population of 100,000 or more. This amounts to 390 directors, comprised of 240 females (61.54 percent) and 150 males (38.46 percent) who were identified and chosen from the *Public Library Data Service (PLDS) Service Report 2003* and the *American Library Directory* (2003–2004).

The study focused on directors of major public libraries because they are the recognized leaders in the field of public library management. For purposes of this study, the 390 public library agencies in 53 states were identified by using those located in the PLDS. Participating libraries surveyed by the Public Library Association for the 2003 PLDS within the states of Vermont, Wyoming, North Dakota, New Hampshire or Maine, West Virginia, and Delaware were not identified as serving populations of 100,000 and as a result are not included (Public Library Association, 2003).

Administration of the Survey

A web-based survey was the method selected for administering the study questionnaire to the identified population of library directors. E-mail and organizational addresses for each director were drawn from the *American Library Directory, 2003–2004*. A paper cover letter including the introduction, purpose, invitation, site address (http://visc.sis.pitt.edu/career_survey), and instructions for survey access was mailed but the specifics of the Computer-Assisted Self-administered Questionnaire (CASQ) were described in the electronic version once the participant accesses the online site.

Respondents were asked to complete the questionnaire within two weeks of receipt of the introductory letter, but the survey remained online an additional week to capture delayed responses from three individuals who were on vacation. Participants were strongly encouraged to answer all the questions and submit the questionnaire on-line and were assured of anonymity in case there were concerns about privacy (Gunn, 2002). Two hundred fifteen completed responses were received (55 percent), including 214 that were useable.

Pilot Study

To test the survey instrument for content and format reliability and validity, a pilot study was conducted. In order for the pretest sample to be of an adequate size to permit generalizations to the population (Powell, 1997), three male and three female directors whose library systems served a population of 100,000 or more were asked to complete the survey. Letters of request were sent to public library directors from Pennsylvania, Iowa, Texas, California, Montana, and Tennessee on June 10, 2004, and the last four of the six responded.

Based on feedback from the pilot participants, the pilot study was successful and an analysis reveals that each of the items measured what they were intended to measure; all of the major definitions and phrases were understood; the questions were interpreted by all of the respondents similarly; and each fixed-question response had an answer, with no questions routinely skipped (Powell, 1997).

Treatment of the Data

Measurable data was reported, coded, and analyzed using SPSS, the statistical package for the social sciences. Comments made in open-ended questions were grouped, coded according to similarities whenever possible, and presented in areas referenced by appropriate research query. Since the numbered responses were manageable and categories were evident, open-ended query analysis was performed using a computerized list allowing groupings.

This study used the χ^2 test of statistical significance to measure the strength of the relationships among the strategies. SPSS produced a variety of results, with one of the most relevant being the listing of the p-value. To facilitate analysis of the relationships among the importance ratings, correlations rather than cross-tabulations, and χ^2 tests of association were used, because the ratings are on a continuous scale. Matrix correlations were used for questions for which the respondents were to rate each factor/strategy using a scale of 1–10 with 1 as very low importance and 10 as very high importance.

The results established the use of selected internal/external factors and strategies by public library directors in their careers; revealed the perceived importance of the internal/external factors and strategies; assisted in the analysis of whether the strategies can be suggested as a developmental tool for public library middle-level managers; and provided a basis for the assessment, formulation and development of a best practices document related to strategies recommended by the directors.

The results contributed to the encouragement of the public library middle-level manager to assess if and how the recommended strategies can best fit into a personal career development plan. The results are also useful to public library administrators in their planning and implementation of leadership development for the middle-level managers.

ANALYSIS AND INTERPRETATION OF THE DATA

Findings

Career Path
Of the 214 respondents, the highest degree earned by 203 (94.9 percent) of the public library directors is a Master's; three also earned doctorates. Seven directors hold a Bachelor's degree as the highest degree earned, and one individual holds a certificate in public administration.

One hundred and ninety-nine (93 percent) of the 214 responding have an earned Master's in library/information science. The additional 29 hold a Master's degrees in public administration (15); business administration (4); history (3); English (2); and biology, education, diversity/psychology, teaching and Spanish (1 each). Twenty-five of these are dual-mastered degrees that are coupled with LIS.

In addition to the Master's of Library/Information Science 17 directors reported holding a total of 25 advanced certificate or specialist degrees in a subject area. There were eight certificates obtained in the library and information field. The additional 17 were in archives, public administration, management, paper preservation, ethnography, human resources, learning disabilities/behavioral disorders, aging and vision loss, gerontology, and vocal music.

Other educational preparation included coursework and/or graduate study in the areas of law, nursing, and sign language as well as various management courses over the years. Two of the three doctorates are held in library/information science with the third in business administration.

A greater amount of diversity in the degree fields was found in undergraduate majors. Pure sciences and business and government majors are least common (math, 2; biology, 1; environmental geosciences and geology, 1; public administration, 3; and government, 1).

The highest concentration of Bachelor's degrees earned was in the fields of English and history. English majors accounted for 17 (20 percent) of the total 84 responses given, and when included as a double major totaled 25 (29.7 percent). History majors ran a close second producing 16 (19 percent) of the total 84 responses given. The remainder of the undergraduate degrees represented are: education and psychology (both at 5), elementary education (3), journalism, political science, philosophy, anthropology, communication arts and Spanish (2 each), and music education, secondary education, home economics, classical languages, German literature, French, speech and theater, fine arts, related art, and liberal studies (1 each).

An undergraduate degree in social sciences (89.3 percent) was the majority field. Administration (i.e., public administration, government, political science) amounted to 6.0 percent of the total and 4.7 percent in the sciences.

Academic Institutions. Two hundred and five public library directors received their library/information sciences degrees from 59 academic institutions in 32 states and Canada. Fig. 2 indicates the regions of the U.S. and Canada where Master's degrees were received.

The top three reported attended institutions are Florida State University with 12 students (5.8 percent of the total number of participants), and both the University of Denver and the University of Wisconsin accounting for 11

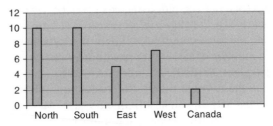

Fig. 2. Regions of the U.S. where Master's Degrees Received.

each (5.4 percent). By state, Pennsylvania produced the most colleges/universities attended even though universities in the eastern region of the United States were the least represented in terms of colleges attended.

The remainder of the survey regarding the Career Path of the directors was concerned with years of experience, number of years as a public library director and years/field of service prior to the directorship. The results given were obtained from 212 participants. From the findings in the survey, the *average*: (a) total years of professional experience is 27.56 years, (b) number of years as a public library director is 13.11 years, and (c) the number of years of professional experience before becoming a director is 13.42 years.

Areas of employment outside of the library field prior to being hired as a public library director and listed by the 82 respondents clearly illustrated two major areas (education at 39 percent and business at 27 percent) with a few other minor ones also indicated.

Factors

Because external factors may work as influences on career success, they also are explored. The four selected external factors for this study were: *gender, age, geographic mobility*, and *luck/serendipity*.

A total of 205 respondents indicated their gender on the survey. Of these, 136 were women (66.3 percent) and 69 were men (33.7 percent). Directors who were sent the letter of introduction and invitation to complete the survey consist of 240 females (61.54 percent) and 150 males (38.46 percent) for a total of 390, meaning that a higher percentage of responses was received from female directors at 56.6 percent (136 women out of a possible 240) than males (69 (46 percent) out of a possible 160) responded to the questionnaire. Of the combined total responses of 207, 136 (66.3 percent) were female directors and 69 (33.7 percent) were males.

Of the 207 responses concerning age, the average number of years at which the participants became the director of the library where they were currently employed was 45.6 years. The youngest was reported as being 22 years old (1 director) and the oldest reported was 65 years old (1 director). The most frequently reported age was 48 years old (17 directors, 8.2 percent).

Relative to career moves and relocations, the data gathered illustrated that the average number of career moves within an institution is 3.92 moves, with the most frequent occurring at three moves (frequency rate of 41). Data also showed that the average number of relocations to a new community was 2.51 relocations with the highest frequency of 43 at 0 times. The average number of moves within the same community was 0.71, with the highest frequency of 128 directors moving 0 times.

Table 1. Summary of Factors and Ratings.

Rating	Ability	Flex.	Determination	Proactivity	Hard work	Personality	Intell.	Enjoyment
1	1			1				3
2		1		3	1			
3		4	3	3	1	2	1	1
4		1	4	6		3	3	2
5	4	6	12	17	3	9	8	15
6	6	12	12	16	7	10	8	9
7	10	28	21	23	12	31	34	30
8	59	57	42	53	41	54	70	46
9	43	37	38	31	51	49	41	33
10	83	58	71	48	89	47	40	63
Total	205	204	204	201	205	205	205	202

As perceived by 205 surveyed subjects, 127 (62 percent) of the directors believed that luck/serendipity factored into their career development. Twenty-three respondents directly claimed being in the right place at the right time. The directors were asked at what point in their careers did they perceive luck/serendipity to have occurred: early in career, mid-career or late in career. All three stages were indicated, but the highest frequency rate occurred early in the directors' career.

Because internal factors as well may influence career success, the following eight selected internal factors are considered: *ability, flexibility, determination, proactivity, hard work, personality, intelligence,* and *enjoyment.* In the questionnaire, the directors were asked to rate the significance of each of the individual internal as well as external factors that influenced their personal career growth. Table 1, a summary comparison table indicates each factor and its rating. Using a scale of 1–10, the rating of 1 illustrates lowest significance and 10 is of highest significance.

Perceived to be the most significant of all of the eight internal factors (by mean) were hard work, having the ability to perform the duties of a director, determination, and flexibility. According to the data collected, the least significant internal factor was proactivity. Fig. 3 includes a visual of the mean for the individual internal factors.

Career Development Strategies

In order to explore successful career development of the public library director, the following strategies were considered for study: *career planning, continuing education, training and development, mentorship, networking,*

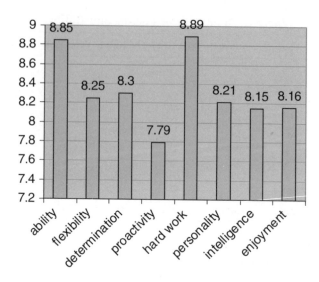

Fig. 3. Mean Significance Rating for Internal Factors.

professional involvement, *recognizing/taking opportunities*, *qualifications*, and *experience*.

Verified by the data, the greatest number of the 202 public library director respondents first learned of the opening for their present position as director through sources other than those listed in this study. Listed by the term *other*, the open-ended 41 responses are summarized into internal sources (23) as the contact was positioned in the system already (five were in the position of assistant director at the time); political sources (10) i.e., state librarian, state websites, city administrators, county judge and mayor's offices; interested community members (2); business contacts; and miscellaneous (5), which included personal friends, just visiting a site, by accident, market awareness, and just sending out a resume.

The responses given to designated sources are indicated in summary Table 2. The highest scoring mean listed for job notification to these directors is former directors recruiting a successor. Noted also are the lowest two sources of position notification to the directors: professional association placement and library school referrals.

Responding to the question as to whether or not those surveyed had a career plan before becoming a director, the collected data showed that of the 195 directors answering, 99 (50.8 percent) did have a career plan and 96 (49.2 percent) did not. The main perceived benefits by the 99 who have a career

Table 2. First Hearing of Opening for Present Position of Library Director.

	Yes	Not Checked
Announcement	37	165
Board of trustees	16	186
Former director recruiting successor	38	164
Library school referral	1	201
Professional association placement	1	201
Publication	36	166
Notification from associate	22	180
Recruiting firm	10	192

plan were coded into the following categories: planning provides focus, helps to set goals, points the individual in one direction, and provides clarity.

There were 62 individuals who both indicate that they did not have a career plan and commented as to whether and how a career plan possibly could have helped them in their career path: 24 stated that it would have been of no help, 17 made comments, 13 were not sure, and eight answers were not applicable.

Sample comments on how a career plan *could have* helped include the following:

- I would have not made one of my moves and instead would have spent another year or two in a previous position. A career plan would have helped me be more systematic in my goals and actions.
- I would have studied the administrative portion of my classes if I would have known I was going to be a director.
- Probably would have helped, but as a female, the concept of a career path was not thought about until the late 60 s.

And those that felt that a career plan would *not* have helped have commented as follows:

- A career plan may have hampered my path. I have looked at lifestyle and family factors in my decision-making. I think that for me the pursuit of the "better deal" would have led me to jump into positions that may not have suited me as well.
- I surely would not hold the position I hold if I had formulated a plan and stuck to it.

Those current directors that had aspired to be an administrator when they entered the profession amounted to 87 (43.5 percent) of the 200 answering the question. One hundred and thirteen (56.5 percent) did not.

Career Choices

Two hundred and two respondents answered the question of what career choices helped them achieve their current position. Choices presented to the respondents included changed library systems (26 percent), acquired additional schooling/certification (17 percent), chose a mentor (14 percent), started entry level and progressed through same system (12 percent), took lateral move (11 percent), left another field to enter library arena (10 percent), and other (10 percent).

Included in the other choices indicated by the directors that were instrumental in achieving their current position were joining professional state and national associations and especially holding office (13 indications given), chosen *by* a mentor (6), willingness to relocate (5), having role models (3), being associate/assistant director first (3), having taken continuing education and management courses (2), having taken a position with less money to gain experience (2), having been coached (2), having taken chances (2), and each of the following was listed once (1): networking, building a reputation, working at a state library, having onsite experience, working hard, taking on unpopular assignments, having a business background, choosing a system for its benefits, learning the system and political structures, and choosing the best and brightest systems to work for.

Career Break

Another distinct element tied into career planning is a career break, whether planned or not. These career breaks were experienced by 66 (33.2 percent) of the total 199 directors that chose to answer this question. Of these, 20 each indicated that the break was planned, with 20 stating the combination response of both yes and no. Reasons given for the break were categorized into two major areas: career related (i.e., incompatibility with board, education, etc.) and family (personal) related to issues such as child birth, spouse relocation, etc. Job/career-related breaks were taken by 28 directors (42 percent) and family-related breaks were taken by 38 (58 percent).

Twenty-five directors (38 percent) of the total 66 who had career breaks took those breaks as a result of motherhood. Of those 25 females, 21 responded as to whether that particular break was an advantage, disadvantage, or neutral to their career. The figure below shows that eight of the female directors thought taking time off for motherhood was a disadvantage to their career, six perceived the break to be an advantage, and seven were neutral.

Sixty-two directors overall chose to answer the question about whether the break was an advantage or a disadvantage to their careers. Thirty-one

(50 percent) respond that the break was an advantage. Sample reasons are as given below:

- This was the cause of my move to the library and of my return to school to get an MLS.
- It was an advantage because it pointed me back to working with smaller libraries where I am happier.
- Just gave me great life experiences which I think always helps.

Nineteen (31 percent) responded that the break was a disadvantage. Sample reasons given follow:

- It was a disadvantage as I felt I had to run fast to catch up.
- I did not work for four years after the birth of my first child. This was definitely not advantageous to my career.
- Took a while to get back to speed especially with the explosion of technology into libraries.

The remainder of the respondents answered as follows: neither yes nor no = 8 (13 percent), somewhat = 1 (1.6 percent), yes and no = 1 (1.6 percent), no disadvantage = 1(1.6 percent), and somewhat = 1(1.6 percent).

The majority of library directors who responded did not take a career break (66.8 percent). Those who did have a planned break (30.3 percent) perceived it to be an advantage to them (47 percent). Most of those who had an unplanned career break did not consider it to be an advantage to their career (28.7 percent).

Before assuming the position of public library director 155 (77.9 percent) answered that they have taken continuing education courses. Of the 162 that answered, 62 (38.3 percent) perceived these courses to be very helpful to their career advancement, 89 (54.9 percent) thought that were somewhat helpful, and 11 (6.8 percent) indicated the courses were not helpful at all. Concerning training and development workshops/seminars, 164 (84.1 percent) directors of the 195 that participated in workshop or seminars perceived them to have helped with their career advancement. Thirty-one (15.9 percent) indicated that the workshops/ seminars did not help.

Subjects that were considered most beneficial are categorized into nine areas. Since the directors were asked to list three of their own chosen subject areas in no particular order, all three of their choices are combined into a total list of 346 responses. Leadership/management/supervision heads the list at 195 responses. The remaining categories were financial development (37 responses); planning and development (36 responses); information technology (28 responses); human resource issues (22 responses); legal issues (nine responses); personal analysis (eight responses); politics (seven responses); and marketing and public relations (four responses) (see Fig. 4).

Of the 193 respondents to the question as to whether or not they have ever had a mentor, 118 (61.1 percent) answered that they have had one. Seventy-five (38.9 percent) replied that they had not. Among the 128 of those who answered the question as to whether they could have achieved their current status without a mentor, 39 (30.5 percent) said that they thought they could, 38 (29.7 percent) said they could not have achieved their current status without a mentor, and 51 (39.8 percent) were undecided. At the time of this study, 106 directors (55.5 percent) of the 191 responding were mentors and 85 (44.5 percent) were not.

When asked whether those surveyed considered networking as a factor in their career advancement, 129 (66.5 percent) of 194 answered *yes, that* they do believe networking assisted with their career development. The remainder of the directors, totaling 65 (33.5 percent), answered *no*.

Those who did respond with the *yes* answer were then asked who they communicated with that assisted with their career climb. Of the 202 responding to this question, 53.5 percent said they communicated with library directors, 35.1 percent with friends, 49 percent with professionals within the organization, 32.7 with professionals outside of the organization, and 11.4 percent said they communicated with others. Listed as others (23 responses)

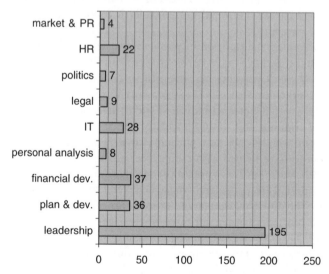

Fig. 4.   Training and Development Participation Categories.

for communication sources were: family, vendors, community members, trustees, former professors, civic/service club members, and "anyone I could find."

The strategy of networking within professional organizations elicited responses from 202 directors. A breakdown of the suggested organizations lists the American Library Association, Public Library Association, Urban Libraries Council, State Library Associations, and other professional organizations. Active participation in these organizations from the 202 directors indicated that the highest numbers of public library directors (173, 85.6 percent) hold a membership in a state library association. The American Library Association was next with 149 (73.8 percent) surveyed directors as members, followed by the Public Library Association at 135 (66.8 percent), the Urban Libraries Council at 49 directors (24.3 percent) and membership in other professional organizations at 44 (21.8 percent).

When asked if there was one particular opportunity that made a difference in their career, 184 directors answered the question. One hundred and twenty-eight (69.6 percent) said *yes* and 56 (30.4 percent) responded with *no*. The comments given are coded into three categories of opportunities: career, personal, and organizational.

For purposes of this study, career opportunities are defined as those that have occurred in the respondent's overall employment development. The responses given amounted to 71 of the total of 128 (55 percent). Personal opportunities apply to situations outside of the working environment that are individual to the respondent (i.e., family, etc.). Personal opportunities amounted to 10 of the total 128 (8 percent). Organizational opportunities applies to those opportunities occurring within the system that the respondent is employed. Respondents submitted a total of 47 of these (37 percent).

A sampling of career opportunities listed appears below:

Career. Going from a small town public library to head up a statewide
project to develop an interlibrary loan code and then working for the
State Library agency as a library development consultant.

Organizational. I had the chance to work under a terrible boss. It made me
work twice as hard. It also taught me a lot about how things should and
should not be done, and reinforced my personal beliefs about the
importance of integrity.

In regard to the final two strategies (qualifications and experience), the results given were obtained from 212 participants. From the findings in the survey, the average: (a) total years of professional experience was 27.56 years, (b) number of years as a public library director was 13.11 years, and

(c) the number of years of professional experience before becoming a director was 13.42 years.

The final question in Section C of the survey asked the respondents to rate each of the career strategies listed by numbering how beneficial they were to their career advancement prior to assuming their current position. The strategies given were: qualifications, experience, professional involvement, networking, mentorship, recognizing/taking opportunities, career planning, training and development, and continuing education.

The directors were instructed to use the number one as very low importance and the number 10 as very high importance. Of the nine strategies, two of the strategies – importance of qualifications and importance of recognizing opportunities were given an importance rating of no lower than 4.

Based on the numbers given by the directors, the importance given to mentorship in terms of how beneficial it was to their career advancement ranked the lowest of all nine strategies; 58.8 percent of the respondents assigned the mentoring process a 5 and below.

Most noteworthy of the strategies are the importance of experience, importance of networking, and the importance of training and development. In each case they were listed with a 50 percent and higher frequency in the 7–10 range of importance.

Both of the strategies importance of professional involvement and the importance of continuing education showed a higher concentration of scores in the 5–8 range. The frequency number for professional involvement included 122 directors (64 percent), and continuing education included 112 (60 percent).

The strategy of the importance of career planning illustrates a score of five being the highest frequency percentage (19.6 percent). The directors appeared to be evenly divided, giving 54.3 percent to a rating of five and below and a 45.6 percent to 6 and above. Table 3 focuses on a summary using the mean score of all of the career strategies listed above.

Career Success

Recognizing/taking opportunities is chosen as the most important career strategy at 32.1 percent of the total 171 valid submissions; training and development (2.3 percent) is of the least of importance; 98 of 166 directors state that there are no additional strategies that have had an influence on their career success other than those mentioned; 68 state that there were.

Relative to their past careers, the directors were asked to choose their most important strategy from the list of the nine indicated above (qualifications, experience, professional involvement, networking, mentorship, recognizing/taking opportunities, career planning, training and development,

Table 3. Perceived Importance of Career Strategies by Frequency Ranking.

Ranking	Qual.	Opp.	Mentor.	Expe.	Networking	Train. and Dev.	Prof. Involv.	Cont. Edu.	Career Plan
1			30	1	10	4	8	11	15
2			17	2	10	6	10	10	22
3			14	2	13	10	10	14	13
4	1	2	14	2	10	9	8	12	14
5	6	7	29	7	30	26	36	29	36
6	5	3	6	8	13	14	19	24	17
7	18	11	18	9	22	39	28	31	22
8	42	46	23	40	35	39	39	28	24
9	29	39	11	48	26	27	17	15	13
10	93	83	15	73	20	17	15	14	8
Total	194	191	177	192	189	191	190	188	184

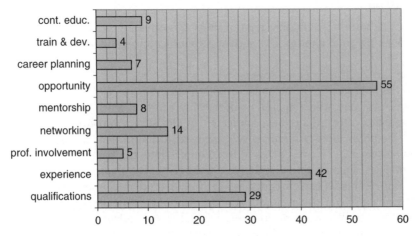

Fig. 5. Strategy Frequency Rate and Percentage of Importance.

and continuing education). They were also asked to indicate how and why the one that they had chosen was beneficial to their career success.

As illustrated in Fig. 5, the collected data showed that recognizing/taking opportunities were chosen as the most important strategy at 32.1 percent of the total 171 valid submissions. Training and development (2.3 percent) was located at the very bottom of the list.

The second part of Section D of the survey asked the directors whether there were any additional strategies that have had an influence on their career success that perhaps are omitted in the nine strategies listed above.

Ninety-eight of 166 directors responded with no and 68 responded with yes. From the 68 answers in the positive, 55 were applicable to the question.

As in the other open-ended questions, the results were coded. The categories of the additional strategies include the strategies that are intrinsic (40 percent) and those that are extrinsic (60 percent).

A sampling of the two types is as follows:

Intrinsic

- A strong professional philosophy
- Being passionate about what you do and communicating that passion to others
- Enjoyment of life in general – achieving a balance of work and play

Extrinsic

- Collaborations, building relationships & motivating skills at all levels
- Making good choices and making situations into good situations

Context to Middle Level Managers
In the final section of the online questionnaire (Section E) the public library directors were asked to list in decreasing priority order what additional strategies, other than those indicated in the survey already, they would advise public library middle-level managers to use in their quest for career advancement. The responses were grouped into the categories of career strategies, organizational strategies, and personal strategies.

For this study, career strategies are those that are used in the respondent's overall employment development. Organizational strategies applies to those used within the operating structure where the respondent is employed. Personal strategies apply to situations outside of the working environment that are individual to the respondent (i.e., family, self, etc.).

Of the total of 246 additional strategies suggested, 95 suggestions (38.6 percent) were coded as personal strategies. There were 84 (34.2 percent) suggested career-related suggestions. And organizational amounts to 67 (27.2 percent). Fig. 6 gives a priority level breakdown.

A representative sampling of the recommended strategies are listed below.

First Priority

Career. Become the position you desire ... act like a senior person, dress like a senior person, go to lunch with the right people, learn how they talk, and

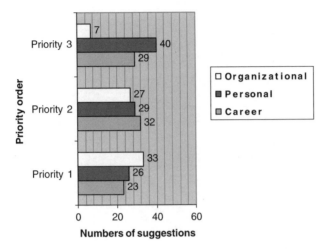

Fig. 6. Priority Level Recommended Strategies by Categories.

visualize yourself in the position. Others will then see you as fitting into the role you aspire to.

Organizational. Broad experience – do not just stay in one track (even if you stay in one library system), e.g., branch and central library, special assignments, move from branch to branch, etc.

Personal. Love what you do and understand the whys of your aspirations.

Second Priority

Career. Broaden your vision of the public library beyond that presented by librarians.

Organizational. Keep current with technological changes.

Personal. Be positive – avoid victim behaviors.

Third Priority

Career. Do regular self-assessments of your own knowledge, skills, and abilities.

Organizational. Be willing to pay your dues by working in a small/medium-sized library as their director.

Personal. Appreciate those things in life that transcend your career.

The final question to the directors from the survey asked them to indicate any obstacles they encountered in their progression to the directorship.

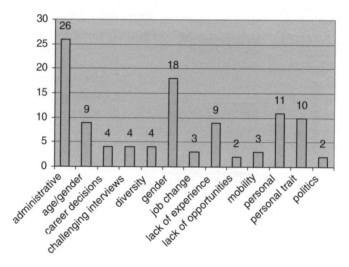

Fig. 7. Obstacles Encountered by Directors.

Forty indicated that they had none, and 105 answered with comments. The obstacles were given as narrative responses, and were coded into the following categories summarized in Fig. 7.

Discussion and Interpretation

The analysis of the findings relative to the sections indicated in the survey concern: career path, internal and external factors, career strategies, career success, and context to middle-level managers. The analysis relates directly to each of the research questions posed in the study and summarizes and interprets additional findings, in particular the correlation of the relationships among the strategies, the correlation of the relationships among the external factors, and the correlation of the relationships between the external factors and the strategies.

The five research questions presented in the study are:

Analysis of Research Question One

What were the career paths of directors of major public libraries?

Examining the educational track of their career paths, data indicated that most directors have an advanced degree in library science with a social sciences background. The doctoral degree did not appear to be a necessity. An acquired background in the field of public or business administration has also not shown to be a necessity but was a chosen preference for a dual Masters' degree. The preference shown for the advanced certificate/specialist degree was in library/information science. All credentials received were from academic institutions within 32 of the States and two from Canada.

The directors were asked how relevant education is to what they are doing now. Of the 210 received, 27.6 percent gave the highest relevance (5) while 5.7 percent gave their education the lowest relevancy rating (1). Concerning the relevancy of education to their current position, the mean is 3.52 thus falling above the middle scale value of 3.0. Therefore, it can be concluded that the majority of directors see their education as having a moderate to high degree of significance.

From the findings in the survey, the mean (a) total years of professional library experience was 27.56 years, (b) number of years as a public library director was 13.11 years, and (c) the number of years of professional experience before becoming a director was 13.42 years. Examining professional library experience as part of the career path taken indicated that 127 of 212 directors responding (59.9 percent) have between 25 and 35 years of experience. Those who have less than 25 years of professional experience amount to 66 (31 percent) and over 35 years equal to 19 (9 percent). Analysis of the data indicated that professional library experience is not always a necessity but that the majority of public library directors did have at least 25 years or more, which includes the years in their present position.

Survey data also showed that, of the 212 directors, one person had been in the directorship for 38 years, and three had been there under one year. The median thus falls at 11.25 years. The highest concentration of directors was at eight years (13 directors), followed by the four-year level (12 directors), then 10 years (11 directors). Indications showed that the majority of current directors had been in their position for at least 11.5 years or more.

Already mentioned is the average number of years of professional experience directors had before becoming a library director as being 13.4 years. However, this amounts to 0.3 percent less than the mean number of years of experience working as a public library director, indicating that most of the work experience was within the library field. The greatest number of public library directors (5.6 percent) reported having 14, 15, and 20 years of professional experience in any field including library/information services before assuming their current position. Surprisingly, this same number of directors (5.6 percent) reported having less than one year of service at the professional level in any field before being appointed to the position of library director.

The analysis indicates that these 5.6 percent could have the library/ information science profession at a pretty substantial level of authority. The possibility also exists that some of these directors could have assumed their position immediately out of library school.

Analysis of the findings also indicated that education was the most common area (39.5 percent) of professional experience outside the library field before directors were appointed to their current positions. Business was shown as second to education (33 percent), encompassing the areas of banking, retail, health care, and ranching, but also including band road manager and doughnut icer. Holding true to the earlier indication in the survey social science undergraduate degree (89 percent), the majority of directors (39.5 percent) began their working experience in the social science fields.

In terms of choices made along their career path, it appears that the majority of respondents changed library systems in order to obtain the directorship (62.9 percent). A few possible considerations for this occurrence are (1) change in organizational culture and dynamics, (2) the organization's lack of "growing their own," (3) adapting new mission and goals, and (4) better opportunities elsewhere. Additional schooling appears to have assisted 40.9 percent of the directors, and mentoring worked for 33.2 percent of them in their career path development.

Even though stories exist of individuals working their way through the same system and progressing to the top position, this choice was taken by only 28.2 percent of the directors and lateral moves were made by 25.2 percent. Those coming from other fields to assume the director's position amount to 7.9 percent.

An analysis of the above then indicates that current directors find that changing library systems is an excellent career choice as they move along their career path.

Analysis of Research Question Two
How do library directors rate the importance of individual external factors on their career success?

The four external factors examined in this study were age, gender, luck/serendipity, and geographic mobility. The directors were asked to indicate the significance of each in influencing their personal career growth.

In assigning a rating to the significance of age as an influence on personal career development, over half (112, 57.5 percent) of the 189 directors assigned it as a 3 or lower. Again, the rating of 1 is the lowest, with 10 being the highest. Even though a few of the directors mention that being too young or too old was an obstacle in their career, age does not appear to be perceived overall as being a significant influence on career success.

Relative to gender, public library directors as a group do not perceive gender to be of major significance in career development. On a significance scale of 1–10 with 1 being the lowest, 61.9 percent assign gender below the median significance number of 5 on a scale of 1–10 as to whether it was an influence on personal career growth. Although listed by some female directors as an obstacle to their career success, the overall indication is that their gender did somewhat influence, yet did not deter them from achieving the director's position.

Examining the significance factor of luck/serendipity, on a scale of 1–10, public library directors most frequently (16.6 percent) assigned 0 the middle, or the 5 rating. Even though 62 percent believed that luck/serendipity factored into their career development only 42 percent believed that it is significant as an external influential career success factor. Of these 127, 45 percent believe that it occurred in their early careers. In addition, 31.9 percent believed that it occurred in the mid-stages and 17.9 percent believed that it played a factor late in their career.

Of the 127 directors (62 percent) who believed that luck/serendipity factored into their career development, 123 responded with an explanation. These responses are grouped into two categories: (1) luck, which is defined for purposes of this study as being in the right place at the right time and (2) serendipity, which is defined as finding something good accidentally. Considering the definitions given above, 57 of the explanations given were due to luck, and 66 were serendipitous. An analysis of the data and the explanations given showed that both luck and serendipity are recognized as factors that exist in career development. See the following examples given by directors.

Luck

I was in the right place as older professionals retired and was prepared to accept greater responsibility.
Being in the right place at the right time when entering the profession and then as each promotion/new job came open.

Serendipity

Career burn out and frustration provided the impetus to apply for a new position. In this regard it was serendipitous.
Librarianship was not my career choice – nursing was. I took a summer job in a medical library, and, from that point on, I have worked in libraries.

Directors rate geographic mobility on a significance scale of 1–10 with 10 being the highest. Of the 190 responses to this question, the highest frequency rate occurs at 1 (lowest significance) with 21.1 percent. A little less than half (49.5 percent) rated geographic mobility as being a significant factor to career development by assigning a value of 6 or more. It can be assumed then that geographic mobility is very slightly less of a significant factor to the overall group of directors than not, keeping in mind, however, that the other 50.5 percent believe it to have little influence on career success.

Analysis of Research Question Two(a)
What are the relationships among the importance ratings of individual external factors?

Because the significance of the four external factors is rated on a continuous scale (1–10) correlations were used to analyze the relationships among the importance ratings. The strongest relationship exists between the significance of age and the significance of gender with the value of 0.546 based on the opinions of 185 respondents. The relationship of the significance of age and significance of geographic mobility may be considered as moderate with variety of significance levels of relationships found between all of the other factors.

Analysis of Research Question Three
How do library directors rate the influence of individual internal factors on their career success?

On the scale of 1–10 with 1 being of very low significance and 10 being very high significance the ranking order based on the mean is as follows, with the rating being significant for all with a 7.79 to 8.89. Internal factors B6.1 through B6.8 are indicated in Table 4.

Even though intelligence and proactivity are at the bottom of the list, they still hold significance rates of 8.15 and 7.79 respectively. Ranking order was given as (1) hard work, (2) ability, (3) determination, (4) flexibility, (5) personality, (6) enjoyment, (7) intelligence, and (8) proactivity.

Although not considered to be a research question for the study, a correlation was performed on the internal factors. Relationships do exist among pairs of internal factors. Three of the strongest correlations seen in this Table 4 were between the pairs of significance of proactivity and determination (0.530), significance of intelligence and ability (0.457), and significance of intelligence and personality (0.439). The weakest was the correlation of the significance of hard work and personality (0.122).

Analysis of Research Question Four
To what extent do library directors report using selected career strategies to achieve career success?

Table 4. Descriptive Statistics/Significance of Factors.

	N	Minimum	Maximum	Mean	Std. Deviation
B6.1 sig. of ability	205	5	10	8.85	1.204
B6.2 sig. of flexibility	204	1	10	8.25	1.647
B6.3 sig. of determination	204	2	10	8.30	1.796
B6.4 sig. of proactivity	201	1	10	7.79	1.977
B6.5 sig. of hard work	205	2	10	8.89	1.350
B6.6 sig. of personality	205	3	10	8.21	1.531
B6.7 sig. of intelligence	205	3	10	8.15	1.414
B6.8 sig. of enjoyment	202	1	10	8.16	1.844
B6.9 sig. of luck/serendipity	193	1	10	4.94	2.716
B6.10 sig. of gender	189	1	10	3.28	2.301
B6.11 sig. of age	188	1	10	3.18	2.078
B6.12 sig. of geographic mobility	190	1	10	5.48	3.225
Valid N (list wise)	172				

Career Planning. 50.8 percent YES

Responding to the question as to whether or not those surveyed had a career plan before becoming a director, the collected data shows that of the 195 answering, 99 (50.8 percent) did and 96 (49.2 percent) did not.

Continuing Education. 77.9 percent YES

Before assuming the position of public library director 155 (77.9 percent) answered that they have taken continuing education courses; 44 (22.1 percent) did not.

Training and Development. 96.5 percent YES

Concerning training and development workshops/seminars, 195 (96.5 percent) participated in workshops or seminars, 164 (84.1 percent) directors of the total perceived them to have helped with their career advancement, while 31 (15.9 percent) indicated that the workshops/seminars did not help.

Mentoring. 61.1 percent YES

Of the 193 respondents to the question as to whether or not they have ever had a mentor, 118 (61.1 percent) answered that have had one. Seventy-five (38.9 percent) replied that they have not.

Networking. 66.5 percent YES

When asked whether those surveyed considered networking as a factor in their career advancement, 129 (66.5 percent) of 194 answered yes that they do believe networking assisted with their career development. The remainder of the directors, which totaled 65 (33.5 percent), answered no.

Professional Involvement. 85.6 percent YES

Active participation in these organizations from the 202 directors is as follows: ALA = 149 (73.8 percent), PLA = 135 (66.8 percent), ULC = 49 (24.3 percent), State Library Associations = 173 (85.6 percent), and other = 44 (21.8 percent).

Qualifications. 94.9 percent YES (Master's degree)

Of the 214 respondents, the highest degree earned by 203 (94.9 percent) of the public library directors was a Master's with three having earned doctorates. Seven directors had a Bachelor's degree, and one individual had a certificate in public administration as their highest degree. In addition to the Master's of Library/Information Science, 17 directors reported holding 25 advanced certificate or specialist degrees in a subject area.

Experience. 59.9 percent Yes (25–35 years)

One hundred and twenty-seven of the 212 directors responding (59.9 percent) have between 25 and 35 years of experience. Those that have less than 25 years of professional experience amount to 66 (31 percent) and over 35 years equal to 19 (9 percent). From the findings in the survey, the average: (a) total years of professional experience was 27.56 years, (b) number of years as a public library director was 13.11 years, and (c) the number of years of professional experience before becoming a director was 13.42 years.

Recognizing/Taking Opportunities. 69.6 percent say YES

When asked if there was one particular opportunity that made a difference in their career, 184 directors answered the question. One hundred and twenty-eight (69.6 percent) said yes and 56 (30.4 percent) responded with a no.

Note that each one of the strategies listed above indicates only that public library directors used them and that the percentage of use ranges from 50.8 for career planning to 96.5 percent for training and development. Research question 4a illustrates how these directors rate the influence these strategies have had on their career success.

Analysis of Research Question Four(a)

How do library directors rate the influence of individual strategies on their career success?

Public library directors were asked to rate each of the following career strategies, indicating how beneficial each has been to their career advancement prior to assuming their current position: qualifications, experience, professional involvement, networking, mentorship, recognizing/taking opportunities, career planning, training and development, and continuing education.

In rank order, the library directors rated the importance of the strategies as follows: (1) qualifications, (2) recognizing/taking opportunities, (3) experience, (4) training and development, (5) networking, (6) professional involvement, (7) continuing education, (8) career planning, and (9) mentorship. Again, although career planning and mentorship are at the bottom of the rating list, they still carry a moderate amount of importance since the scale of ranking is 1–10 and both fall above the 5.0 range.

A few possible reasons were offered by the directors to indicate why career planning and mentoring are at the bottom of the strategy list. Sample comments are given: "Back then, we didn't think about career planning;" and "I don't quite know what is meant by having a mentor ... is a coach the same thing?" The mean rating is indicated in Table 5, and Table 6 illustrates the perceived importance of career strategies by frequency ranking.

Analysis of Research Question Four(b)
What are the relationships among the importance ratings of individual strategies?

Because the significance of the nine career strategies was rated on a continuous scale (1–10), correlations were used to analyze the relationships among the importance ratings. A matrix structure was examined to show that a relationship does exist between pairs of individual strategies. Note that this correlational study does not establish causal relations between variables.

The strongest correlation seen was between the importance of continuing education and the importance of training and development (0.693). The next strongest was between the importance of networking and the importance of professional involvement (0.650). The weakest relationship occurred between the importance of networking and qualifications (−0.023).

Cross-tabulations showing the tests of association among the strategies were also calculated. Note that the cross-tabulations of the strategies included were ones that were shown to have had a significant relationship by the information gathered. Variables found not to be highly correlated were eliminated from further consideration in this research question, while variables that were highly correlated were used to prompt further examination.

Table 5. Mean Rating of Strategies.

	N	Minimum	Maximum	Mean	Std. Deviation
C15.1 importance of qualifications	194	4	10	8.85	1.382
C15.6 importance of recognizing opportunities	191	4	10	8.83	1.370
C15.2 importance of experience	192	1	10	8.58	1.747
C15.8 importance of training and development	191	1	10	6.77	2.228
C15.4 importance of networking	189	1	10	6.38	2.616
C15.3 importance of professional involvement	190	1	10	6.29	2.389
C15.9 importance of continuing education	188	1	10	5.99	2.469
C15.7 importance of career planning	184	1	10	5.32	2.576
C15.5 importance of mentorship	177	1	10	5.10	2.956
Valid N (list wise)	170				

Table 6. Perceived Importance of Career Strategies by Frequency Ranking.

Ranking	Qual.	Opp.	Mentor.	Expe.	Networking	Train. and Dev.	Prof. Invol.	Cont. Edu.	Career Plan
1			30	1	10	4	8	11	15
2			17	2	10	6	10	10	22
3			14	2	13	10	10	14	13
4	1	2	14	2	10	9	8	12	14
5	6	7	29	7	30	26	36	29	36
6	5	3	6	8	13	14	19	24	17
7	18	11	18	9	22	39	28	31	22
8	42	46	23	40	35	39	39	28	24
9	29	39	11	48	26	27	17	15	13
10	93	83	15	73	20	17	15	14	8
Total	194	191	177	192	189	191	190	188	184

The test of association among the strategies is among the following factors. Directors:

- acquired additional schooling/certification and left other field to enter the library arena
- took lateral moves and changed library systems
- changed library systems and started at entry level and progressed through same system
- had a career plan and aspired to be an administrator upon entering the profession
- had a career plan and perceived networking to be a factor
- took continuing education courses and had a mentor
- took continuing education courses and served as a mentor
- took continuing education courses and perceived networking as a factor
- had a mentor and now serves as one to others
- had mentor and perceived networking was a factor in their development
- had a mentor and had one opportunity that made the biggest difference
- now serve as a mentor and perceived networking as a factor

Acquired Additional Schooling/Certification and Left other Field to Enter the Library Arena. The results indicate that from the 202 respondents, participants who left another field to enter the library arena were more likely to acquire additional schooling/certification than participants who did not leave another field to enter into library work (68.8 percent of the former group acquired additional schooling compared to 38.2 percent of the latter group). The research did not ask whether the additional schooling/certification was necessary, but only verified that it had been done.

There was a significant association between acquiring additional schooling and leaving another field to enter the library arena shown by the results of the χ^2 test of association. With this value being less than 0.05, the results indicated a p-value of 0.017 serving as evidence that the observed association reflected a real relationship between the two strategies.

Took Lateral Move and Changed Library Systems. Results indicated that the 202 participants who changed library systems were more likely to take a lateral move than participants who did not change library systems (29.9 of the former group took a lateral move as compared to 17.3 percent of the latter group). Since the directors were not questioned as to why they changed library systems, one could speculate that the individual needed to move over and out in order to move up in another organization.

There was also a significant association between changing library systems and taking a lateral move. The results of the χ^2 test of association indicated the *p*-value of 0.047, showing a real relationship existing between the values.

Changed Library Systems and Started Entry Level and Progressed Through Same System. The 202 participants who started at the entry level and progressed through the same system are less likely to change library systems than those who did not (26.3 percent of the former group changed library systems as compared to 77.2 percent of the latter group). No reason was given, but one might conclude that loyalty to the organization as well as retirement benefits could have been possible motivating factors to remain within a system.

There was significant association between starting at entry level and progressing through the same system and changing library systems shown by the results of the χ^2 test of association. The significance indicate by *p*-value was 0.000. This *p*-value, being less than 0.05, served as evidence that the observed association between starting at entry level and progressing through the same system and changing library systems reflected a real relationship.

Had a Career Plan and Aspired to be an Administrator upon Entering the Profession. The 194 participants who aspired to become an administrator when entering the profession were more likely to have a career plan than those who did not aspire to become administrators (64.3 percent of the former group had a career plan as compared to 40 percent of the latter group). These two strategies have a rather obvious connection even without the determination through the test of association of the cross-tabulation process. However, this significant association between directors aspiring to become administrators when entering the profession and the directors having a career plan does show a *p*-value of 0.001 in the χ^2 tests showing a real relationship.

Had a Career Plan and Networking was a Factor. Results indicated that the 188 respondents who considered networking to be a factor in career development are more likely to have a career plan than participants who do not (55.1 percent of the former group are more likely to have a career plan as compared to 39.3 percent of the latter group). This relationship illustrated that networking is considered a strategy in the career planning process. Results also indicated a significance because the *p*-value is 0.043.

Took Continuing Education Courses and Ever having a Mentor. Participants who ever had a mentor, from the 192 respondents, were more likely to take continuing education than those who never had a mentor (85.6 percent of the former group took continuing education courses as compared to 64.9 percent of the latter group). The possibility exists that this could have been a result of the mentor's influence. A possibility also exists that because the mentor has taken these courses (see next strategy relationship) there is a perceived value and a suggestion passed on to the mentee.

The observed association between ever having a mentor and taking continuing education courses reflected a real relationship. Results of the χ^2 test of association indicated a significance with the *p*-value being 0.001.

Took Continuing Education Courses and Serving as a Mentor. Participants, who are now serving as a mentor, from the group of 190 respondents, are more likely to take continuing education than those who never have served as a mentor (84 percent of the former group took continuing education courses as compared to 70.2 percent of the latter group). Noteworthy here is that in both cases, a respectable number of directors have taken continuing education courses. The possibility exists that within the mentoring process, the director (mentor) achieves self-awareness to increase education levels both for self-improvement and for the benefit of the mentoring relationship.

The observed association between directors now serving as mentors and taking continuing education courses reflected a real relationship. Results of the χ^2 test of association indicated a significance with the *p*-value being 0.024.

Took Continuing Education Courses and Networking was a Factor. Results indicated that from the 193 participants who believe networking to be a factor are more likely to take continuing education courses than participants who do not believe networking was a factor in career development (85.2 percent of the former group took continuing education courses as compared to 61.6 percent of the latter group). One possible indication of this relationship points to the assumption that perhaps through networking, continuing education courses are discovered and the value (or not) is related.

The observed association between networking as a factor and taking continuing education courses reflected a real relationship. Results of the χ^2 test of association showed evidence indicating a significance with the *p*-value being 0.000.

Ever having a Mentor and Now Serving as a Mentor. Results indicated that, from the 190 respondents, participants who are now serving as a mentor are more likely to have had a mentor than participants who did not ever have a mentor (78.3 percent of the former group are more likely to have a mentor as compared to 41.7 percent of the latter group). This relationship illustrated that when the value of mentoring is recognized, the practice is continued. The majority of those who are mentored will mentor. The analysis of this finding can have an impact on the creation of a formal mentoring process with the implications that not everyone can/should become a mentor.

Ever having a Mentor and Networking was a Factor. Results from 193 show that the participants who believe that networking is a factor in career development are more likely to ever have had a mentor than those who do not believe networking is a factor. (67.4 percent of the former group has had a mentor as compared to 48.4 percent of the latter group.) One possible assumption here is that, through networking with other professionals, the mentoring process could have been indicated in the survey as a possible successful career development strategy. There was nothing in the data gathered, however, to be able to prove a causal relationship, only that a relationship exists between these two strategies.

The observed association between networking as a factor and ever having had a mentor reflected a real relationship. Results of the χ^2 test of association indicated a significance with the p-value being 0.011. This p-value is less than 0.05 served as evidence that a real relationship exists.

Ever having a Mentor and having One Opportunity that Made the Biggest Difference. Results indicated that the participants who believe there was one opportunity that made the biggest difference in their career are more likely to have had a mentor than participants who do not believe that there was one opportunity that made the biggest difference in their career. (67.2 percent of the former group have had a mentor as compared to 50.9 percent of the latter group.) Although not specified as a causal relationship, mentoring could have been the venue through which the opportunity was recognized/ presented and seized. In any case, a relationship exists between the two strategies.

The results of the χ^2 test of association showed that there is a significant association between the directors believing there was one opportunity that made the biggest difference in their careers and ever having had a mentor. The results indicated a significance with the p-value being 0.037.

Now Serving as a Mentor and Networking was a Factor. In the final set of cross-tabulations, the results indicated that the participants who believe that networking is a factor are more likely to be now serving as a mentor than participants who do not believe that networking was a factor in their career development. (64.6 percent of the former group are more likely to be now serving as a mentor as compared to 37.5 percent of the latter group.) What can be assumed here is that networking and mentoring both factor into the career development of directors and, therefore, could be passed on to their protégés in the mentoring relationship.

The observed association between networking as a factor and now serving as a mentor reflected a real relationship. Results of the χ^2 test of association indicated a significance with the *p*-value being 0.000, serving as evidence that a real relationship exists.

Analysis of Research Question Four(c)
What are the relationships between importance ratings of individual external factors and the importance ratings of individual strategies?

Given the correlation matrix below, the strongest relationship exists between recognizing opportunities and geographic mobility (0.286), indicating either that opportunities existed outside the library system which caused a move, or that an opportunity was recognized after the move occurred. In either case, 49.5 percent perceived geographic mobility to be a significant factor giving it a rating of 6–10 (scale of 1–10 with 1 being the lowest).

Relating to Table 7, mentorship and luck/serendipity (0.238) and networking and geographic mobility (0.236) proved to have the next strongest relationships between them. The weakest relationship occurred between professional involvement and luck/serendipity (−0.002).

Analysis of Research Question Five
Which career strategies are recommended by library directors to assist middle-level managers in the successful pursuit of their careers as future library directors?

As indicated by Table 8, the collected data showed that recognizing/taking opportunities was chosen as the most important strategy at 32.1 percent of the total 171 valid submissions. Indicated above in research question 4, 69.6 percent of the responding directors believed recognizing/taking opportunities played a significant role in their career growth. Note that even though 96.5 percent participated in workshops or seminars and 164 (84.1 percent) directors perceived them to have helped with their career advancement, training and development (2.3 percent) was located at the very bottom of the list as a recommended strategy.

The findings indicated that, in addition to the "given" responses, the directors were asked to offer additional strategies that they would advise

Table 7. Summary of Significance of External Factors.

	C15.1 Imp. of Qual.	C15.2 Imp. of Exper.	C15.3 Imp. of Prof. Involve.	C15.4 Imp. of Networking	C15.5 Imp. of Mentor.	C15.6 Imp. of Rec. Oppor.	C15.7 Imp. of Career Plan.	C15.8 Imp. of Train. and Dev.	C15.9 Imp. of Cont. Edu.
B6.9 sig. of luck/ser	-0.053 183	-0.168* 181	-0.002 180	0.018 179	0.238** 170	0.035 180	-0.133 177	-0.021 180	0.020 177
B6.10 sig. of gender	-0.123 178	-0.056 176	0.024 175	0.158* 174	0.060 165	0.061 175	0.076 172	0.025 175	0.014 173
B6.11 sig. of Age	0.054 177	0.099 175	0.047 174	0.208** 173	0.064 164	0.124 174	0.164* 171	0.073 174	0.101 171
B6.12 sig. of geog. Mobil.	0.041 180	0.187* 178	0.165* 176	0.236** 176	0.152 165	0.286** 177	0.154* 171	0.179* 178	0.202** 175

*Correlation is significant at the 0.05 level (2-tailed).
**Correlation is significant at the 0.01 level (2-tailed).

Table 8. Frequency and Percentage of Director Recommended Career Strategies.

Strategy	Frequency	Percentage
Qualifications	21	17
Qualifications and experience*	6	
Qualifications and professional involvement*	1	
Qualifications and taking opportunities*	1	
Experience	41	24.5
Experience and opportunity	1	
Professional involvement	3	2.9
Professional involvement and experience*	1	
Professional involvement and networking*	1	
Networking	13	7.6
Mentorship	8	4.6
Recognizing/taking opportunities	55	32.1
Career planning	7	4.1
Training and development	3	2.3
Training and development and continuing education*	1	
Continuing education	8	4.6

*Combination given by directors. Added into both categories.

middle-level public managers to use in their quest for career advancement. The responses were grouped into the categories of career strategies (i.e., pick a career objective and work toward it); organizational strategies (i.e., study business trends and carry them out in the job); and personal strategies (i.e., critical self-evaluation.)

Of the total of 246 additional strategies suggested, 95 of them (38.6 percent) were coded as personal strategies, 84 (34.2 percent) were career-related, and 67 were organizational strategies (27.2 percent). These results showed that this group of directors believed that personal strategies took priority.

SUMMARY AND CONCLUSION

Summary

Because the best path for middle-level managers aspiring to become public library directors is not known, the purpose of this study was to investigate selected factors and strategies that could contribute to the leadership and successful career development of current public library directors. Career development strategies both used and recommended by the library directors were explored in order to provide a possible pathway for the middle-level manager. More specifically, this study examined:

(1) the career paths of major public library directors,
(2) the significance of external factors and strategies in shaping the careers of a selected group of current public library directors,
(3) obstacles incurred along the directors' career path, and
(4) strategies the library directors recommended that middle-level managers should apply to enhance their career development.

The results of each of the researched elements are shown in this summary. Because of how the questions were phrased, (open-ended or closed) comparisons cannot be made in all cases.

Career Paths of Major Library Directors
Three figures are provided in this section to offer comparative summaries relating to career paths of the public library directors: educational levels, aspirations to enter the administrative field and age at which the participants became library directors. Others, such as mobility, career planning, professional membership, mobility, etc., are included in the following sections as factors and strategies.

The majority of directors in this study, 203 of 214 indicated that he or she holds an advanced degree in library science (94.9 percent). Illustrated by Fig. 8, studies have shown that at least 79 percent of directors since 1985 hold at least an MLS. Research by Chatman (1992) reflects 37 of the 38 (97.3 percent) as reporting an MLS or better, Haycock and McCallum (1995) reflect 23 of 28 respondents (82.2 percent) with an MLS and Greiner (1985) 78 percent holding an MLS. This is not surprising in that many director positions require the Master's degree in Library Science, and not necessarily because the MLS degree was chosen over others.

Indicated in Fig. 9, studies showed that librarians had a downturn in their desire to become directors, and then an upswing occurred after 2000. This data (numbers/percentages of librarians aspiring to become administrators) cannot be generalized without further examination of additional studies. Thus it is noted as a recommendation for future study.

In addition to aspirations and education, the age at which public library directors acquired their position illustrates another path taken. Comparing Greiner's study (1985) and this research (Golden, 2005) the currently surveyed directors appear to have acquired their position at a later point in

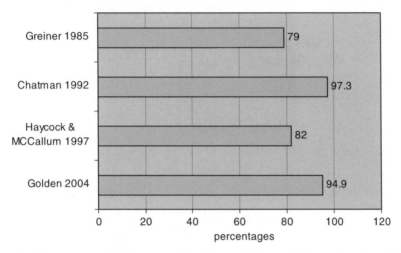

Fig. 8. Percentages of Directors with Advanced Library Science Degrees (MLS or Better).

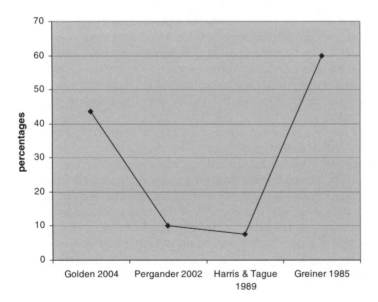

Fig. 9. Percentages of Librarians Aspiring to become Administrators.

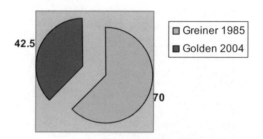

Fig. 10.   Age at Becoming a Director: 44 Years or Younger (Shown in Percentages).

their careers specifically over the age of 44 – in comparison to 19 years ago (Fig. 10).

Summarizing the career paths of library directors researched by this study then, three conclusions have been made: the majority of library directors obtained an MLS or higher; there appears to be a resurgence of those aspiring to become administrators, and librarians are becoming directors at a later age.

Significance of External Factors and Strategies in Shaping the Careers of a Selected Group of Current Public Library Directors
External Factors. In summarizing the significance of luck/serendipity, gender, age, and geographic mobility, the most important seems to be geographic mobility. Because of the structure of the question and the way it was posed to participants in the various studies, Table 9 indicates the summary results in a variety of topics/percentages. Yet, the indication here is that a high percentage of directors did indeed move in order to enhance career development.

There are two primary findings focusing on mobility found in this study. The first indicates that participants who changed library systems are more likely to take a lateral move than participants who did not change library systems. The second finding shows that participants who started at the entry level and progressed through the same system are less likely to change library systems than those who did not start at the entry level and progress through the same system. Geographic mobility is perceived in this study as very slightly less of a significant factor to the overall group of directors than not.

Age, the second external factor, does not appear to be perceived as being a significant influence on director's career success. This is illustrated in Table 10.

Gender did somewhat influence, yet was not a deterrent to, achieving the director's position. The strongest relationship exists between the significance

Table 9. Summary of Director Geographic Mobility: Specific Research Studies.

Study	Geog. Moves to New Comm. (%)	No. of Geog. Moves	Instit. Moves (%)	No. of Instit. Moves	Moves within an Inst. (%)	No. of Moves within an Institution	Position to Position Moves (%)	No. of Pos. to Pos. Moves
Golden (2004)	49.2							
Haycock and McCallum (1997)	50	1 or less	60	5 or more	42.3	1-3	75	5-7
Harris and Tague (1989)		1.42 average		2.01 average				
McNeer (1985)	100	Moved to accept current position						

Table 10. Age/Gender Factor Significance in Researched Studies.

Study	Age Significance (%)	Gender Significance(%)
Greiner (1985)	4	10
Harris and Tague (1989)	n/a	8
Farmer and Campbell (1998)	0	0
Golden (2004)	1 of highest significance	0.5 of highest significance

of age and the significance of gender. This relationship illustrates that the directors who believed gender to be of a less significant factor in career development also believed age to be of a less significant factor.

To summarize the role of luck and serendipity, a variety of descriptions were used by the studies. Ferriero (1982) finds that 46 percent perceived luck to be of significance to their success; Greiner (1985) finds that timing/luck was a relevant factor in career progression; women were more likely than their male counterparts to acknowledge the role of serendipity in upward mobility (Harris & Tague, 1989); luck was ranked second along with experience as a factor affecting career success in Farmer and Campbell's 1998 study; and in this study, 62 percent of public library directors believed that luck/serendipity factored into their career development. However, even though luck/serendipity factored into their career development (and early in the career) directors perceived it to be not a significant external influential career success factor.

Internal Factors. In the analysis and interpretation section by the public library directors as to the influence on career success the ranking order was as follows: (1) hard work, (2) ability, (3) determination, (4) flexibility, (5) personality, (6) enjoyment, (7) intelligence, and (8) proactivity. From the above list, Farmer and Campbell's (1998) results have shown ranking order for four of the same factors: (1) hard work, (2) ability, (3) personality, and (4) determination. As indicated in the purpose of this study, no further research was planned for these factors.

Strategies. All of the directors applied the career strategies presented in this study to their own career development. Each strategy was used by at least 50 percent or more: training and development 96.5 percent, qualifications 94.9 percent (Master's degree), professional involvement 85.6 percent, continuing education 77.9 percent, recognizing/taking opportunities 69.6 percent, networking 66.5 percent, mentoring 61.1 percent experience 59.9 percent (25–35 years), and career planning was used by 50.8 percent.

Relative to the benchmarking studies, the following data were collected as a summary to be used as a centralized comparison point for the reader. Again, noted are the differences in the studies and the queried items.

Continuing education
Haycock and McCallum (1997): 80 percent (16)
Harris and Tague (1989): 27 percent (7)
Activity in professional associations
National
Haycock and McCallum (1997): 80 percent (23)
Chatman (1992): 100 percent (45)
Harris and Tague (1989): 27 percent (7)
Greiner (1985): 90 percent (288)
Local and State
Harris and Tague (1989): 38 percent (10)
Greiner (1985): 93 percent (297) in state organization/50 percent (160) regional
Mentoring
Haycock and McCallum (1997): 60 percent (17)
Chatman (1992): 50 percent (23)
Harris and Tague (1989): 46 percent (12)
Greiner (1985): 50+ percent (160)
Publishing
Haycock and McCallum (1997): 39 percent (11)
Chatman (1992): 63.1 percent (24)
Harris and Tague (1989): 85 percent (22)

Strategy Relationships
Comparison figure charts indicate the major relationship statements involving career strategies. No comparisons have been made between the results of this study and the other studies since the objectives of this one was to establish only those results currently being assessed. Correlation statements among the strategies of career planning, continuing education, training and development, mentorship, networking, professional involvement, recognizing/taking opportunities, qualifications, and experience correlation statements are given to summarize data presented earlier in the findings and interpretation section.

Data presented can be summarized as follows: the strongest correlation seen is between the importance of continuing education and the importance of training and development (0.693). The next strongest found was between the importance of networking and the importance of professional involve-ment (0.650). The weakest relationship occurred between the importance of networking and qualifications (−0.023).

Also critical to this study are the additional relationships found *between significant strategies only* presented by matrices in the findings and inter-pretation section. These relationships are presented to illustrate to the mid-dle-level manager which ones have occurred together most often by public library directors as indicated. By investigating the correlation of these fac-tors and strategies, the value and role of the relationship has been estab-lished in accordance with research question 4b. They are listed as follows:

Relative to Career Planning

- Participants who *started at the entry level and progressed through the same system are less likely to change library systems* than those who did not start at the entry level and progress through the same system.
- Participants who *aspired to become an administrator* when entering the profession are more likely to *have a career plan* than those who did not aspire to become an administrator.
- Participants who *left another field to enter the library arena* are more likely to acquire additional schooling/certification than participants who did not leave another field to enter into the library work.
- Participants who *changed library systems* are more likely to take a *lateral move* than participants who did not change library systems.

Relative to Networking

- Participants who consider *networking* to be a factor in career develop-ment are more likely to have a career plan than participants who do not consider networking to be a factor.
- Participants who believe *networking* to be a factor are more likely to take *continuing education courses* than participants who do not believe net-working was a factor in career development.
- Participants who believe that *networking* is a factor in career development are more likely to ever *have had a mentor* than those who do not believe networking is a factor.
- Participants who believe that *networking* is a factor are more likely to be now *serving as a mentor* than participants who do not believe that net-working was a factor in their career development.
- Participants who believe there was *one opportunity that made the biggest difference in their career* are more likely to *have had a mentor* than

participants who do not believe that there was one opportunity that made the biggest difference in their career.

Relative to Mentoring

- Participants who had a *mentor* are more likely to take *continuing education courses* than those who never had a mentor.
- Participants who are now serving as a *mentor* are more likely to *take continuing education courses* than those who never have served as a mentor.
- Participants who are *now serving as a mentor* are more likely to *have had a mentor* than participants who did not ever have a mentor.

Obstacles

Administrative causes are shown to be the major reason obstacles were encountered along the directors' career paths. These tended to stem from those externally caused as well as those due to internal conditions. The following list presents the obstacles categorized by real numbers (frequencies).

Administrative, Administrative – external conditions, Administrative – internal conditions, Administrative – supervisor (26)
Age, Age/gender (9)
Career decisions (4)
Challenging interviews (4)
Diversity (4)
Gender (18)
Job change (3)
Lack of experience (9)
Lack of opportunities (2)
Mobility (3)
Personal, Personal – education, Personal – family, Personal – physical attributes (11)
Personal trait (10)
Politics (2)

In the comparison studies regarding career obstacles, gender discrimination is indicated in the survey by Harris and Tague (1989). Gender is indicated in the survey by Haycock & McCallum (1997) where it reportedly played a role particularly in the number of years to the directorship. Greiner in 1985 also found that 44 percent (39) had encountered no obstacles to their career progression.

Strategies Recommended

Library directors suggested strategies for middle-level managers to apply to enhance their career development. Strategies were rated both as recommended and as important. Those strategies that were recommended are those that the directors suggest to the middle-level managers to use. The important strategies are those which directors consider to have been of importance in their own career.

Directors were asked to rate the strategies. And as such the ranking order is also produced. The recommended strategies by the directors are given in decreasing priority order as follows: (1) recognizing/taking opportunities, (2) experience, (3) qualifications, (4) networking, (5) mentorship, (6) continuing education, (7) career planning, (8) professional involvement, and (9) training and development.

In rank order the library directors rated the importance of the strategies as follows: (1) qualifications, (2) recognizing/taking opportunities, (3) experience, (4) training and development, (5) networking, (6) professional involvement, (7) continuing education, (8) career planning, and (9) mentorship.

Director Profiled

Based on the summarized data of the findings, if the mean numbers are actually applied to create the silhouette of a current public library director participant of this study, the profile would indicate a public library director, with an advanced degree in library science, who became a director at the later age of 45 or older, and whose career was not deterred by age or gender discrimination. This director has approximately 27.56 years of professional experience and has been a director for about 13.11 years. Along the career path, the director has moved 3.9 times within the working institution and has relocated 2.5 times to a new community.

Completing the profile based on highest frequency rate, this director had a career plan but did not aspire to become a library administrator. The current position was learned of through a former library director recruiting a successor.

This director has been mentored and is also mentoring. However, the belief is that the current career status could have been achieved without a mentor. He or she belongs to the state library organization primarily and then to the national association, and considers networking as a factor in career advancement particularly with library directors. Continuing education courses have been taken, and luck and serendipity did have a role in the career process as well.

This director believes that hard work, ability, and determination were three major internal factors affecting his/her career development, and that training and development, qualifications and professional involvement are the three top strategies that got him/her the current position. This director also recommends recognizing/taking opportunities, experience, and qualifications as the top three strategies. He or she has had one particular opportunity that made a difference in career development.

Strategies Profiled
The investigation of strategies and factors in this study should provide the middle-level managers with not only strategies used by the directors, but with the importance these strategies had in the career development of the directors. In addition to use and importance to their own careers, the priority rankings of these strategies are given by directors in an attempt to assist middle-level managers with their career path.

Focusing on the main problem of this research (recommended best path for middle-level managers aspiring to become public library directors), a closer look at the summaries listed by Table 11 and Fig. 11 enables certain conclusions to be drawn.

The first observation is that the three strategies of obtaining the necessary qualifications, recognizing/taking opportunities, and experience are all essential strategies (listed more than once in the top three rankings). Note that

Table 11. Rank-Order Strategies.

Rank	Use of Strategies	Most Important Strategy	Beneficial Strategy
1	Training and development	Recognizing/taking opportunities	Qualifications
2	Qualifications	Experience	Recognizing/taking opportunities
3	Professional involvement	Qualifications	Experience
4	Continuing education	Networking	Training & development
5	Recognizing/taking opportunities	Continuing education	Networking
5		Mentorship	
6	Networking		Professional involvement
7	Mentorship	Career planning	Continuing education
8	Experience	Professional involvement	Career planning
9	Career planning	Training & development	Mentorship

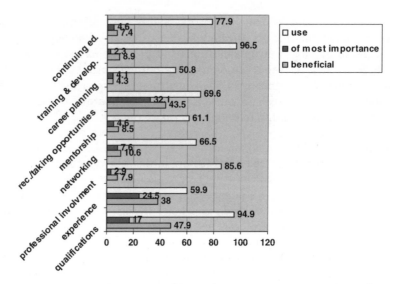

Fig. 11. Frequency Percentage of Strategies: Use, Importance and Beneficial.

the directors have used all three, gave them a high importance rating and recommended them for middle-level managers. Neither experience nor qualifications are a surprise since many times they are a requirement of the position. Recognizing/taking opportunities is an obvious strategy as well; however, what is interesting is that it ranks number one as a recommendation of all of the nine selected strategies.

Observed also is that mentorship was ranked as a number 5 recommended strategy, particularly since the importance of it to the directors' own career development was ranked low (9). It may be concluded that with little recognizable use (7) in comparison to the other strategies, mentoring sustained very little importance. Or it may be the lack of recognition of the mentoring process. As one of the directors in the study revealed, "I learned a lot from individuals ... by observing or through the opportunities they provided for me. I would not have called them mentors. ... but you have not clearly identified what you define as a mentor." Sheldon points out that the library leaders interviewed in her study said that "right out of library school, and very often while in school, they were advised, pushed, and offered positions...(implying mentorship)" (Sheldon, 1991, p. 53). Perhaps the interest level can be elevated.

Data reflected in Table 11 (Rank-order strategies) and Fig. 11 (Frequency percentages of strategies: use, importance and benefit) show that the directors have received a significant amount of training and development (number 1 ranking for use). As Hendry illustrated in the managerial literature, there is a need to train and develop "first-class library managers who will become the future directors of large multi-disciplinary departments, inside or outside the conventional framework of local government" (Hendry, 1996, p. 356).

But the directors give training and development an average ranking of importance (4) and also list it at the bottom of the recommended list (9). Perhaps this is due to a growing disenchantment with the conventional educational and training programs that are offered within their organizations. Murray pointed out "Often the content of these courses are aimed at the average person and an insult to an experienced professional" (Murray, 2001, p. 23). In addition many times there is also no follow up nor is there any type of reinforcement by the supervisor.

Career planning is ranked low on use (9), importance (8), and recommended priority list (7). Perhaps the directors were agreeing with the belief of Myers (1995) that because the traditional career ladder has been destroyed by downsizing an individual may need alternative ways to get where they want to go with no fixed paths established.

Professional involvement is ranked as the third strategy for use, yet is lower in importance (6) and close to the bottom as a recommended strategy (8). This finding aligns with the findings of the study done by Harris and Tague who observed that the library directors responding to their study reported that participation in professional associations, publishing, or holding more advanced degrees did not seem to offer any quick routes to success. "Several of the directors had reached the top of their profession in spite of these factors that are often indicated in the survey as significant career development strategies in librarianship" (Harris & Tague, 1989, p. 129).

Surprisingly, networking was ranked lower in use (6) than in importance ranking (5) and as a recommended strategy (4). Not shown by the directors' ranking of use was a point indicated in the survey by Kouzes and Posner (1995) which found that the literature revealed all leaders were already in a network of relationships by the very nature of the position. However, by ranking networking as a number 4 for recommendation purposes, it appears that the directors agree with Kotter who found in his study of general managers that "developing effective lateral relationships is one of the critical job challenges and a key predictor of job success" (Kotter, 1982, p. 50).

Given a moderate ranking by the directors for use, (4) continuing education is listed lower (7) in the importance ranking and again given a moderate ranking (5) as a recommended strategy. By not assigning the lowest of rankings, the directors fell into place with the literature that points out that given the pace of change in the field, aspiring managers need to make a commitment to lifelong learning. The only job security lies in being more talented tomorrow than you are today (Peters & Austin, 1985).

Conclusion

Contributions

Career development strategies both used and recommended by the library directors were explored in order to provide a possible pathway for the middle-level manager. By examining the career paths of directors of major public libraries and the significance of career development external factors and strategies in shaping their careers, this study addressed all three areas and produced a comparison of factor/strategy use vs. importance vs. suggested use. It is the outcome of this comparison that is a most important component of this study because of its applicability of use in the "real" world.

This study encourages the public library middle-level manager to assess if and how the recommended strategies can best fit into a personal career development plan. By looking at the priority listing of recommendations, the manager is armed with the knowledge that recognizing and taking an opportunity possibly could be one of the most beneficial strategies to be applied to the pursuit of career success. In addition perhaps focusing on continuing education rather than training and development would prove to be more effective. These middle-level managers are encouraged to examine the career path taken by the surveyed library directors to compare, contrast, and evaluate their own career ladder in terms of geographic mobility, changing library systems, taking lateral moves, and career break possibilities.

This research is also useful to public library administrators in their planning and implementation of leadership development for the middle-level managers. As their surveyed colleagues have shown, the list of career strategy use, benefit and recommendations is a desirable tool for guidance in the creation of a successful career developmental pathway. What became evident while analyzing the data, as well as grouping the comments and recommendations, is that public library directors generally agree that this study is important in showing public library middle-level managers how the directors achieved their positions ("I very much like the way that this study is crafted – I think that it is vitally important that those of us in leadership positions share how we got here and what we've learned – and that we can learn from all of our colleagues.").

The directors also believe that this study can assist the middle-level managers in filling the positions as the baby boomers retire ("Good to see this type of research. Who will lead our libraries as the boomers retire? This is, in essence, asking who will take the challenge of ensuring and defining the future of the public library!"). The statements quoted here come from the last question on the survey (Comments and Suggestions) and give an added element of context to the perceived importance of the study.

Final Statement on Results
This study began as a proposal to question whether mentorship was the primary factor necessary to assist in leadership development for the public library middle-level manager. However, the study expanded to include other strategies researched in the literature: training and development, qualifications, professional development, continuing education, recognizing and taking opportunities, networking, experience, and career planning.

Findings of this study show that basing future symposia, training modules, and guidance to the middle-level manager only on the mentoring process would have severely limited access to higher-level priority recommended strategies. Mentoring is one of many, but certainly not the predominant one selected by the surveyed directors. Mentoring being heavily used by 61.1 percent of the directors, given a beneficial rating by 8.5 percent of the directors, yet recommended by only 4.6 percent tells the researcher as well as the practitioner that other strategies ought to be examined for use first – but only after a needs assessment of the targeted audience has been performed.

As there are additional strategies listed as high usage, of low benefit, and not highly recommended the need for future study in the field of library leadership and management exists. Selecting three of the most obvious of these strategies (training and development, professional involvement, and career planning) the practitioner needs to examine what factors actually should be applied when considering personal career success. Application of the recommended strategies first would be a priority as suggested by this study. For the researcher, among other challenges, the possibility presents itself to pursue the cause of the high use and low recommendations given.

Recommendations for Future Study
Resulting from this study there are issues that have presented themselves as avenues for further research. Recommended topics for future exploration are:

• A study of gender differences with regard to the use, importance of, and the recommendations made for selected strategies.

- Gender as it also relates to career planning. The directors who hold their positions now are products of the 1960s and 1970s. The idea behind this further research is drawn from a statement made by one of the directors who commented: "I liked the survey. But I think many of the females that graduated in the 60s/70s were not given information about planning their life concerning a career. Library school did not teach anything about managing people."
- Both informal and formal methods of mentoring by and for public library directors. The need exists to explore the meanings of both types giving the directors a definition of the process clarifying the possible confusion with coaching or supervision. Very possibly during their entry into their current positions, formal/informal mentoring could have been only for those individuals considered by the administration as high flyers.
- Follow up research on the middle-level managers' response to the strategies recommended to them in this study by the current library directors.
- A further examination of various training and development components currently being developed between academic institutions and public libraries.
- The further exploration as to whether or not an MLS is a desirable element for directors.
- Additional research into whether there has been a resurgence in the leadership aspirations of librarians? If so, what is the cause/effect?

By examining these suggested items for future study and using the resultant data and analysis of this research paper, the intent is that a twofold purpose has been served. First is that organizations will use the outcomes to assist with achieving their goals of filling the leadership gap within their ranks by focusing on strategies and factors helpful to the middle-level manager. The second purpose is to guide the middle-level manager in acknowledging how previous library directors have achieved career success, thus serving as a point of reference in offering direction for their own career development.

REFERENCES

American Library Directory. 56th ed. (2003–2004). New York: R.R. Bowker.

American Management Association. (1993). Downsizing: Down but not out. *Management Review, 82*(12), 6.

Bailey, M. J. (1982). *Supervisory and middle managers in libraries*. Metuchen, NJ: Scarecrow Press.

Barter, R. R. (1994). In search of excellence in libraries. *Library Management, 15*, 4–15.

Bell, C. R. (1998). The Mantle of Mentorship. *Security Management, 42*(1), 26–33.

Bernthal, P. R., Rioux, S. M., & Wellins, R. W. (2004). *The leadership forecast: A benchmarking study.* Bridgeville, PA: HR Benchmark Group. http://www.ddiworld.com/pdf/cpgn53.pdf

Chatman, E. A. (1992). The role of mentorship in shaping public library leaders. *Library Trends, 40*, 492–512.

Curran, W. M. (2003). Succession: The next ones at Bat. *College & Research Libraries, 2*, 134–141.

Davies, R. (1995). Integrating and organizations: An introduction to team management systems for career professionals. *Librarian Career Development, 3*, 4–9.

Evans, G. E., Ward, P. L., & Rugaas, B. (2000). *Management basics for information professionals.* New York: Neal-Schuman Publishers, Inc.

Farmer, J., & Campbell, F. (1998). Continuing professional development and career success: Is there a causal relationship? *British Library Research and Innovation Report 112.* West Yorkshire, UK: British Library Research and Innovation Center.

Ferriero, D. S. (1982). ARL directors as protégés and mentors. *Journal of Academic Librarianship, 7*(6), 358–365.

Giesecke, J. (2001). *Practical strategies for library managers.* Chicago, IL: American Library Association.

Goldberg, B. (2000). *Age works: What corporate America must do to survive the graying of the workforce.* New York: The Free Press.

Golden, J. (2005). *The role and contribution of strategies and factors in the career successes of public library directors.* Unpublished doctoral dissertation, University of Pittsburgh, Pittsburgh, PA.

Greiner, J. M. (1985). A comparative study of the career development patterns of male and female library administrators in large public libraries. *Library Trends, 34*, 259–289.

Griffiths, J.-M., & King, D. W. (1994). Libraries: The undiscovered national resource. In: M. Feeny & M. G. Londo (Eds), *The value and impact of information* (pp. 79–116). London: Bowker & Saur.

Gunn, H. (2002). Changing the survey process. *First Monday*, No. 12. http://firstmonday.org/issues/issue7_12/gunn/index.html

Hall, D. (1996). *The career is dead-long live the career.* San Francisco, CA: Jossey-Bass.

Harris, R. M., & Tague, J. M. (1989). Reaching the top in Canadian librarianship: A biographical study of sex differences in career development. *Library Quarterly, 59*, 116–130.

Haycock, K., & McCallum, L. (1997). Urban public library directors: Who are they? Where did they come from? *Feliciter, 43*(1), 34–37.

Hendry, J. (1996). On the fast track or the road to nowhere. *The Library Association Record, 98*, 357–359.

Johnson, I. M. (1999). Catching the tide: Environmental pressures for an emphasis on management in the library and information sciences curriculum. *Library Management, 20*, 317–332.

Katz, R. N., & Salaway, G. S. (2003). *Information Technology Leadership in Higher Education: The Condition of the Community*, Key Findings of a study for EDUCAUSE Center for Applied Research (ECAR). Report availability via www.educause.edu/ecar/.

Kotter, J. P. (1982). *The general managers.* New York: Free Press, p. 50.

Kouzes, J. M., & Posner, B. Z. (1995). *The leadership challenge: How to keep getting extraordinary things done in organizations* (p. 323) San Francisco, CA: Jossey-Bass.

McAnally, A. M., & Downs, R. B. (1973). The changing role of directors of university libraries. *College and Research Libraries, 34*(2), 103–125.

McNeer, E. (1988). The mentoring influence in the careers of women ARL directors. *Journal of Library Administration, 9*(2), 23–32.

Mech, T. (1989). Public Library Directors: A Career and Managerial Profile. *Public Libraries, 28*(4), 228–235.

Mintzberg, H. (1975). The manager's job- folklore and fact. *Harvard Business Review, 53*, 61.

Moran, B. B. (1992). Introduction. *Library Trends, 40*(3), 377–380.

Murray, M. (2001). *Beyond the myths and magic of mentoring.* San Francisco, CA: Jossey-Bass.

Myers, W. S. (1995). Navigating your career path. *Women in Business, 47*, 25.

Pergander, M. (2003). Experiences of early career public library directors. *Public Libraries, 42*(4), 252–254.

Peters, T., & Austin, N. (1985). *A passion for excellence: The leadership difference.* London: Collins.

Powell, R. R. (1997). *Basic research methods for librarians.* Greenwich, CN: Ablex Publishing Corporation.

Public Library Association. (2003). *Public library data service statistical report 2003.* Chicago, IL: The American Library Association.

Riggs, D. J. (1997). What's in store for academic libraries? Leadership and management issues. *Journal of Academic Librarianship, 23*, 2–8.

Sayles, L. R. (1993). *The working leader: The triumph of high performance over conventional management principles.* New York: The Free Press.

Sheldon, B. E. (1991). *Leaders in libraries: Styles and strategies for success.* Chicago, IL: American Library Association.

Sicker, M. (2002). *The political economy of work in the 21st century: Implications for an aging American workforce* (pp. 55–72). Westport, CT: Quorum Books.

Stueart, R. D., & Moran, B. B. (2000). *Library and information center management* (6th ed). Greenwood Village, CO: Libraries Unlimited.

Stueart, R. D., & Moran, B. B. (2002). *Library and information center management* (6th ed.). Greenwood Village, CO: Libraries Unlimited.

Thomas, R., & Dunkerley, D. (1999). Career downwards: Middle managers' experiences in the downsized organization. *British Journal of Management, 10*, 157–169.

Ward, P. L. (2000). Trends in library management. *Library Review, 49*(9), 436–442.

Wessel, D. (1993). The outlook: Is it jobless growth, or just slow growth? *The Wall Street Journal,* (E), November 1, A1.

White, H. S. (1987). Oh where have all the leaders gone? *Library Journal, 112*(16), 69.

APPENDIX. CAREER SUCCESS SURVEY

Questionnaire to Public Library Directors

Section A. Career Path

1. What is your highest level of education attained? (check all that apply)

    ___ Bachelor's Degree. List major _____

    ___ Master's degree in library/information science _____

    ___ Master's degree in subject area. List area _____

    ___ Advanced certificate or specialist degree in library/information science

    ___ Advanced certificate or specialist degree in a subject area. List area _____

    ___ Doctorate in library/information science _____

    ___ Doctorate in a subject area. List area _____

    ___ Other (please specify) _____

2. In your opinion, how relevant was your education to what you are doing now?
    Please assign a number below to indicate the relevance using a scale of 1 to 5 with 1 as very *low* relevance and 5 as very *high* relevance.

    ___ Relevance number

3. If you received a library degree, please name the academic institution: _____

4. What is the total number of years, including the current year, of your professional library experience?

    ___ Number of years

5. How many years have you been in the position of Public Library Director?

    ___ Number of years

6. How many years of service at the professional level in any field (following a Bachelor's, Master's or Doctorate degree) did you work before you were appointed to the position of library director?

    ___ Number of years

7. If you worked outside of the library field before being appointed to the position of public library director, in what field(s) were you employed? (ex. business, education, social work, healthcare, etc.)

_____

_____

Section B. Internal/External Factors

1. At what age did you become the director of the library in which you are currently employed?

_____ Years old

2. What is your gender?

_____ Female _____ Male

3. Previous to achieving your position as library director:

a) How many **total** career moves have you made within institutions? (A *career* move is defined here as an action taken by an individual with regard to one's professional lifework. Implies a change of position, job, and/or title, and/or responsibilities.)

_____ Number of total career moves within institutions

b) How many times have you geographically relocated to a new community because of a career move?

_____ Number of geographical relocations to a new community

c) How many times have you moved from one institution to another within the same community?

_____ Number of moves from one institution to another within the same community

4. Do you believe that luck/serendipity factored into your career development?

_____ Yes _____ No

If Yes, please explain: _____

_____

5. If luck/serendipity did factor into your career development, at what stage did this occur? (check all that apply)

_____ early _____ middle _____ late

6. Both internal and external factors may work as influences on career success. In the table below please rate the significance of each individual factor in influencing your personal career growth on a scale from 1-10.
NOTE: 1 is of very *low* significance, 10 is of very *high* significance.

Internal Factors	Significance (1-10)	External Factors	Significance (1-10)
Ability		Luck/serendipity	
Flexibility		Gender	
Determination		Age	
Proactivity		Geographic Mobility	
Hard Work			
Personality			
Intelligence			
Enjoyment			

7. Are there any additional factors (either internal or external) that have had an influence on our career success that were omitted in the question #6 table above?

   Yes   _____ No

If Yes, please indicate them here:

_____

Section C. Career Strategies

1. Where did you first learn of the opening for your present position as director? (check one)

   _____ Announcement

   _____ Board of Trustees

_____ Former director recruiting successor
_____ Library school referral
_____ Professional association placement
_____ Publication
_____ Notification from associate
_____ Recruiting firm
_____ Other (Please specify)

2. Did you have a career plan before becoming a director? (A *career plan* is defined here as a design formulated for pursuing one's professional lifework. Plan may be altered as career progresses.)
_____ Yes _____ No
If Yes, how was career planning beneficial to your career success?
Please explain:

_____

If No, how would a career plan have helped you in your career path?

_____

3. When you entered the profession did you aspire to be a library administrator?
_____ Yes _____ No

4. What career choices did you make that helped you achieve your current position? (check all that apply)
_____ Chose a mentor
_____ Acquired additional formal schooling/certification
_____ Took a lateral move to position oneself for a career climb
_____ Changed library systems
_____ Left another field to enter into the library arena
_____ Started entry level and have progressed through the same system
_____ Other. Please specify:

_____

5. Have you ever had any career break(s)? (A *career break* is defined here as a separation, interruption, interval or pause in the performance of one's professional lifework.)

    _____ Yes   _____ No

If Yes:

Was it planned?

    _____ Yes   _____ No   _____ Both yes and no

    _____ What were the reasons for the break(s)? (please specify)

    _____

Did it/they advantage or disadvantage your career? (please explain)

    _____

6. Have you taken continuing education courses prior to assuming your present position?

    _____ Yes   _____ No

7. If you have taken continuing education courses how helpful were they to your career advancement? (Please check one)

    _____ Very helpful   _____ Somewhat helpful   _____ Not at all helpful

8. Have there been training and development workshops/seminars that have helped you in your career advancement?

If Yes, please list the subject areas that were most beneficial to you:

    _____

    _____

    _____

9. Have you ever had a mentor?

    _____ Yes   _____ No

10. If you have/have had a mentor, do you believe you could have achieved your status without one?

    _____ Yes   _____ No   _____ Undecided

11. Are you now serving as a mentor?

    _____ Yes   _____ No

12. Was networking a factor in your career advancement?
    ___ Yes ___ No
    If Yes, who did you communicate with that assisted with your career climb? (check all that apply)
    ___ Library directors
    ___ Friends
    ___ Other professionals within the library organization
    ___ Other professionals outside of the library organization
    ___ Other (please specify):
    _____

13. In which professional organizations do you actively participate? (check all that apply):
    ___ American Library Association
    ___ Public Library Association
    ___ Urban Libraries Council
    ___ State library association
    ___ Other (please specify)
    _____

14. Was there one particular opportunity in your career that made the biggest difference?
    ___ Yes ___ No
    If Yes, please explain:
    _____

15. Rate each of career strategies listed below by numbering how beneficial they were to your career advancement prior to assuming your current position. Please use the number 1(one) as very *low* importance and 10 (ten) as very *high* importance.

Career

Strategy (1 to 10)	Level of Importance
Qualifications	
Experience	
Professional Involvement	
Networking	
Mentorship	
Recognizing/	
Taking opportunities	
Career Planning	
Training and Development	
Continuing Education	

Section D. Career Success

1. From the list of career strategies in question #15 choose your most important one and indicate how/why this one was beneficial:

_____

_____

2. Are there any additional strategies that have had an influence on your career success that were omitted in the question #15 table above?

_____ Yes _____ No

If Yes, please indicate them here:

_____

_____

Section E. Context to Middle Level Managers

1. What additional strategies (other than those listed in Section C Question 15 above) would you advise middle-level public library mangers to use in their quest for career advancement? (list in decreasing priority order)

a) _____

b) _____

c) _____

2. What obstacles did you encounter in your progression to the directorship?

_____

_____

_____

Comments and Suggestions:

_____

_____

_____

ACADEMIC LIBRARIAN'S CAREER CHOICE

Jeff Luzius

INTRODUCTION

There is currently a shortage of academic librarians in the United States. This shortage is affecting staffing levels at libraries and making it increasingly difficult to fill positions. Pollock (2002) reported that libraries across the nation are facing the same dilemma, "how to fill the growing number of vacancies in the ranks of professional librarians" (p. 94). There are several explanations for this trend. There is a phenomenon known as the graying of the profession. A large number of academic librarians are nearing retirement age and new librarians will be needed to replace them. Crosby (2001) stated that "many experienced librarians are expected to retire, switch occupations, or leave the occupation permanently for other reasons. This will create about 39,000 job openings for new librarians between 1998 and 2008" (p. 9). Wilder (2000) reported, "In demographic terms, librarianship in North America is a profession apart. Librarians are, as a group, substantially older than those in comparable professions, and they are aging at a much faster rate" (para. 1). Lynch (2002) reported that over 20% of the librarians currently employed in the United States will reach age 65 by 2014.

Another relatively new situation is the competition for academic librarians. Dolan and Schumacher (1997) stated, "Opportunities have never been better for the librarian in a non-traditional setting. The Internet and cutting-edge information technology have created new jobs" (p. 68). Librarians now

Advances in Library Administration and Organization, Volume 23, 245–262
Copyright © 2006 by Elsevier Ltd.
ISSN: 0732-0671/doi:10.1016/S0732-0671(05)23006-7

have several job choices outside of the traditional library setting to consider. Kaufman (2002) states, "It appears that, in recent years, smaller percentages of students pursuing graduate degrees in library and information science have moved into traditional libraries. New opportunities in the private sector, albeit slowing slightly but temporarily in the current economy, appear to be luring more graduates with the promise of interesting work and robust salaries" (para. 4).

The number of graduate schools that award the Master's degree in library science (MLS) has declined in the past two decades. During the past 20 years ALA went from accrediting 83 graduate programs in the United States, Canada, and Puerto Rico to 58 (O'Neill, 2002). Stieg (1991) explains that library science programs were closed because "They have few sources of outside funding and a relatively limited market for the kind of research they might sell. Their alumni are not likely to make fortunes and become generous benefactors" (p. 270).

Librarianship has historically been a female dominated profession. In today's society women are going into a much wider variety of careers though and are leaving a shortage in occupations such as teaching, nursing, and librarianship. While women are branching out into new careers, librarianship remains a female dominated profession. The latest statistical data shows that women hold 83.4% of the jobs in the field (U.S. Census Bureau, 2003).

Proof of the librarian shortage lies in the number of job openings and difficulty that libraries are having filling advertised positions. Judith Robinson, professor and chair of Library and Information Studies at SUNY Buffalo is quoted as saying, "Administrators of school, university, and public libraries are beating the bushes to locate qualified applicants to fill thousands of vacancies. Many urban libraries can't staff new branches, and small-town libraries, sometimes hobbled by lower salaries, can remain unstaffed for years" (Jacobson, 2002).

O'Connor and Marien (2002) studied the job market for business librarians for one year and examined 96 job searches. They found that applicant pools averaged just 7.7 minimally qualified librarians per position and that 70% of the employers were dissatisfied with their pools. The top three reasons for their dissatisfaction were the quantity, quality, and the qualifications of the candidates (2002). ALA's (2004) conference placement statistics indicate that there were more job openings posted then the number of job applicants at their mid-winter and annual conferences from 1998 to 2002.

LITERATURE REVIEW

Pollack (2002) surveyed graduate students enrolled in three MLS programs in the state of Texas to determine their career interests. Three hundred thirty-nine students completed the survey. Close to twenty percent, 19.74%, indicated that they wanted to pursue work in an academic library followed by 15.52% at a special library, and 12.76% at a public library. The most important characteristic when deciding to apply for a job was the work environment, 40%, followed by geographic location at 26.46%.

Carmichael (1992) studied male librarians and the feminine image. Four hundred eighty-two male librarians participated in the study. The librarians were asked to rank order reasons why they entered the profession. Over 56% (56.75) indicated a love of books, 45.80% indicated previous experience in libraries, and 17.23% indicated accident or happenstance. Librarians in the study were also asked about the male librarian stereotype. Nearly 60% of the respondents confirmed the existence of a stereotype. They indicated effeminate (probably gay) as the most pervasive stereotype followed by a lack of social skills and a lack of ambition. Carmichael believed that "the survey confirms the existence of problems associated with the male librarian image and gender issues within the profession" (p. 436). Simpson (2004) conducted a similar study where she interviewed males in female dominated professions. She found that male librarians choose their career due to their enjoyment of working with books and information.

The Chronicle of Higher Education (1981) surveyed 187,000 college freshmen in 1980 and found that 0.0% had any desire to become librarians (p. 7). Genoni and Greeve (1997) surveyed graduating high school students in Australia on their perceptions of librarians and librarianship. They found that the career choice of librarian ranked at the bottom of the list and "is extremely unattractive in terms of either material or psycho-social rewards" (p. 301).

Dewey (1985) studied MLS students at the University of Indiana over a three-year period to determine why they chose librarianship as their future career. The study consisted of 287 students, 29.9% of the students were influenced by a librarian while 15.9% were influenced by current MLS students. The reasons for choosing the school: academic rank, 55.4%; in-state tuition, 36.5%; lived in the area, 28.4%. Dewey believes that "The results of this questionnaire reaffirm the primary importance of librarians as influential in the career choice of individuals at one large nationally based library school" (p. 22).

Heim and Moen (1988) conducted a major research project on MLS students' attitudes, demographics, and career aspirations. They surveyed all the MLS students in the United States in 1988. The survey was broken into four sections and dealt with the choice of an MLS program, attitudes toward the profession, education and work background, and information about the students and their families. Heim and Moen found that "The typical student currently enrolled in a program of library and information science education is part-time, geographically place-bound, white, female in her mid-thirties with an undergraduate degree in English or education" (p. 185). The students' undergraduate majors were English 18.5%, Education 16.4%, and Social Sciences 15.7%. They found that the average length of time between the baccalaureate degree and enrolling in their MLS program was 10 years. Of the MLS students, 26.9% already possessed a Masters degree prior to starting their MLS held the Master's in Education, 23.3% in Arts and Humanities, and 10% in the Social Sciences. Overall, 21% of the MLS students already had earned a Master's degree. The work experience of the MLS students indicated that 52% of all respondents had worked in libraries prior to enrollment. Forty percent of the respondents held non-library employment. Teaching accounted for 30%, administrative support for 20%, management 10%, and sales 10%. The decision to enroll in a MLS program was made largely (62% of respondents) after completing their Bachelor's degree and while working. Eighty-one percent of the students were female and 19% were male. Age ranges indicated mostly adult learners with the highest number of respondents falling in the following groups: 20% were age 25–29, 19% were 30–34, 19% were 35–39, and 17% were 40–44.

In the 1980s, Nancy Van House (1988) conducted a study to investigate library school students' decisions to enter librarianship. Van House surveyed students entering the MLS program at the University of California-Berkley in 1982, 1983, 1984, and 1985. The most frequent answer was "liked (or thought would like) working in a library," followed by "wanted a career, marketable skills." The third most cited answer was "interest in studying the subject" followed by "like working with people."

Magrill (1969) conducted a study on the occupational image of librarians and how it affects the choice to become a librarian. She compared MLS students' view of librarianship to the views of graduate students with majors in education, political science, journalism, and sociology. The study consisted of instruments designed to measure occupational stereotypes, occupational values, and library work activities. Respondents included 130 MLS students and 248 students with other majors. The two groups had similar occupational values. The MLS students ranked librarians and librarianship higher then the non-MLS students on 32 scale items. Magrill found that non-MLS students picture librarians as individuals with little money, low social status, low social popularity, and little opportunity for advancement. Magrill also found that the MLS students had a more favorable image of librarians and librarianship.

David (1990) researched occupational interests and personality types of librarians. She compared academic librarians with two other types of librarians in the state of Michigan. The other two types were database and automation librarians and senior system librarians. A total of 232 respondents returned the survey. The Strong Interest Inventory was used to determine personality type. David found that "Librarians are a homogeneous occupational group with very similar occupational likes and dislikes, even when they belong to differing specialties within the profession" (p. 126). She found no significant difference between the different sub-groups of librarians. David did find that librarians had moved from the Conventional personality type to the Artistic personality type on the Strong Interest Inventory when compared to the original placement of careers when the inventory was created. David (1990) stated, "the media and the public continue to portray librarians as conventional and conservative, and this is the stereotypical image that many hold of librarians even today" (p. 124).

Scherdin (1989) researched librarians and information professionals in order to determine if there was a personality difference between the two groups. She distributed the American College Testing (ACT) Interest Inventory and a job activity questionnaire in order to compare librarians and information professionals. She found that there was no significant difference between librarians who were members of ALA and information professionals who were members of American Society for Information Science (ASIS). Scherdin (1994) also conducted another study that dealt with the personality types of librarians. She administered the Myers–Briggs Type Indicator (MBTI) instrument to a random sample of librarians who were members of ALA and Special Libraries Association (SLA). The MBTI is "an inventory of preferences that indicate a person's innate predispositions on four dichotomous scales" (p. 126). The scales are extraversion (E) vs. introversion (I), sensing (S) vs. intuition (N), thinking (T) vs. feeling (F), and judging (J) vs. perceiving (P). Scherdin distributed the MBTI to 1600 librarians and found that the rating of ISTJ was the most popular at 16.5% followed by INTJ at 11.5% and INTP at 9.1%. The respondents were also asked for reasons why they engage in their occupation, "I like to perform the activities it requires" ranked the highest followed by "I can use my best talents," and "I can make an important contribution." Scherdin concluded that "The fact that 63% of librarians have Introverted preferences has importance for the profession. While Extraverts show their first or best function to the outside world, Introverts save their best function for the inner world of ideas" (p. 148).

Elizabeth Gail McClenney wrote a thesis in 1989 that asked the question "why do students choose careers in information and library science?" (McClenney, 1989. p. 1). McClenney surveyed students from three graduate programs in the state of North Carolina to collect information on the students' career choice motivation. She found that a majority of the respondents chose to pursue the career because they liked the field. She also found a significant number of individuals wanted to change careers and that a librarian was the most influential factor in the decision-making process.

Whitten and Nozero (1997) conducted a study on second and third career reference librarians in Nevada to see what impact the librarians' background had on their librarian positions. Twenty-six librarians completed their survey and 21 were deemed second or third career librarians. Nine of the librarians came to the field from an education background. Whitten & Nozero state, "This is not surprising, since the educational and service goals associated with the teaching profession are also a component of librarianship" (p. 199). They also found that the librarians that mentioned the importance of customer service skills "were more likely to have come from business and government background than from education" (p. 198).

Deeming and Chelin (2001) posed the research question "why do people change careers to become professional librarians?" (p. 13). Their sample consisted of 20 librarians who had changed careers in order to become college librarians. Deeming and Chelin identified five key issues from their survey results. The key issues were (1) drift versus active choice; (2) previous career; (3) context of life as a whole; (4) influence of other people; and (5) nature of work. The issue of drift versus active choice demonstrated the extent to which librarianship was actively considered as a potential career and revealed that some librarians actively sought out the career while others found it serendipitously (2001). The previous career issue showed that "for some, how they felt about their previous career was a major factor in the decision to change" (p. 18). The context of life as a whole issue "included areas such as the desire to use existing skills, practical life considerations such as family and location and attitudes to life in general" (p. 18). The nature of library work and influence of other people showed that current librarians influenced their career choice. Deeming and Chelin found that "the majority of respondents (85.8%) were "very satisfied" or "satisfied" with their career change to librarianship" (p. 19).

Mosely (1999) studied African-American law school students in the state of Florida on their perception of law librarianship. Fifty-six students completed surveys for the study. Mosley found that 91% of the students indicated that no one had ever talked to them about being a librarian during their college years, and 76% indicated that, even if given a scholarship, they would not be willing to study librarianship (1999). Mosley also found that 83% of the students indicated that "Librarianship may be a good career choice for some people, but it is not a good career choice for me" (p. 233).

Bello (1996) researched the career selection of librarians in Nigeria and looked at three sets of factors. The first factors studied were the choice of librarianship as being influenced by family, friends, or the mass media. The second set of factors studied were the influence of professional reasons such as stability, security, and social status. The third set of factors studied was the influence of one's special ability or aptitude (1996). Bello sent out a questionnaire to librarians and received 68 responses that were useable. Bello was able to accept two of the three hypotheses about the influences of becoming a librarian. Both the influence of family and friends and the influence of professional factors proved to be significant factors. The influence of one's special abilities or aptitude did not prove to be a significant reason.

Afolabi (1996) researched Holland's typological theory and how it applies to librarians and their choice of career. Holland's theory is that an individual's choice of vocation is partly due to personality. Afolabi based his research on this theory and surveyed 20 current librarians to discover what they felt was the dominant personality type of librarians. Eighty percent of the librarians chose the dominant personality type of social, followed by investigative and then enterprising (1996). Afolabi also went a step farther within the career and looked at different areas of college librarianship and why certain personality types would fare better in different areas of the library. An example of this is in reader services departments of libraries where it was ranked by 90% of the respondents as a social environment involving frequent interaction with library users. "It therefore follows that librarians working in this environment should exhibit social orientation" (p. 20).

Houdyshell, Robies, and Hua (1999) researched the career choice of librarians along with their job satisfaction. They found that "three hundred eight librarians (62%) had worked in a library environment before obtaining their library degree." Of the 500 librarians surveyed 82% said the intellectual challenge was a large part of the attraction to become a librarian, and 95% also said the opportunity to be part of a service-oriented profession was important. They concluded from their research "the bottom line seems to be that most people who chose to enter the profession did so primarily because of a genuine appreciation for the pursuit of knowledge and information and for helping others pursue the same" (p. 21).

Buttlar and Caynon (1992) surveyed minority librarians to ascertain the factors that influenced them to choose a career in librarianship. They found that minority and non-minority role models, minority librarian mentors, and the availability of minority scholarships all were significant factors in influencing minorities to choose librarianship. Respondents to their survey ranked the three most important reasons for becoming a librarian. The number one reason was "had a mentor," number two was "began as paraprofessional," and three was "like the work that librarians do" (1992).

Hackenberg (2000) investigated who chooses science and technology librarianship as a career in 2000. A survey was developed and distributed to librarians employed in the science and technology area. Hackenberg found that the majority of sci-tech librarians fell into the position due to special circumstances and because it was the only opening at the library. Hackenburg did find that almost 60% of the respondents came into their science and technology positions with some type of science background.

Fikar and Corral (2001) surveyed non-librarian health professionals who went on to become librarians to determine what influenced their career choice and why they left their original position. Many of the respondents cited "burn out" as a reason for leaving their health career while an interest in libraries, computers, and information retrieval was stated as a reason for choosing to go into librarianship.

Julian conducted a study of full-time library science students at George Peabody College in 1979 to determine why the students chose librarianship as a career. Two areas that Julian looked at where the effect library-related experiences had upon their career choice and when the individuals made their career choice. Eighty-seven percent of the respondents indicated that they had worked in a library prior to working on their graduate degree in library science. Forty-five percent of the respondents chose librarianship sometime after college with an additional 23% making the decision during their senior year in college (Julian, 1979).

METHODS

The purpose of this study was to identify motivating factors that influence the decision of individuals to pursue careers as academic librarians and to gather background demographic information on the academic librarians.

The sample for this study consisted of academic librarians employed at Association of Research Libraries (ARL) institutions in the United States and librarians who belong to the Association of College & Research Libraries (ACRL). There are currently 123 libraries in ARL. The study excluded the public libraries, health and other special libraries, and academic libraries in Canada. This left 99 college libraries in the United States for the study. Thirty-nine libraries opted to participate in the study, which led to a total of 453 respondents from ARL. Six hundred one librarians responded from ACRL, bringing the total sample to 1054.

Data collection was accomplished by employing a Web-based survey instrument. A Web-based survey was deemed the most feasible means of data collection. It is reasonable to expect all academic librarians to have access to a computer connected to the Internet. The survey instrument was composed and posted on the WWW by using the online survey software company SurveyMonkey. SurveyMonkey allows researchers to design surveys and post them to their website. Respondents are directed to the website by email. The emails contain a hyperlink that points the respondents' web browser to the uniform resource locator (URL). Respondents are able to complete and submit the survey electronically from their Web browser. In this study three listservs were used to distribute the survey: the ARL Dean Listserv, the ACRL College Library liserv, and the ACRL University Library listserv.

RESEARCH INSTRUMENT

The survey was designed to gather demographic information on the academic librarians and to identify career choice motivation factors of academic librarians. The survey is composed of two sections. Section one contained demographic background, education, and vocation questions. The questions asked about gender, age, ethnicity, education level, year degrees were attained, and prior work experience. Education questions sought to discover the year in which the Bachelor's degree and MLS were earned and if any additional degrees were earned. Vocation questions sought to discover prior careers, length of time spent in those careers, and prior work experience in a library setting, and when the choice was made to become an academic librarian. Section two consisted of 17 Likert Scale questions, which focus on the respondents' career choice motivation. The questions asked the respondents to rate a set of factors on how much these influenced their decision to become an academic librarian. The 17 Likert Scale items were assigned a numerical value to each response. The responses were (1) no influence, (2) slight influence, (3) moderate influence, (4) high influence, and (5) extremely high influence.

The computer software program Statistical Package for the Social Sciences (SPSS) was used to analyze the data. Data analysis began with a tabulation of the demographic information collected in section one of the survey to provide a detailed description of the respondents. Frequency distributions and percentages were calculated for each item.

RESULTS

The gender and ethnicity of the respondents were as follows: 793 were female (76%) and 244 were male (24%). Ten were American Indian (0.01%), 23 were Asian (2%), 34 were African-American (3%), 24 were Hispanic (2%), and 969 were Caucasian (90%) (Tables 1 and 2).

Respondents were asked about their undergraduate degrees and level of education when they started their MLS as well as when they completed their degrees (Tables 3 and 4). English was the highest ranking major with 200 respondents followed by History with 153 respondents, Foreign Language with 72 respondents, Biology with 57 respondents, and Education with 50 respondents (see Table 5). Two hundred seventy-eight respondents indicated that they had completed their Bachelor's degree followed by 81 respondents with a Master's degree, 59 respondents with a Bachelor's degree plus graduate

Table 1.   Gender of Respondents.

	n	%
Female	793	76
Male	244	24
Total	1037	100

Table 2.   Ethnicity of Respondents.

	n	%
American Indian	10	1
African-American	34	3
Asian	23	2
Hispanic	24	2
White	969	92
Total	1060	100.0

Table 3.   Year Respondents Finished their Undergraduate Degree.

Year	*n*	%
1960–1964	54	5
1965–1969	141	14
1970–1974	195	19
1975–1979	154	15
1980–1984	109	11
1985–1989	113	11
1990–1994	140	13
1995–1999	105	10
2000–2004	26	2
Total	1037	100

Table 4.   Year Respondents Finished their MLS.

Year	*n*	%
1960–1964	12	1
1965–1969	48	5
1970–1974	107	10
1975–1979	139	13
1980–1984	106	10
1985–1989	132	13
1990–1994	132	13
1995–1999	178	17
2000–2004	184	18
Total	1038	100

Table 5.   Undergraduate Majors.

Rank	Major	*n*
1	English	200
2	History	153
3	Foreign Language	72
4	Biology	57
5	Education	50
6	Psychology	48
7	Political Science	34
8	Liberal Arts	26
9	Communications	24
10	Business	21
11	Philosophy	9

coursework, 20 respondents with a doctorate, three respondents with a Juris Doctorate, and one respondent with a Specialist degree (see Table 6). Nine hundred eighteen (89%) indicated that they completed their degree on campus, 30 (3%) through distance learning (DL), and 89 (8%) through a combination of both (see Table 7).

Four hundred thirty-nine (43%) indicated that academic librarianship was their first full-time career while 592 (57%) indicated that they worked in a prior career (see Table 8). Teaching ranked as the top choice with 129 respondents followed by library assistant with 57 respondents (see Table 9). Seven hundred twenty-seven respondents (71%) indicated that they worked in a library prior to pursuing their MLS and 303 (29%) did not work in a library (see Tables 10 and 11). The type of library that individuals worked in is displayed in Table 12; respondents could select more then one choice.

Table 6.   Level of Education when started MLS.

	n	%
Bachelors	653	64
Bachelors + coursework	149	15
Masters	186	18
Specialist	1	−1
Juris Doctorate	4	−1
Doctorate	31	3
Total	1024	100

Table 7.   How MLS was Completed.

	n	%
On campus	918	89
Distance learning	30	3
Combination	89	8
Total	1037	100

Table 8.   Academic Librarianship as First vs. Second Career Choice.

	n	%
1st career	439	43
2nd career	592	57
Total	1031	100

Table 9. First Careers of Academic Librarians.

Rank	Career	n
1	Teaching	129
2	Library assistant work	57
3	Special librarianship	21
4	Researcher	19
5	Secretarial work	19
6	Sales	17
7	Military	13
8	Writing	12
9	Management	11
10	Insurance work	9

Table 10. Length of Time Spent in First Career Other than Academic Librarianship.

Years	n	%
1–5	344	53
6–10	128	24
11–15	69	12
16–20	32	5
21–25	20	2
26–30	14	2
31–35	11	2
Total	618	100

Table 11. Respondents who Worked in a Library Prior to MLS.

	n	%
Library	727	71
Non-library	303	29
Total	1030	100

Section two consisted of 17 Likert Scale questions, which focus on the respondents' career choice motivation. The questions asked the respondents to rate a set of factors on how much these influenced their decision to become an academic librarian (Table 13). The 17-Likert Scale items were assigned a numerical value to each response. The responses were (1) no influence, (2) slight influence, (3) moderate influence, (4) high influence, and

Table 12.   Type of Library Worked in Prior to MLS.

Type of Library	n
School	105
Public	204
Academic	503
Special	99
Total	911

Table 13.   Age Respondents became Academic Librarians.

Age	n	%
20–24	188	18
25–29	327	31
30–34	229	22
35–39	109	10
40–44	79	8
45–49	70	7
50–54	28	3
55–59	11	1
60–65	1	0
Total	1042	100

(5) extremely high influence. The highest-ranking score from the career choice factors was "Liked the college setting" with a mean of 4.23 on a five-point scale. This was followed by "Thought you could do a good job" with a mean of 4.13, "Intellectual stimulation" with a mean of 4.13, "Work Environment" with a mean of 3.94, and "enjoy research" with a mean of 3.87. The results from this section are given in Table 14.

DISCUSSION

The results of this study show the lack of diversity among academic librarians. The field is overwhelmingly made up of female Caucasians. Adkins and Espinal (2004) explain that this situation has a negative effect on the field: when people of color do not see themselves represented in libraries, they may not approach the librarians. They may not even approach the library.

Over half of the librarians identified in this study worked in another career prior to becoming academic librarians, and yet there is no difference

Table 14. Career Choice Factors of Academic Librarians.

	Mean	Standard Deviation	Minimum	Maximum
Parents	1.73	1.07	1.00	5.00
Family	1.94	1.134	1.00	5.00
Other librarians	3.06	1.38	1.00	5.00
Job opportunities	3.43	1.03	1.00	5.00
Job security	2.93	1.21	1.00	5.00
Salary	2.15	1.08	1.00	5.00
Benefits	2.58	1.16	1.00	5.00
Work environment	3.94	0.94	1.00	5.00
Enjoy helping	3.80	1.12	1.00	5.00
Enjoy research	3.87	1.18	1.00	5.00
Love books	3.46	1.27	1.00	5.00
Work with technology	2.71	1.33	1.00	5.00
Intellectual stimulation	4.13	1.02	1.00	5.00
College setting	4.23	0.97	1.00	5.00
Thought you could do a good job	4.13	0.94	1.00	5.00
Length of MLS	2.12	1.32	1.00	5.00
Distance learning	1.25	0.76	1.00	5.00

between any of the groups in their motivation when choosing academic librarianship as a career. Individuals are attracted to the career for the same reasons; they like the environment and the work itself. The challenge remains to introduce the career to as many people as possible.

The present study's findings support those found by Heim and Moen (1988). They found that 62% of librarians made the decision to enroll in an MLS program after completing their Bachelor's degree and while working. This study found 78% of the respondents made the decision after completing their Bachelor's degree.

Recruitment efforts should concentrate in two directions; one, advertising the career to as many people as possible and two, recruiting individuals who are already working in the library. The career field has historically drawn individuals from the library ranks but with the current shortage and pending retirements that will affect the field it is now time to increase recruitment efforts outside of the library.

RECOMMENDATIONS

The first recommendation is to do a better job of advertising the career to young people. Only 22 respondents (4.9%) indicated that they made the decision to become academic librarians during their K-12 years. Academic libraries need to reach out to the K-12 student population and inform students about academic librarianship. Reese and Hawkins (1999) state, "We need to target outreach programs to the full range of the population, starting with junior and senior high school students" (p. 62). One such program is underway at Cornell University in Ithaca, NY. Cornell University Library implemented a recruitment program in 2002 titled the Cornell University Library Junior Fellows Program. This program introduced high school students of color to academic libraries and librarianship (Revels, LaFleur, & Martinez, 2003).

The second recommendation is to do a better job of advertising the career to the general public. Bosseau and Martin (1995) state, "Librarianship may be termed an 'accidental' profession – a profession populated overwhelmingly by people who discovered it while detouring from some other planned career" (p. 198). Fifty-five percent of the respondents in this study worked in another career prior to becoming an academic librarian. It seems many individuals do not discover the career until later in life after having worked in another career.

The third recommendation is to increase the number and amount of financial incentives for graduate studies in library science. Personal earnings, student loans, and family support ranked as the three highest choices as to how the respondents financed their MLS. There are several scholarships currently being offered by IMLS for potential graduate students and these opportunities should be expanded. Academic libraries should offer library science scholarships to staff members who are interested in becoming professional librarians. Seven hundred twenty-seven (71%) respondents indicated that they worked in a library prior to pursuing their MLS. Berry (2003) states, "schools have neglected recruiting too long. They never looked at the para-professional potential. They need to attract new librarians from the reservoir of candidates who are working in libraries" (p. 8).

The fourth recommendation is to increase the recruitment efforts toward minorities. Camila Alire sums up the importance of the minority librarian by stating that minority librarians can identify with people in the minority community; assist in the outreach efforts to serve minority residents; and serve as role models for minority children using the library (Alire, 1996). There are currently national efforts underway to recruit minority librarians into the field, but these need to be expanded. Several academic libraries offer minority residency programs that introduce under-represented librarians to research libraries. While these programs help jump-start the career of new minority librarians, they need to take the program a step farther. Additional programs need to be implemented that offer scholarships paired with employment opportunities. New programs should be implemented that pay for the individual's MLS and then offer the residency program. The fifth and final recommendation is to go about recruiting new librarians with data from this study in mind. The librarians who completed this survey have shown us what was important to them when they chose the career. We need to advertise the career as one where you can help people, do research, work with the latest technology, and enjoy the benefits of the college environment. The next step is to use this data to recruit the next generation of librarians.

REFERENCES

Adkins, D., & Espinal, I. (2004). The diversity mandate. *Library Journal, 129*(7), 52–55.

Afolabi, M. (1996). Holland's typological theory and its implications for librarianship and libraries. *Librarian Career Development, 4*(3), 15–21.

Alire, C. A. (1996). Recruitment and retention of librarians of color. In: S. G. Reed (Ed.), *Creating the future: Essays on librarianship* (pp. 126–143). Jefferson, NC: McFarland & Company.

American Library Association (ALA). (2004). *ALA placement center statistics*. Retrieved August 23, 2004, from http://www.ala.org/ala/hrdr/placementservice/placementcenter.htm

Bello, M. A. (1996). Choosing a career: Librarian? *Librarian Career Development, 4*(4), 15–19.

Berry, J. N. (2003). Recruit new librarians at work. *Library Journal, 128*(2), 8–9.

Bosseau, D. L., & Martin, S. K. (1995). The accidental profession. *The Journal of Academic Librarianship, 21*(3), 198–199.

Buttlar, C., & Caynon, W. (1992). Recruitment of librarians into the profession: The minority perspective. *Library and Information Science Research, 14*(3), 259–280.

Carmichael, J. V. (1992). The male librarian and the feminine image: A survey of stereotype, status, and gender perceptions. *Library & Information Science Research, 14*, 411–446.

Crosby, O. (2001). Librarians: Information experts in the information age. *Occupational Outlook Quarterly, 44*(4), 2–15.

David, I. M. (1990). A study of occupational interests and personality types of librarians. *Dissertation Abstracts International, 51*(08), 2555A (UMI No. 9029617).

Deeming, C., & Chelin, J. (2001). Make your own luck: A study of people changing career into librarianship. *New Library World, 102*(1160/1161), 13–25.

Dewey, B. I. (1985). Selection of librarianship as a career: Implications for recruitment. *Journal of Education for Library and Information Science, 26*(1), 16–24.

Dolan, D. R., & Schumacher, J. (1997). New jobs emerging in and around libraries and librarianship. *Online, 21*(6), 68–76.

Fikar, C. R., & Corral, O. L. (2001). Non-librarian health professionals becoming librarians and information specialists: Results of an Internet survey. *Bulletin of the Medical Library Association, 89*(1), 59–67.

Freshmen characteristics and attitudes (February 9, 1981). Chronicle of Higher Education, p. 7.

Genoni, P., & Greeve, N. (1997). School-leaver attitudes towards careers in librarianship: The results of a survey. *The Australian Library Journal, 43*(6), 288–303.

Hackenberg, J. M. (2000). Who chooses sci-tech librarianship? *College & Research Libraries, 61*(5), 441–450.

Houdyshell, M., Robies, P. A., & Hua, Y. (1999). What were you thinking? If you could choose librarianship again, would you? *Information Outlook, 3*(17), 19–24.

Jacobson, J. (2002). A shortage of academic librarians. *The Chronicle of Higher Education.* Retrieved August 14, 2004 from http://chronicle.com/jobs/2002/08/2002081401c.htm

Julian, C. A. (1979). *An analysis of factors influencing the career choice of librarianship.* ERIC Document # 191448.

Kaufman, P. T. (2002). Where do the next "we" come from? Recruiting, retaining, and developing our successors. *ARL Bimonthly Report 221.*

Lynch, M. J. (2002). Reaching 65: Lots of librarians will be there soon, *American Libraries,* pp. 55–56.

MaGrill, R. M. (1969). Occupational image and the choice of librarianship as a career. *Dissertations Abstract International, 31* (02), 776A (UMI No. 7013404).

McClenney, E. G. (1989). *Why students choose careers in information and library science: Factors that affect the decision-making process.* Unpublished master's thesis, University of North Carolina at Chapel Hill, Chapel Hill, NC.

Moen, W. E., & Heim, K. M. (1988). *Librarians for the new millennium.* Chicago, IL: American Library Association.

Mosely, M. (1999). Perceptions of African-American law school students toward law librarianship as a career choice. *Journal of Academic Librarianship, 25*(3), 232–234.

O'Connor, L., & Marien, S. (2002). Recruiting quality business librarians in a shrinking market. *The Bottom Line: Managing Library Finances, 15*(2), 70–74.

O'Neill, A. (2002). Cited in Jacobson, J. A shortage of academic librarians. *The Chronicle of Higher Education.*

Pollack, R. D. (2002). A marketing approach to recruiting librarians. *The Acquisitions Librarian, 28,* 93–115.

Reese, G. L., & Hawkins, E. L. (1999). *Stop talking, start doing: Attracting people of color to the library profession.* Chicago: American Library Association.

Revels, I., LaFleur, L. J., & Martinez, I. T. (2003). Taking library recruitment a step closer: Recruiting the next generation of librarians. *Reference Librarian, 39*(82), 157–159.

Scherdin, M. J. (1989). *Measuring interests of library and information professionals using the American College Testing (ACT) Interest Inventory.* Dissertation Abstracts International, 51 (01), 9A, (UMI No. 9010329)

Scherdin, M. J. (1994). Vive la difference: Exploring librarian personality types using the MBTI. In: M. Scherdin (Ed.), *Discovering librarians: Profiles of a profession* (pp. 125–156). Chicago, IL: Association of College & Research Libraries.

Stieg, M. F. (1991). The closing of library schools: Darwinism at the university. *Library Quarterly, 61*(3), 267–272.

U.S. Census Bureau. (2003). Employed civilians by occupation, sex, race and Hispanic origin: 1983 and 2002. Table no. 615. *Statistical Abstract of the United States: 2003* (p. 399). Washington, DC: U.S. Census Bureau.

Van House, N. A. (1988). MLS students' choice of library career. *Library and Information Science Research, 10,* 157–176.

Whitten, P. A., & Nozero, V. A. (1997). The impact of first careers on "second career" academic reference librarians: A pilot study. *The Reference Librarian, 59,* 189–201.

Wilder, S. J. (2000). The changing profile of research library professional staff. *ARL Bimonthly Report,* (208/209).

WILL THEY STAY OR WILL THEY GO? PREDICTORS OF ACADEMIC LIBRARIAN TURNOVER

Linda K. Colding

INTRODUCTION

During the 2001 Association of College and Research Libraries (ACRL) conference, members were asked what they thought were the most pressing issues for academic libraries. As a result, the Focus on the Future Task Force was created and charged to study these concerns. One of the top seven issues was the recruitment, education, and retention of librarians (Hisle, 2002). Retaining librarians by preventing turnover has become one of the leading issues in academic libraries.

In a recent article, Rogers (2003) asserted the profession of librarianship, in general, faces a difficult time in recruiting and retaining librarians. With the "graying" of the profession, retirement follows. With the difficulty in recruiting replacements for those retiring librarians, administrators are faced with shrinking staffs. Turnover of any kind could spell disaster for library services and the public it serves.

In addition to recruiting and retention problems, library administrators are facing another problem. State budgets are being reduced at a rapid rate. According to Armone, Hebal, and Schmidt (2003), more than half of the states have reduced their appropriations to higher education in the 2002–2003 fiscal year. This is a trend that will likely continue if the economic situation in the United States overall fails to make substantial improvements.

Advances in Library Administration and Organization, Volume 23, 263–280
Copyright © 2006 by Elsevier Ltd.
ISSN: 0732-0671/doi:10.1016/S0732-0671(05)23007-9

Therefore, with budgetary problems, library administrators must be concerned when their employees are thinking of leaving because of the possibility of permanently losing positions when librarians actually turn over.

Copious amounts of research concerning turnover and turnover intentions are available for administrators and human resources managers to apply to their organizations. This is not a groundbreaking research topic. So why conduct further research? The answer is easy. When it comes to research concerning turnover intentions in the field of librarianship, very little research exists.

The purpose of this research is to fill the gap concerning turnover intentions of librarians serving in public university libraries. This study investigates whether the leading causes of turnover, as found in the classic meta-analysis of Cotton and Tuttle (1986), apply to academic librarians working in public university libraries. The causes of turnover investigated are those specifically found to be applicable to white-collar, non-managerial, service-oriented, and professional employees – characteristics of these librarians. This research also investigates the leading causes of turnover found by Allison and Sartori (1988) in their study of librarians at the University of Nebraska. In essence, this research attempts to replicate the findings of Cotton and Tuttle (1986) and Allison and Sartori (1988).

Literature Review

This literature review first considers the causes of turnover found in the two studies used for this replication study and continues with a brief examination of the causes of turnover intentions in librarians. It concludes with the theoretical explanations for turnover.

Turnover Causes: Previous Studies

Owing to the enormous number of articles and books about turnover and turnover intentions, Cotton and Tuttle's (1986) meta-analysis was used to discuss previous research concerning the leading causes of turnover and turnover intentions. Cotton and Tuttle analyzed 120 data sets to determine the strengths and weaknesses of turnover studies. They determined there were three categories and 26 predictors of turnover. The first category is external correlates and includes employment perceptions, unemployment rate, accession rate, and union presence. The second category is work-related correlates and includes pay, job performance, role clarity, task repetitiveness, organizational commitment, overall job satisfaction, satisfaction with pay, the work itself, supervision, coworkers, and promotional opportunities. The third category investigated by Cotton and Tuttle is personal correlates, which include age, tenure, gender, biographical information, education, martial status, number of dependents, aptitude and ability, intelligence, behavioral intentions, and met expectations.

Of the preceding predictors of turnover, Cotton and Tuttle found the following to be the strongest: employment perceptions, union presence, pay, overall job satisfaction, satisfaction with the work itself, pay satisfaction, satisfaction with supervision, age, tenure, gender, education, number of dependents, biographical information, organizational commitment, met expectations, and behavioral intentions. The strongest predictors relevant to white collar, non-managerial, service, and professional employees are employment perceptions, union presence, satisfaction with the work itself, overall job satisfaction, number of dependents, and pay. With the exception of union presence, which has limited application to academic libraries, these variables were investigated in this research.

Allison and Sartori's (1988) study identified the factors contributing to professional librarian turnover at the University of Nebraska – Lincoln (UNL) between 1974 and 1984. They administered their survey to librarians currently employed at the UNL library. Thirty librarians responded, representing a response rate of 67%. They also administered a survey to librarians who had left the UNL library between 1974 and 1984. Of those librarians, only 28 of 51 responded. Although this study is an excellent starting point for librarian turnover research, the sample size is quite small.

Allison and Sartori found 28 factors that were considered important in making the decision to stay or leave. Of those 28, the top six factors for those who left include career goals, future salary prospects, competence of supervision, decision-making opportunities, stimulating work, and relationship with coworkers. The top two factors, career goals and future salary prospects, were incorporated into this study. Moreover, longevity, specifically less than five years at an institution, proved to have the strongest association with employee mobility and was also investigated.

CAUSES OF TURNOVER IN LIBRARIES

Beyond the Allison and Sartori (1988) work, there are but a few articles that have been published concerning turnover in libraries in general and fewer yet that deal with specifically academic libraries. A search in library literature did not produce any new articles since 2000. Most of the articles were descriptive in nature and dealt with turnover of librarians between the mid-1980s and 1990s.

Descriptive Literature

Throughout the 1990s and beyond, anecdotal articles appear throughout library literature. One article suggests transferring employees to other departments to reduce turnover in the organization (Transfers down turnover, 2000). In another article, Armour (2000) suggests ways to deal with stress before it leads to burnout and turnover. Stress management activities, including retreats and meditation rooms, were suggested. One organization introduced a stress survival class, which included employees meeting with physicians, nutritionists, massage therapists, and psychiatrists. Overall, very little descriptive literature addresses the causes of turnover and turnover intentions of librarians, much less academic librarians.

Empirical Research

Richard Rubin (1987) wrote his doctoral dissertation on public librarian turnover in moderately large and large public libraries in seven Midwestern states. Data were obtained from 31 public libraries and 421 individual turnovers during a five-year period, 1980 through 1984. One finding of the dissertation is that the turnover for full-time professional librarians is rather low when compared to other professions. The rate of turnover was 8.7 percent. Price (1977) stated that professional and technical workers turnover was 13 percent, turnover among white-collar workers was 19 percent, and turnover in service organizations stood at 21 percent. Librarians are far below those rates according to Rubin. Also, Rubin reported no statistical difference in turnover rates of men and women; although previous turnover studies found that women left more often than men. Rubin found that gender was not a good predictor of librarian turnover.

Rubin (1986) has published several articles over the years on turnover. One such article was concerned with librarian turnover rates in three moderately large public libraries in Ohio. These libraries include the Akron-Summit County Public Library, the Public Library of Columbus and Franklin County, and Dayton–Montgomery County Public Library. Two surveys were used to gather data. The Voluntary Turnover Activity Form gathered data, such as demographic information and the destination of the employee after quitting, on each full-time librarian who voluntarily left between 1980 and 1984. The Summary Data Form gathered general hiring and staffing activity of full-time librarians during the five-year period. Unlike the findings in his doctoral dissertation, this study found that females left the workforce in greater numbers than expected. Family reasons are listed most often for turnover. Also interesting to note is that movement to other library positions was not significant.

Several factors of Rubin's work limit comparison for this study. Rubin's work on turnover deals with public librarians, not academic librarians. Also Rubin's research measured librarian turnover for any full-time library employee, not just individuals holding a Masters degree in Library Science. For the purpose of this research, the term "librarian" refers to an individual holding at minimum a Masters degree in Library or Information Science. Library staff and/or non-degreed individuals were not considered for this study. Rubin himself states that the limitations of his study include a sample that was not randomly drawn, the small number of males included, making statistical analysis difficult, and the fact that no attempt was made to analyze individual psychological reasons for leaving the job.

James Neal began his research into librarian turnover in the early 1980s and presented the results of a study concerning library support staff turnover (Neal, 1982). A survey of Association of Research Libraries (ARL) members reveals that support staff turnover is a major problem for 30 percent of the 65 respondents. In fact, two of the libraries responded that a lack of turnover is the problem. But it is important to remember that this study deals with staff, not librarians in academic libraries.

Collins (1989) researched professional staff turnover in medium to large-sized academic health sciences libraries for her thesis. In her study, she again pointed to the lack of literature concerning librarian turnover. Collins surveyed 65 health science libraries to determine the amount of turnover over a two-year period. Of the 50 responding libraries, 14 percent of the responding libraries had no turnover during that time. The average turnover rate was 11.13 percent. This figure is far less than Price's turnover rates for professional workers, white-collar workers, or service organizations. While Collins investigated the turnover rates of these libraries, she did not examine the turnover intentions of individual librarians.

Throughout the 1990s, research on librarian turnover and turnover within the profession continued to be modest. Henry, Caudle, and Sullenger (1994) studied the relationship between tenure and turnover among academic library directors. They did not examine other causes of turnover in their study. Surveys were sent nationwide to library directors of colleges and universities with at least five professional librarians. Ninety-four surveys were returned for a 76 percent response rate. The study found that tenure track require-ments had no significant effect on turnover in academic libraries.

Koenig, Morrison, and Roberts (1996) also studied turnover in university library directors. Their study investigated the effect of faculty status on turnover and job satisfaction. Surveys were sent to 108 of the 120 ARL directors. The twelve library directors not included in the study were not at academic libraries, and it was deemed inappropriate to include them. In this study, the researchers found turnover to be unrelated to faculty status.

Although turnover literature in libraries is concentrated in the United States, the subject has surfaced elsewhere in the world. Moyo (1996) studied library staff turnover at the University of Zimbabwe. The turnover rate for professional librarians at the library between 1991 and 1993 was an un-precedented 55 percent. The reasons given for their departures include working conditions, anomalies in university salary scales, lack of staff de-velopment programs, expansion of the private sector in Zimbabwe, the lift-ing of South African sanctions, and the opening of two new universities (the last three items relate to employment perceptions). While such reasons as South African sanctions are unique to that region, many of the reasons for turnover that existed in Zimbabwe can be found at public university li-braries in the United States.

THEORETICAL EXPLANATIONS OF TURNOVER

Because this research attempts to replicate the findings of the Cotton and Tuttle (1986) meta-analysis and Allison and Satori's (1988) research on at a university library, several theories and various logic provide the basis for the hypotheses tested. Many of the explanations for turnover are grounded in motivational theories developed in the 1960s. These include expectancy theory, job satisfaction theory, and equity theory (Vroom, 1964; Herzberg, 1966; Adams, 1963).

Expectancy theory explains how employment perceptions cause turnover. When individuals perceive that there are other positions available and ex-pect that they could be easily obtained, the odds increase that they will consider leaving their current position. Porter and Steers (1973) also noted that when an individual's work expectations are not substantially met, the individual is more inclined to withdraw.

The theoretical literature on job satisfaction also provides explanations for turnover and intentions to turnover. March and Simon (1958) stated the greater the dissatisfaction, the more likely the individual will withdraw and position will turn over. In contrast, the more satisfied a worker is, the stronger the force on him or her to remain on the job and the less the likelihood of his or her leaving.

Much of the explanation of why pay leads to turnover is based on equity theory and the research of J. Stacey Adams (1963). Simply stated, when an individual gives something, she/he will receive something in return. If the return is less than expected relative to other employees with comparable inputs to an organization, the resulting inequity will cause dissatisfaction and tension. The tension that is created from pay inequities, in turn, is relieved through the motivation to turn over.

Theories of individual sexism and dependent care responsibility suggest that gender affects whether one will remain in a job or turn over. Women still bear a disproportionate responsibility for raising children and caring for dependents such as elderly parents. As a consequence, they are more likely than men to quit work to assume such responsibilities. Often perceived as being the secondary income earners in a family, women are also more likely than men to quit their work in order to follow their spouse to a more lucrative position or more promising career.

Similarly, the number of dependents also has an effect on turnover. It was assumed in previous studies (Federico, Federico, & Lundquist, 1976; Viscusi, 1980) that along with dependents comes family responsibilities. Individuals with many dependents stay in their current jobs in order to provide children continuity in schools, friendships, and extracurricular activities. In turn, single and divorced individuals without children are not tied down and feel freer to move to other positions.

Lack of longevity, or tenure, is also an empirical explanation for turnover. Employees with less time invested in organizations are purportedly more inclined to leave organizations. Many times, employees with less tenure are in early career stages and are looking for other jobs that are more lucrative or more compatible with their needs or interests.

Career goals also affect whether an individual intends to turn over. If the career goals have not or cannot be met or satisfied in the present position, the individual will move to another position in order to meet those goals (Porter & Steers, 1973).

METHODOLOGY

This section describes the methodology used to determine the reasons why some librarians consider leaving their positions and/or profession.

Based on the leading causes of turnover from the Cotton and Tuttle (1986) meta-analysis and the Allison and Sartori (1988) study, 10 independent variables were selected. Cotton and Tuttle's (1986) meta-analysis demonstrated many variables associated with turnover. Their leading predictors relevant to white collar, non-managerial personnel were selected for the purpose of this study. The hypothesized predictors of turnover were employment perceptions, lack of longevity, pay, overall job satisfaction, satisfaction with the work itself, gender, and number of dependents. The remaining independent variables were drawn from Allison and Satori's (1988) study. They include career goals and future salary prospects. The dependent variables in this study are intent to turn over and stay within the profession of librarianship and intent to turn over and leave for another profession. A model of predictors of librarian turnover is presented in Fig. 1.

A questionnaire was developed and was administered to 300 public university librarians. Because this study was a replication study of the previous work of Cotton and Tuttle (1986) and of Allison and Sartori (1988), questions selected for this survey came directly from those studies whenever possible. In some cases, the wording of the questions was modified to fit the profession of librarianship. The survey contained 60 questions. Fifty-three questions asked the participant to provide the extent of one's agreement with a statement. The remaining questions asked the participant to provide demographic information.

The survey was designed to determine the attitudes of librarians regarding many facets of their job and career and whether they were considering

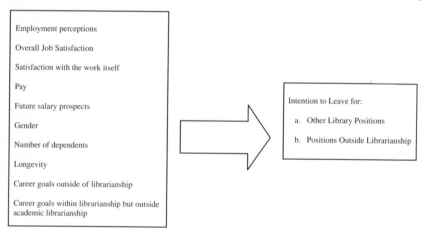

Fig. 1. Predictors of Librarian Turnover.

leaving their current position, library, and/or profession. Except for those questions gathering demographic data, the questionnaire consisted of items with which the sample indicated the strength of their agreement on a scale of one to five, with one indicating strong disagreement and five indicating strong agreement. In addition, "Inapplicable" was given as an option for respondents to use when the statement did not apply. Instructions on how to take the survey were provided at the beginning of the survey. Respondents were instructed to click the circle that best indicated the strength of their agreement. The seven questions asking for demographic information required the respondent to type in a number or click on a circle to provide information such as tenure, gender, and the type of library in which they were employed.

A mailing list from ACRL, Instruction Section (ACRL/IS) was obtained to select participants for the survey. On request, ACRL/IS narrowed the list of approximately 1,700 members to 1,000 members by deleting organization and company members, as well as librarians living outside the United States. Because membership in ACRL/IS is open to librarians nationally, efforts were made to randomly select librarians from each state.

Although the ACRL/IS mailing list contained 1,000 members, only 300 librarians were selected for the study. This number was selected because it provided a large enough sample for the purposes of conducting data analysis and constituted a research project that could be managed by one person within a reasonable time frame.

An online survey was determined to be the best method of gathering data for this study. The survey population, public university librarians, regularly uses computers and email in their positions. Whether preparing and teaching library instruction classes, providing reference services, or communicating via email with internal or external colleagues, librarians work with computers daily and are very familiar with computer functions. An online survey was also selected because data could be gathered quickly and at a low cost.

Three hundred cover emails were sent to the participants asking them to take the online survey. The cover email provided general information about the research, confidentiality provisions, and how further information could be obtained. Two weeks after the initial request for participation, an initial follow-up email was sent to the participants. This email also served as a "thank you" to those participants who had already responded. The final follow-up email was sent two weeks later.

Once the results were received, the data were prepared and coded for entry into the SPSS program. The coding scheme assigned higher values for responses that signified a more positive attitude toward the survey items.

The more positive the response, the higher the number. Using a Likert scale of five responses, a 5 designated the "Strongly Agree" choice. Consequently, a response of "Agree" was designated 4, "Neutral" was designated with 3, "Disagree" was designated with 2, and finally "Strongly Disagree" was designated with 1. Responses that were marked as "Inapplicable" were coded "0". When responses were not provided, the item was given 9. Once the data were entered into the SPSS program, zeros and nines were treated as missing values by the SPSS program. Reverse coding was necessary for several survey items to ensure valid measurement of the survey scales.

SPSS version 11.5 software was used to analyze the responses to the survey. Frequencies were run to determine how librarians' perceptions were distributed along the Likert scale and to determine if data were appropriately coded. Factor analysis and scale reliability analysis were used to determine the construct validity and reliability of the survey. Pearson correlation and multiple regressions were used to determine the validity of the hypotheses.

Three hundred emails were sent to selected public university librarians requesting they participate in the survey. With the survey available for only one month, 189 out of 300 librarians responded. A response rate of 63 percent was obtained and was considered reasonable for the purpose of generalization.

FINDINGS

The survey included seven demographic questions. Of the seven, the final question was used to confirm the respondents were public university employees. All 189 participants responded that they were public university librarians.

The demographic items revealed the respondents were overwhelmingly female (73.5 percent), a figure that was only slightly different than the gender figures available from the ARL. According to the ARL, male librarians make up approximately 35 percent of librarians working in academic libraries (Kyrillidou & O'Connor, 2002).

The average respondent was middle-aged (44.2 years) with the youngest respondent being 25 years and the oldest being 63 years. The respondents had worked in their current positions for an average of six years, with the shortest longevity being one year and the longest being 38 years. Likewise, the respondents had worked in their current library for an average of nine years, with the shortest longevity being one year and the longest being 38 years. The number of dependents of the participants ranged from none to

Table 1. Respondent Profiles.

Demographic	Data
Percent female	73.50
Percent male	25.90
Average years of age	42.20
Average years in current position	6.00
Average years in current library	9.00
Average dependents	0.89
Percent tenured or tenure track	63.50

six. The average number was 0.89, with more than half (52.4 percent) of the respondents having no dependents. Nearly two-thirds of the respondents (63.5 percent) were tenured and/or on tenure track (Table 1).

The next step in the data analysis involved testing the reliability of the scales created for each variable measured by more than one item. Cronbach's coefficient alpha was used to test the reliability of the scales. A principle component factor analysis was also run for each set of scale items in order to determine if any items should be removed for the purpose of enhancing reliability and construct validity.

Individual hypotheses were initially tested through Pearson correlations. Pearson correlations were calculated for each of the independent variables and both of dependent variables. Pearson correlations indicate that overall job satisfaction, satisfaction with pay, and future salary prospects have statistically significant *negative* associations with intentions to leave the library profession. These associations are also moderately strong. In turn, career goals outside librarianship have statistically significant *positive* relationships with intentions to leave the profession. This relationship is also quite strong.

Pearson correlations further reveal that overall job satisfaction and satisfaction with the work itself have strong, statistically significant *negative* associations with intentions to turnover but stay within library work. Satisfactions with pay, satisfaction with future salary prospects, and longevity have modest to moderately strong significant negative associations with intentions to turnover but to stay within librarianship. Moreover, career goals within librarianship but outside academic librarianship have moderately strong *positive* correlations with intentions to turnover but to stay within library work.

To control the effects of all independent variables and to determine a more parsimonious model of predicting intent to turn over in public university librarians, multiple regressions between the two dependent variables and independent variables were conducted. The independent variables were regressed on each of the dependent variables. Should any of the independent variables be removed and the regression analysis run again, the results might be different.

A multiple regression indicated that perceptions of employment opportunities elsewhere and satisfaction with the work itself have a modest to moderately strong negative associations with intentions to leave the profession of librarianship. Career goals outside the field of librarianship, in turn, have a strong positive relationship with intentions to leave the profession. When all of the independent variables are regressed, the greater the perceptions of career goals outside of librarianship, the greater the intent to leave the profession. Likewise, the lower the employment perceptions and the satisfaction with the work itself, the greater the intent to turn over. Overall, the independent variables also explain a substantial amount of variance ($r^2 = 0.54$) in intentions to leave the profession of librarianship.

A second multiple regression revealed that overall job satisfaction, satisfaction with the work itself, and satisfaction with future salary prospects have negative relationships with intentions to turnover but stay within librarianship. The unstandardized coefficient for overall job satisfaction is also quite large. By contrast, career goals within librarianship but outside academic librarianship have a moderate positive association with intention to leave but stay within librarianship. When all of the independent variables are regressed, the greater the perceptions of career goals within librarianship but outside of academic librarianship, the greater the intent to leave but stay within librarianship. Likewise, the lower the overall job satisfaction, the lower the satisfaction with the work itself, and the lower the satisfaction with future salary prospects, the greater the intent to leave but stay within librarianship. Overall, the independent variables also explain a substantial amount of variance ($r^2 = 0.54$) in intentions to attrite but stay within librarian work.

Finally, multiple regression reveals that employment perceptions and satisfaction with the work itself are negatively related to intentions to leave the library profession. Career goals outside the field of librarianship are positively related to intentions to leave the library profession. Multiple regression also reveals that overall job satisfaction, satisfaction with the work itself, and satisfaction with future salary prospects have negative relationships with intentions to turnover but stay within librarianship. Career goals outside librarianship have a positive association with intention to leave but stay within librarianship.

DISCUSSION

Overall Findings and the Studies Replicated

The overall findings reveal that career goals outside the field of librarianship are the most consistent predictor of turnover intentions. Overall job satisfaction, satisfaction with future salary prospects, and goals within librarianship but outside academic librarianship are also fairly consistent predictors of turnover intentions.

Cotton and Tuttle (1986) found the strongest predictors of turnover to be employment perceptions, pay, overall job satisfaction, satisfaction with the work itself, tenure (longevity), gender, and number of dependents. The research findings presented here therefore replicate only two of the seven leading predictors of turnover from Cotton and Tuttle's meta-analysis.

When the research findings are compared to the results of the Allison and Sartori (1988) survey, more similarities are found. However, it is important to note that no statistical analysis was run on the Allison and Sartori survey results. They only report how often each respondent answered a question. Allison and Sartori found that career goals and future salary prospects were the two leading causes of turnover of librarians at the University of Nebraska Library. With few exceptions, the research results confirm the findings of Allison and Sartori that turnover intentions are affected by future salary prospects and career goals.

IMPLICATIONS OF THE RESEARCH

For far too long library administrators have neglected the study of librarian turnover in public universities. This study should serve as a reminder and wake-up call to those administrators that turnover cannot, and should not, be neglected. When administrators address turnover factors, librarians are less likely to leave their positions and the library patron is well served. Librarians also have some responsibility for their turnover. When applying for and accepting positions, they should be sure that the position meets their needs both professionally and personally. While needs and preferences change and grow over the years, librarians should periodically evaluate and become aware of their personal and career preferences. Not only is this helpful to the librarian, it is important for the library organization and the patrons which it serves.

Specifically to reduce intentions to leave the profession, library administrators need to address career goals outside librarianship, satisfaction with the work itself, and career goals within librarianship but outside academic libraries. To reduce intent to leave the current position but stay within librarianship, library administrators need to address overall job satisfaction, career goals outside librarianship, and satisfaction with future salary prospects.

Creating an environment in which the librarian feels comfortable and can contribute to the organization should increase overall job satisfaction. Providing a mix of intrinsic and extrinsic rewards, such as supervisory praise, recognition awards, and interesting work assignments and projects might also enhance an employee's overall job satisfaction. To help ensure job satisfaction, librarians can make the employer aware of their interests, skills, and abilities at the time they were being hired. Likewise, the employer should ensure that the position announcement is accurate and reflects the true needs of a position to avoid having an unqualified librarian or someone who does not fit the announcement to apply for the position.

To reduce turnover, administrators need to discern the factors that enhance overall job satisfaction and satisfaction with the work itself. This initially may involve drawing from the body of empirical research on the determinants of overall job satisfaction and satisfaction with the work itself. Ideally, this might involve the conduct of additional research to discern the determinants of job satisfaction that are idiosyncratic to academic libraries.

To increase a librarian's satisfaction with the work itself, administrators can endeavor to decrease feelings of being overwhelmed by the amount and/or the repetitiveness of the work though exploring innovative ways in which the tasks can be accomplished.

Library administrators can also ensure that there are opportunities for librarians to develop and enhance their career goals within libraries. Career development could include increasing support for participation in professional conferences where librarians can network with others in their profession and learn about and discuss the latest technology and public service issues. Administrators might increase internal career development by increasing support for library-related sabbaticals and time off for personal growth.

During employment interviews, administrators can provide a realistic job preview that helps prospective academic librarians discern whether their career goals can be met through librarianship. To reduce turnover, these findings also suggest that during the election processes, administrators must be resolved to uncover whether the career aspirations of applicants are consistent with the career opportunities in academic librarianship. Going beyond asking applicants about their career goals, administrators must discern whether the educational preparation, work histories, and professional activities of applicants are indicative of a commitment to a career in academic librarianship.

To reduce turnover through enhancing future salary prospects, administrators can submit budgets to their universities that accurately reflect the expectations of their personnel. Pay and benefit packages should also be made as attractive as possible and tailored to the individual needs of librarians. Salary prospects might also be enhanced through fundraising efforts to endow salaries. In addition to salary endowments, endowments and/or awards might be created for professional travel that would defray personal expenditures for travel. Public university library administrators must also become involved in efforts to lobby their state legislatures in order to increase appropriations for salaries and benefits. Library administrators must partner with university administrators to increase the prospects for attractive salaries.

In addition to its practical implications, this research has several academic implications. As noted in the literature review, there is very little empirical research concerning turnover among academic librarians. The research and findings of this study generally extend the external validity of Allison and Sartori's (1988) research. In turn, the findings generally delimit the external validity of the broader body of research on turnover. Only one variable – overall job satisfaction – from Cotton and Tuttle's (1986) meta-analysis demonstrates any consistency in predicting turnover intentions of the nationwide population of academic librarians. Overall, the factors that tend to encourage turnover in academic libraries appear to be unique to academic libraries. As such, addressing turnover intentions of librarians on the basis of the findings from the larger body of turnover research outside librarianship would most likely prove to be ineffective.

RECOMMENDATIONS

Because there is so little research about academic librarian turnover, there is much for future researchers to explore about the topic. This study barely touches the surface when it comes to research on librarian turnover. It examined academic librarians serving the public. Future research should expand the collection of data to include other academic librarians, such as those serving in acquisitions, cataloging, collection management, and automation services. These librarians play an essential role in the function of academic libraries and are often overlooked because they are not working with the public.

Although this research tests many of the predictors of turnover as determined by Cotton and Tuttle (1986), future turnover research on academic librarians should be conducted using criteria more applicable to higher education and university faculty. While two of the leading causes of turnover, according to Allison and Sartori, were included in this study, criteria specific to academe might provide further insight to the reasons academic librarians consider leaving their positions and/or the profession. This would include conducting research similar to that of Henry et al. (1994). In their research on library directors, they tried to determine whether if the tenure-track requirements caused turnover in library directors. Future research should be expanded to include whether tenure-track requirements cause academic librarians to leave their positions and/or the profession.

In addition to investigating tenure, burnout might be explored as a possible explanation of turnover of academic librarians. The effect of burnout on turnover has been studied in many other professions. The professions of education and social work closely resemble librarianship because they are dominated by women and are service oriented. Because burnout has been determined to cause turnover in those professions (Jackson, Schwab, & Schuler, 1986; Drake & Yadama, 1996), it is possible it could cause turnover in librarianship.

Beyond investigating intentions to turnover, future research on librarians might investigate actual turnover. The examination of turnover records, exit interviews, and absenteeism records might provide administrators with specific information on the causes of turnover in libraries. It could also provide information needed to develop human resource programs and policies for their organization.

In addition to academic libraries, other public library institutions should be examined. Rubin conducted his turnover research in public libraries, but it appears that no one has expanded this valuable research. Rubin's research concerning librarian turnover was limited to the Midwest and could also be expanded to other regions and the entire country.

Another consideration for future researchers is data collection methods. The data for this research was obtained through an online survey. When surveying librarians, this proved to be an effective method to collect the data. Librarians, no matter what area or type of the library they work, are very computer savvy. The online survey also minimized costs and timesaving.

CONCLUSION

In 1929, Charles H. Compton (Compton, 1929) stated that labor turnover in libraries was a serious problem. More than 75 years later, Compton's statement still holds true and should be a concern to library administrators. Moreover, with the graying of the profession, turnover rates could dramatically increase. Library administrators must be prepared to handle this human resource issue with complete confidence. Knowing the predictors of turnover intentions should help administrators prepare for and prevent turnover. This awareness will only enhance the profession of librarianship, public universities, and the population served.

REFERENCES

Adams, J. S. (1963). Toward an understanding of inequity. *Journal of Abnormal and Social Psychology, 67*(5), 422–436.

Allison, D. A., & Sartori, E. (1988). Professional staff turnover in academic libraries: A case study. *College and Research Libraries, 49*(2), 141–148.

Amone, M., Hebel, S., & Schmidt, P. (2003). Another bleak budget year. *Chronicle of Higher Education, 49*(17), A21–A22.

Armour, S. (2000). Employers urge workers to chill out before burning out: Moves aimed at cutting turnover. *Library Personnel News, 13*(1–20), 12–13.

Collins, L. J. (1989). *Professional staff turnover in medium-to-large sized academic health sciences libraries.* Unpublished master's thesis. University of North Carolina at Chapel Hill, Chapel Hill, North Carolina.

Compton, C. H. (1929). Comparison of qualifications, training, demand and remuneration of the library profession with social work. In: J. S. McNiece (Ed.), *The library and its workers; reprints of articles and addresses* (pp. 127–138). New York: H. W. Wilson Company.

Cotton, J. L., & Tuttle, J. M. (1986). Employee turnover: A meta-analysis and review with implications for research. *Academy of Management Review, 11*(1), 55–70.

Drake, B., & Yadama, G. N. (1996). A structural equation model of burnout and job exit among child protective services workers. *Social Work Research, 20*(3), 179–187.

Federico, S. M., Federico, P. A., & Lundquist, G. W. (1976). Predicting women's turnover as a function of extent of met salary expectations and biodemographic data. *Personnel Psychology, 29*, 559–566.

Henry, E. C., Caudle, D. M., & Sullenger, P. (1994). Tenure and turnover in academic libraries. *College and Research Libraries, 55*(5), 429–435.

Herzberg, F. (1966). *Work and the nature of man.* Cleveland: World Pub. Co.

Hisle, W. L. (2002). Top issues facing academic libraries. *College and Research Libraries News, 63*(10), 714–715, 730

Jackson, S. E., Schwab, R. L., & Schuler, R. S. (1986). Toward an understanding of the burnout phenomenon. *Journal of Applied Psychology, 71*(4), 630–640.

Koenig, M., Morrison, R., & Roberts, L. (1996). Faculty status for library professionals: Its effect on job turnover and job satisfaction among university research library directors. *College and Research Libraries, 57*(3), 295–300.

Kyrillidou, M., & O'Connor, M. (Eds) (2002). *ARL annual salary survey, 1999–2000*. Washington, DC: Association of Research Libraries.

March, J. G., & Simon, H. A. (1958). *Organizations*. New York: Wiley.

Moyo, L. M. (1996). Library staff retention strategies in the face of accelerated turnover: University of Zimbabwe case. *International Information and Library Review, 28*(2), 105–119.

Neal, J. G. (1982). Staff turnover and the academic library. In: G. B. McCabe & B. Kreissman, (Eds), *Foundations in library and information science* (Vol. 17, Part a, pp. 99–106). Greenwich, CT: JAI Press (Options for the 80s: Proceedings of the second national conference of the association of the college and research libraries).

Porter, L. W., & Steers, R. M. (1973). Organizational, work, and personal factors in employee turnover and absenteeism. *Psychological Bulletin, 80*(2), 151–176.

Price, J. L. (1977). *The study of turnover*. Ames, IA: Iowa State University Press.

Rogers, M. (2003). Tackling recruitment. *Library Journal, 128*(2), 40–43.

Rubin, R. (1986). A pilot study on employee turnover rates of librarians in three moderately large public libraries in Ohio. *Journal of Library Administration, 6*(4), 89–105.

Rubin, R. (1987). A study of employee turnover of full time public librarians in moderately large and large size public libraries in seven Midwestern states. *Dissertation Abstracts International, 48*(07) (UMI No.8721746).

Transfers turn down turnover. (2000). *Library Personnel News, 13*(1–2), 14–15.

Viscusi, W. K. (1980). Sex differences in worker quitting. *The Review of Economics and Statistics, 62*(3), 388–398.

Vroom, V. (1964). *Work and motivation*. New York: Wiley.

CASE EXAMINATION OF DECISION-MAKING FACTORS: DO FACULTY AND LIBRARIANS AGREE ON CRITERIA UPON WHICH TO CANCEL JOURNALS?

James H. Walther

INTRODUCTION

Scholarly communication in the U.S. has been closely examined in the past two decades by librarians because of the acceleration in costs of serial, scholarly communication. Specific disciplines of research have increased at unprecedented rates, namely the areas of scientific, technical, and medical (STM) publishing.

The problem of price increases of journal subscriptions has reached unprecedented heights. Price for journal subscriptions climbed an average of 147 percent from 1986 to 1996; specifically, the calculated average serial subscription for research library materials increased by 9.5 percent a year for over a decade (Case, 1998). Granting that these statistics will continue to climb, cancellations of journals will only become more commonplace, yet unsuccessful in meeting the goal of containing costs.

The Association of Research Libraries in their *Serials Pricing Project* (1989) highlighted seven elements in publishing that may be partially

Advances in Library Administration and Organization, Volume 23, 281–331
Copyright © 2006 by Elsevier Ltd.
All rights of reproduction in any form reserved
ISSN: 0732-0671/doi:10.1016/S0732-0671(05)23008-0

responsible for journal price increases. These are publisher–market behavior (duplicate pricing structures of publishers that charge U.S. libraries more than libraries of other countries); exchange-rate differentials; growth in published research; competition in the academy; publisher domination by market segment; journal-publishing economics (namely, fewer libraries or a narrower market); and finally, the mergers and acquisitions of smaller presses to create a handful of giant, commercial publishers. While each of these may be more dramatic in certain libraries, each is a relevant cause of the current problem.

The solution to the increasing expense, consistently used throughout the past two decades, has been to cancel journals. These cancellation decisions are usually made by using a list of factors upon which to evaluate the journal collection, which is then forwarded to the faculty for consultation on the decision (Budd, 1998). But, faculty involvement in journal cancellations is sometimes seen only as an opportunity to object to scheduled cancellations from the librarians, and, at some institutions, university administrations have not wanted the library to discuss specific journal cancellations with the faculty (Stephens, 1993).

At the same time that journal costs were rising, the overall economy of higher education tightened (Hamaker, 1993; Paul, 1984). A university administration could no longer provide a library collection–development budget that was increasing at the same rate as the annual renewals of library journals, and librarians had to look for other ways to provide information, namely through resource sharing, in order to cancel journal subscriptions (Kaser, 1995). By the 1990s, sizeable journal cancellation projects were occurring at a time when library collection–development budgets were in decline or when there were no increases to the overall library budget (Cummings, Witte, Bowen, Lazarus, & Ekman, 1992; Hawkins, 1998; Tenopir & King, 2000). Therefore, what librarians came to grapple with was an environment in which the library budgets were held hostage by the spiraling financial needs of the journal collection, a problem known to librarians as the "serials crisis" (Okerson & Stubbs, 1991; White, 1988).

Costs of journals during the 1980s and 1990s continued to accelerate and created what could be identified as a science of journal cancellations. Identified characteristics of this new economy of journals were (1) the two-tiered, differential pricing structures, one structure for libraries and another price for individuals; (2) different library rates for specific, targeted countries; (3) the varying factors in the weakening of the U.S. dollar; and (4) the substantial, yearly incremental increases of sci-tech journals (Astle & Hamaker, 1988).

As these inflationary increases became commonplace in scientific publishing, a more prominent issue was the growing role of foreign business entities and their impact on the scholarly publishing marketplace (Okerson, 1986). As these foreign monopolies grew, so did the problem of differing library rates for specific, targeted countries. The nature of these systemic problems were exacerbated by (1) the reduction of cheaper, nonprofit scholarly society publication houses and (2) the emergence of monopolies in publishing by academic subject area, especially within the sciences (Mattlage, 1999). This collapsing of competition in the scientific publishing marketplace is one of the current, essential problems facing libraries purchasing scientific, technical, and medical research today.

While faculty have been seen to be extremely loyal in suggesting specific journals for purchase and cancellation (Hamaker, 1993), their needs are still high, especially in the sciences. The competition to be published increases in the scientific literature, and new publications are developed from established journals as a way to meet new, growing areas of research, a trend called "twigging" (Richards, 1991). However, the trend is not seen in the humanities, where competition increases, but few specialized journals develop (Bieber & Blackburn, 1993).

With these growing expectations for a large and diverse medical journal collection, faculty expect journals to be annually renewed and new journal titles in emerging fields to be added in anticipation of new, committed readers (Walker, 1998). Both of these expectations will inhibit the cancellation of journals (Stankus, 1985). A compounding problem is finding a strategy to make cancellations across subject areas equitably, yet unfairly as some areas of research are more heavily invested in journals (Williamson, 1985). Faculty involvement is crucial in this process, and it is within these dynamic and difficult constructs that journal collections must be built.

WHY LIBRARIANS WITH FACULTY?

As the academic library plays the role of both intermediary and adjudicator of collection, purchases, and cancellations, faculty involvement in library resource decisions is not only commonplace, but essential to making these campus decisions (Atkinson, 1993).

Faculty involvement in cancellation of projects is often enhanced by a thorough explanation of the depth of the financial problems confronting libraries as a result of journal pricing (Barstow, 1993). Literature on scholarly communication pricing starts with the initial studies of journals by Fry and White (1976) and *Scholarly Communication: The Report of the National Enquiry* (1979), which creates the historical foundation for any examination of scholarly communication issues. Fry and White (1976) researched library budgets and the shifting of fiscal resources from monograph purchases to maintain journal collection purchases. The 1979 Report posed several research questions, including how scholarly information was dispersed through publishing channels during times of financial difficulty.

Both of these studies set the stage for an understanding of the continued scholarly communication problems that academic institutions would face in the following decades. As these problems became more intensified, communicating the issues of purchasing journals and promoting campus and national involvement of faculty in the discussions have been championed as solutions in the field of academic library administration (Madison, 1999).

As a result of accelerated journal costs and the inability of library budgets to keep pace, libraries have been forced, and are continuing to cancel journals to deal with financial problems. As the financial inability to purchase journals continues, librarians work with the knowledge that previous journal cancellations have been ineffective in completely controlling these price escalation and related problems, yet it is crucial that faculty involvement in making these cancellation decisions continue. Even as academic libraries have become an essential part of the modern university's complex social system, serving as the "nodes" in the scholarly communication process (Dain, 1990), library journal budgets have not retained their percentage of overall university expenditures, and the library collections across the academy are in continual risk of cancellation.

The situational problem has the essential elements of (1) constant increase in journal prices (Case, 1998, 2001) and (2) exceptional growth of published information. The general expansion of research and research fragmentation (twigging) usually occurs in developing areas of thought, where new journals explore issues of new perspectives from existing journals (Nisonger, 1998).

Constant Increases in Prices

The price of journal subscriptions climbed by an average of 147 percent from 1986 to 1996. As price increases became solidified on campus, during this same period book costs increased by 63 percent and the Consumer Price Index by 41 percent (University of Virginia, 1999). Since 1986, the calculated average serial subscription for research library materials increased by 9.5 percent each year (Case, 1998). For libraries purchasing STM journals, fields in which journals are the predominate form of information delivery,

Table 1. Current Increases in Science, Technical, and Medicine (STM) Journals.

Field of Study	Price per Title (2001)	% of Change 1997–2001
Biology	$1,064.33	34.53
Botany	$ 790.28	25.93
Chemistry	$1,918.09	34.29
General science	$ 830.55	48.30
Health sciences	$ 728.14	38.89
Technology	$1,013.34	42.18
Zoology	$ 866.03	39.21

Source: Born and Van Orsdel (2001).

the data are considerably worse. Comparing what library budgets were able to purchase in 1986, library budgets would need an increase of 70 percent to purchase the same share of library materials in 1998 (Association of Research Libraries, Association of American Universities, & Pew Higher Education Roundtable, 1998).

By the late 1990s, libraries purchasing in science, technology and medical fields were spending 30 times more on journal collections than they did in 1970, yet the volume of journal information collected was demonstratively smaller because of cancellations (Table 1; Cox, 1998). The difficult issue for the academy is that journals are an ongoing financial commitment, unlike one-time budget expenditures. When journal expenditures continue and increase, the predictions of averages are difficult to budget. The Association of Research Libraries now predicts that by 2020 their average member library will pay $1,632 per journal per year (Kyrillidou, 2000). For the hard sciences, especially medicine, it can be demonstrated that these averages are measurably higher (Table 2).

Growth of Published Research

The rates of both published articles and the number of overall faculty conducting research have substantially increased in the past quarter century (Bentley & Blackburn, 1990; Blackburn & Lawrence, 1996). This ties directly to the problem of more scholars attempting to publish, which then results in expanded avenues for publication. In a setting in which academic units examine the number of publications produced by faculty to determine productivity for advancement, publishing venues have become more specialized and more numerous, and more taxing on the research collections in those libraries supporting high-producing departments (Gardner, 1991).

Table 2. High-Priced Journal Subscription Prices, FY2000.

Journal Title	2000 Price	Publisher
Brain Research	$16,344.00	Elsevier
Journal of Comparative Neurology	$14,995.00	Wiley
Nuclear Physics B	$12,113.00	Elsevier
Tetrahedron	$11,624.00	Elsevier
Journal of Applied Polymer Science	$11,570.00	Wiley
Chemical Physics Letters	$ 9,029.00	Elsevier
Journal of Polymer Science Part A: Polymer Chemistry	$ 8,535.00	Wiley
Journal of Polymer Science Part B: Polymer Physics	$ 8,535.00	Wiley
Physics Letters B	$ 7,595.00	Elsevier
European Journal of Pharmacology	$ 7,329.00	Elsevier
American Journal of Medical Genetics	$ 6,995.00	Wiley
Gene	$ 6,974.00	Elsevier

Source: Create Change (2000).

Most disciplines have seen an expansion in the size of given publications, demonstrated by higher page counts and additional issues (Bieber & Blackburn, 1993). This phenomenon has deepened since there is competition to publish quality journals, and other journals are concerned with developing a reputation in the field (Williamson, 1977; Ziman, 1980). Science has the additional onus of having a preference for journal publication because of the need for speed in scientific discovery and publishing (Richards, 1991). All of these expansive issues in publishing only make the problems of an expanding journal collection more difficult to control.

Purpose of this Study

The purpose of this two-tiered study is to (1) find factors that faculty and librarians will find agreeable and accept for selecting journals for cancellation and (2) identify how faculty input into the decision-making process of canceling journals is viewed and used by librarians. The conceptual framework of this study attempts to address the window of unexamined instances in which effective faculty involvement in journal cancellation projects has occurred. It is not known whether members of the faculty even agree upon the factors that librarians use to cancel journals (Hawthorn, 1991; Sapp & Watson, 1989), let alone want to be engaged in this process.

What is needed in the academy is a way to identify and develop a shared vocabulary for making decisions on journal cancellations. Faculty governance has long been involved in library governance (Budd, 1998). One model of governance in higher education is consensus building on campuses, where the collegial decision-making model is used (Tierney, 1999). Today, although multiple priorities exist in academic institutions, academic integrity and inquiry are still the focus of higher education. Even though libraries are a basic part of these cultural values, they also have a managerial nature that may be in conflict with the autonomous culture of the faculty (Berberet & McMillin, 2002). Placed in the context of this study, the managerial focus of canceling journals may be in direct contradiction to the expansive, self-managed culture of the faculty role.

This study examined whether faculty approach the factors used in journal cancellation differently from librarians using the same factors. Organizational decision-making has several theorists; however, East's (1997) work has been chosen as the theoretical framework for this study of faculty and library decisions within an educational organization. East's topologies of decision making are built upon the theories of Odiorne (1969) and Drucker (1966). The "four primary constraints that impinge upon the organizational decision-making process in higher education" will be used exclusively in this study. These decision constraints are time (temporal proximity), text (information), context (environment), and constituents (stakeholders).

While journal cancellation projects may seem like routine, process-ridden activities, decision makers are often affected by these constraints. Without such constraints, faculty might participate differently in decisions (East, 1997), such as in assisting with canceling journals. Despite these constraints, Hanson (1981) found successes when the library administration contributed to the process of canceling journals, and library staff provided the leadership and vision to meet the financial objectives that journal cancellations were intended to meet. Hanson continues, noting that faculty involvement is cited as a crucial element to accomplishing the goals of the library's cancellation project and, furthermore, it was faculty contact via departmental contact that was especially important. The examination of these issues continues.

Since decisions such as these do affect the research capacity and long-term research viability of the institution (Dow, Meringolo, & St. Clair, 1995), an investigation of the cancellation factors should be tied to the faculty on campus and the decision-making constraints they face (East, 1997). In journal-cancellation projects, it is still unknown to what level the lack of faculty participation is due to organizational constraints, such as questioning whether faculty's input will be used.

RESEARCH QUESTIONS

Research suggests that librarians make journal cancellations with the rationale that factors such as citation reports, language of publication, price, subscription availability, coverage by indexing and abstracting services, and use are valid and agreed upon decision-making variables (Bourne & Gregor, 1975; Broadus, 1985).

- From the perspective of faculty and librarians, are the factors used by librarians to cancel journals sufficient to inform librarians in the decision-making process for canceling journals?
- How is faculty input in the decision-making process gathered and used to inform librarians in their decision-making process for journals?

Significance of the Study

Finding agreeable factors for faculty to accept in deciding on journal cancellations would significantly add to what librarians in higher education know about the decision process and provide a common basis in evaluating the factors. This study aimed to illustrate what various factors may indicate about the faculty's understanding of and agreement to the process of canceling journals.

If librarians, in the spirit of continuing a collegial culture in the academy, include faculty in the decision-making process for canceling journals but do not take the faculty's needs truly into consideration, a dissonance exists, or is created. Why are the faculty consulted for their input in such a case and why should they cooperate (Schwartz, 1998)? The current structure of continual cancellations does not illuminate what we know about the decision process of canceling journals.

This research gives an illustrative example of how faculty are included in library decisions. Faculty and librarians must use the contextual understanding of the decision-making process, namely for collections assessments involving faculty. Fussler and Simon (1961) point out that previous library usage is an indication of future library usage. Such usage and evaluative information was essential to this study. By involving the faculty in the evaluation of the factors used to cancel journals, librarians can learn how faculty use the library and whether they agree with the librarians' cancellation criteria, which in turn further provides information on how to maintain a journal collection that best fits the needs of the faculty and greater research community.

If librarians and faculty do have differing decision-making processes in place, and faculty are included in library decisions, what must be known about faculty influence on the final decisions? The significance of these findings is the identification of how faculty regard the usage of factors in a valuative instrument utilized in libraries for the cancellation of journals. Johnson (1983) offered that, as the journal collection problems grew more common on campuses, faculty were involved to provide justification for journals; however, the common pattern followed by librarians was to use the evaluative justification as a faculty *opinion* and to allow librarians themselves to retain the right to make the final decision. Allowing faculty, as an external committee, to be involved in a fuller process of developing recommendations may be the best strategy for creating a valued journal collection (Tallman & Leach, 1989).

Need for the Study

Within this system of escalating costs and reduced access, researchers still demand the widest variety of scholarly journals. Colleges and universities have rich histories of the "publish or perish" mentality, where colleagues count the number of research results published as a measure of evaluation (Creswell, 1986). Such an environment only increases the demands on library journal collections, given a greater need for the journal collection to facilitate further faculty research (Harrington & Grice, 1992).

Among the substantial numbers of procedural examinations and case studies of journal cancellations (Metz, 1992; Stephens, 1993), it remains clear that librarians are looking for useful information to assist in the process of selecting and canceling journals. While librarians have used these studies of cancellations to develop useful techniques to cancel journals in academic libraries, the evaluation of faculty interpretation of the factors used to cancel journals has not been fully exploited.

Librarians and faculty in the academy are stakeholders in the decision to cancel journals. Decisions have consequences, and a better understanding of the factors used to make decisions will only enhance library decision-making. Therefore, this study attempted to (1) provide faculty with a further understanding of how librarians are attempting to work effectively with the dilemma of providing journals within tight, budgetary constraints and (2) further the use of a valuative factor, which may prove to be an effective procedural tool for librarians. As a descriptive study, which will further a previously used instrument, this research further illuminates how cancellation factors are viewed by faculty. Fallon and Young (1983), Milne (1990), and Neame (1986) all concur that it is useful to include faculty members in the decision-making process, especially in attempts to create a dialogue with faculty on these issues. Yet, the dialogue is ineffective if not based on the overall problems and not matched with an effective assessment of whether the factors used to evaluate journal collections are agreed upon or, at least, useful.

The study attempted to provide librarians with a working knowledge of how much similarity or dissonance exists between faculty's and librarians' view of the factors used to procedurally decide which journals to cancel. As library users, faculty are essential to naming which journals are needed for their teaching, research, and service (Broadus, 1985). Additionally, there is a growing interest and research in the process of making decisions about journals in institutions of higher education (Hamaker, 1993). Findings such as these inform members of both groups, faculty and academic librarians, as well as the greater higher education community, by providing insight into how decisions are made. The study provides a successful, new framework and dialogue between faculty and librarians as faculty are made more aware of the financial barriers to collection management issues in libraries. Without such organizational knowledge, the long-term effects of these barriers may include inhibiting the growth and health of the academy and knowledge as a result of the continued, rising costs of published research today (Case, 2001; Lawal, 2002).

SUMMARY

In summary, as journal budgets in academic libraries continue to diminish in relationship to the acceleration in journal costs, library administrators must more closely examine university expenditures for library collections. Journals, due to their growing portion of the library budget, are often under constant risk of cancellation or non-renewal.

To more fully understand the issue, this study was designed to find agreed upon factors to use for selecting journals for cancellation and also to how faculty input in the decision-making process is used by librarians to make these cancellation decisions. This study demonstrates areas of similarity and differences between faculty and librarians, and concludes with a checklist of ways these two groups can work together on these critical issues.

LITERATURE REVIEW

Role of the Faculty

Of greatest interest to higher education may be the degree to which faculty are involved in the decision making about journals. In examining why faculty are not playing a substantial role, Atkinson (1995) found they are regularly consulted, but they are not responsible for building library collections, namely because of time and subject bias. In research into the academic environment of canceling journals, it appears that the lack of a functional deselection model is one of the many problems facing librarians and faculty (Broude, 1978). Where decisions were made by librarians based on models created to cancel journals, these decisions to cancel journals correlated poorly with the choices faculty would have made based on the same variables (Stenstrom & McBride, 1979). The varying degree to which faculty were involved in the decision-making processes make it necessary to understand (1) more about the cancellation process and (2) the faculty's view of cancellation factors, which is equally crucial and timely now.

There is a considerable range of faculty involvement in journal cancellation projects in academic libraries. One concern is to avoid contacting the faculty too often and ask only when truly needed (Durey, 1976). Another study acknowledges the political advantages to involving faculty in the process (Fry & White, 1979), including knowing more fully what research faculty are involved in and what curricula are being taught on campus. And, last, there is a need to find a balance of faculty involvement and not allow final decisions to be held under faculty control (Nisonger, 1998; Slote, 1982).

Research indicates that faculty–librarian collaboration could expand beyond selection and cancellation of library materials; however, so far the quantity of faculty–librarian contact has received little attention (Kotter, 1999). With improved relations between the two groups and librarian's and faculty's knowing each other's daily concerns, the relationship may become more productive and less contentious (Sapp & Watson, 1989). As cancellation projects continue, librarians could be viewed more as an advocate for faculty research materials rather than a detriment to faculty's access to journals.

In trying to keep the faculty involved in the process of maintaining an academic journal collection worthy of their research, librarians often solicit faculty to rate journals by lists or by factors, as well as to choose which journals are worthwhile for their specific research interests (Tucker, 1995).

Faculty inclusion in decisions may be both advantageous to the library by providing librarians with a sense of the journal needs of faculty (Perkins, 1990), and at the same time giving the academy the benefit of cost containment for journals.

Since faculty are often asked their opinion in this process rather than given the opportunity to make the final decision for canceling journals, it is of interest to both librarians and faculty to determine the best way to include them in this process, rather than simply to assume that faculty involvement is always solicited (Grefsheim, Bader, & Meredith, 1983). Librarians are often working without enough faculty input to make informed decisions about what is needed in their libraries. Several studies note faculty members' resistance to the way in which librarians decide what materials to cancel, namely applying low-use indicators and canceling what they assume are unused library materials (Hubbard & Williams, 1989). It is expected that with more strategy in the process, faculty will become full partners in the decision-making process and assist librarians in these decisions.

Costs and Medical Journals

Cost, although commonly the deciding factor, should not be the exclusive factor in determining when to cancel a journal, especially without including other measures and factors (Bader & Thompson, 1989). Viewing journal cancellation as a dynamic mixture of factors for consideration might present a more realistic picture of the many elements that faculty might consider when asked to offer input on which journals to cancel. However, in practice, research shows that the cost of specific journals is the reason that specific titles are commonly selected for cancellation (Chrzastowski & Schmidt, 1993, White, 1980; Yocum, 1989).

Librarians and researchers concur that in evaluating collections, among the factors that should be utilized are cost data matched with usage statistics and citation impact studies (Metz & Cosgriff, 2000). New financial models illuminate an essential problem associated with scientific, technology, and medical (STM) units publishing. As scientific, technology, and medical (STM) journals accelerate in cost, faculty drop their personal subscriptions, preferring library-provided subscriptions (Tenopir & King, 1997). Therefore, as faculty lose access to their personal journal subscriptions, library journals become a crucial link to access. Then, as libraries cancel these publications because of the continual price increases, the list of total

Table 3. A Hypothetical Example of Journal Price Increases.

Circulation below 2,500	100 subscriptions cancelled	Price increases $6.00 per subscription
Circulation of 500	100 subscriptions cancelled	Price increases $186 per subscription

Source: Tenopir and King (2000).

subscribers declines, and the remaining libraries subscribing to these expensive journals are forced to pay even higher prices.

Statistics of how publishing costs for journal subscriptions can quickly increase in response to canceling subscriptions in libraries and by individuals can be found in the following illustration. As the publishing companies attempt to remain profitable, these losses from cancellations are pushed on to the remaining subscribing libraries (Table 3).

Cancellation

Research on journal cancellation is conducted in four frameworks: (1) studies of journal-usage measures, (2) studies of cost indexes, (3) procedural studies and determining factors for canceling journals, and (4) studies of the long-term outcomes and consequences of canceling journals. In each type of study, librarians' efforts have focused on canceling journals and examined whether these efforts accomplished cost savings.

Studies of Journal-Usage Measures

Studies on journal use usually focus on the benefits or cautions of exclusively using journal-usage data as a measure for canceling. Representatives of these cautions are Nisonger (2000), naming the *Journal Citation Reports* of the Institute for Scientific Information (ISI) as a "useful tool that can assist research librarians in the serials [journals] decision-making process…but, in conjunction with other traditional factors" (p. 273). Kovacs (1989) concurs, offering that multiple criteria should be considered when canceling journal titles, pointing out that journal rankings or impact factors are just one factor to consider when canceling journals.

Francq (1994) employs a usage-cost relational index measure, which allows for a formula to be applied on two measures rather than on exclusive factors. Research illuminates how librarians use multiple factors to cancel journals, but the problems in canceling journals continue without a matched understanding of how the faculty view these factors or cancellation methods (Broude, 1978).

A study of journals at Wichita State University (WSU) examined usage in relationship to the goal of reducing overall costs of journals in the library. With an eye on cost information and inviting faculty input, the library was able to ground its entire project in efforts to educate the faculty on (1) the intensity of the journal cost problems, (2) the economic factors on campus, and (3) the general trends in scholarly communication. This study found that faculty see serious problems in the procedures utilized by librarians to develop cancellation lists and also found that their faculty expressed resentment toward the lack of library funding available to support established academic programs (Hubbard & Williams, 1989). Librarians and researchers often find a gap between what is purchased and what is used in libraries (Schoch, 1994). For faculty, the results of shelf studies or nonuse studies alone are often not seen as valid factors for cancellation. Neame (1986) also points out that faculty often do not agree with the librarian's reliance on studying whether specific journal issues have been used by faculty and think that librarians should not cancel journals based on real or perceived nonusage of the journal collection by faculty.

Studies of Cost Indexes
Cost indexes and price studies are best summarized in the annual studies in *American Libraries* and *Library Journal*, where the annual U.S. periodical prices are reported. These indexes are subject breakdowns of costs of scholarly journals available and purchased in a given year. Other research examines price and publisher efforts, such as identifying the rate of the price increases over the years (Marks, Nielsen, Petersen, & Wagner, 1991). Librarians call for the application of price studies, contrasting the unit costs of journals across disciplines and showing cost-per-use or cost effectiveness of journals (Astle, 1993). Such price studies, especially longitudinal studies, prove valuable when reviewing journals and making cancellation decisions.

Cost indexes in relationship to the proposed study are valuable since they document how specific journals have increased in price from year to year. Journal unit costs increased by an overall 147 percent from 1986 to 1996, whereas books increased by only 65 percent from 1986 to 1998 (Case, 1998; Tenopir & King, 2000). Libraries could not keep pace with these increases, and throughout those years they purchased approximately 6 percent fewer journals and 26 percent fewer books (Kohl, 2001; Tenopir & King, 2000).

Procedural Studies and Determining Factors Used to Cancel Journals
The most common type of cancellation study in the literature is the third type of study, the procedural case study. Representative examples of this

research are found in Schoch and Abels (1994) and Segal (1986). Schoch and Abels examined the process of journal cancellation by developing a valuative instrument. To counter criticism of methodologies used by librarians creating title lists for faculty to review, Schoch and Abels examined the viability of creating and implementing a valuative instrument for use in canceling journals on campus. Their instrument was developed to assist in providing faculty with useful information for making collection and cancellation decisions. Their instrument employs nine factors upon which to evaluate journals (1) costs, (2) citedness, (3) authority, (4) currency, (5) language, (6) physical characteristics (graphics and legibility), (7) indexing, (8) in-library use, and (9) availability (elsewhere) (Schoch & Abels, 1994, p. 48). Their instrument takes into consideration the difficult problem of making further cancellations to already lean journal collections and attempts to work with faculty's need for information in how to assist in journal cancellation decisions.

The procedural cancellation research in the literature often describes how the problem of costs was dealt with in individual libraries (Clark, 1987), often including the need for faculty–librarian communication. Yet, within this type of research, it becomes clear that academic libraries have a value in their unique and diverse collections, and by canceling these resources, the growth of knowledge in higher education is blocked (McCarthy, 1994). The cancellation literature often gives procedural steps, such as which departments to include and when to automate (Metz, 1992). Yet, the literature does not fully evaluate the role of the involved faculty (Farrell, 1981), but merely suggests librarians' need to initiate faculty contact on these issues.

Studies of the Long-Term Outcomes and Consequences of Canceling Journals
The fourth type of examination of these problems is the study of the long-term outcomes and consequences of canceling journals. By examining STM journal cancellations, it was found that libraries were moving toward the development of a two-tier system in which academic libraries would be able to offer substantial collections in the social sciences and humanities, while their basic and hard sciences would suffer a loss of securing intellectual capital in journals (Yocum, 1989).

In studying factors considered for journals cancellation, White (1980) found that over 80 percent of what is predominately canceled is unique to the canceling academic library. With White's research findings, matched with the budgetary shifts and economic trends in libraries, it has become all too common to shift financial resources from book budgets to journal budgets to maintain journal collections (McCabe, 2001). Previously successful techniques, such as eliminating duplicate copies of the same journal title, have long since been exhausted (Chrzastowski & Schmidt, 1993). Initial rounds of journal cancellations forced libraries to make cancellations that were mainly seen as inconvenience measures involving a lack of immediate access to journal articles (White, 1980), possibly due to the elimination of multiple subscriptions to specific journal titles. However, recent research on cancellations indicate that smaller academic libraries will be unable to meet the intellectual needs of their users because collections continue to shrink with each price increase (Lawal, 2002).

Scientists need current information, and journals are an essential part of their information-seeking behavior. Researchers have found a doubling of available scientific information in scholarly journals approximately every 15 to 17 years (Tenopir & King, 2000). To support research and teaching, faculty must have continual access to this growing stream of published research. Specifically, science researchers rely heavily on journal collections (Branin & Case, 1998), especially for information that is considered cutting edge (Lawal, 2002).

Thus, the long-term effects of canceling may be the elimination of the uniqueness of each academic collection. Research on cancellation projects demonstrates substantial changes in the library collections of academic and research libraries for current and future users (Okerson & Stubbs, 1991). One study explored whether canceling activity across five academic libraries revealed decisions to cancel the same or similar journals (Chrzastowski & Schmidt, 1993). The findings in the initial study concluded that libraries in the study had retained high-use, essential titles. However, by their second study, Chrzastowski and Schmidt (1997) pointed out that libraries were canceling an exceptionally higher number of journal titles unique to each library. Faculty should be concerned with journal cancellations essentially because there is the possibility that some journals will be held by only a few libraries. Even some journals exclusively collected by a few libraries may now be targeted for cancellation (Bennion, 1994).

Academic libraries deciding to cancel journals in relative isolation may be canceling journals of value to other academic libraries and to their faculty. In examining librarians involved in canceling journals, researchers studied (1) the similarity of cancellation selections and (2) the typical cost of a serial title canceled. Relevant to this study, it was found that science and medicine are highly targeted areas for title cancellations (Chrzastowski & Schmidt, 1993). In their follow-up study (1997), it was found that science journals, namely those in the Library of Congress Class Sections of science, medicine, agriculture, and technology, are indeed "at-risk" journals. This study went on to report that over 71 percent of canceled dollar amounts come from these collection areas.

DECISION MAKING IN ACADEMIC
LIBRARY SETTINGS

Decision Making as Applied to Journal Problems

What is examined here are not the models found in decision making, but the participation and how the information produced in such participation creates a dialogue and informative vocabulary for members of the decision-making groups. Paul (1984), in examining the scholarly communication problems, found that faculty and librarians existed in competing states. Faculty exist in the *publish* or *perish* mode, while librarians were forced to evaluate access to individual journal titles rather than purchasing holdings of all journals available (Atkinson, 1993). In this new reality, faculty and librarians must work together on these issues; this will give faculty a better opportunity to become involved in the process of journal collection management issues.

Nutt (1990) compared different decision-making case situations, finding that managers have conflict, ambiguity, and uncertainty that they must deal with and find ways to respond to. He also found that after a stage of problem identification and option evaluation, decision makers can take time to evaluate assumptions and search for missed opportunities. It seems that the problem of scholarly communication and journal cancellation fits in well with Nutt's model, in that, the problem is clearly identified, the alternatives (cancellations) have been identified, and it now comes time to evaluate assumptions and search for missed (or new) opportunities. Perhaps librarians' more fully involving faculty in factor evaluation for journal cancellation is one such missed opportunity in higher education decision-making.

Throughout organizational research, the same situation can be viewed by multiple decision models (Allison, 1971), yet Nutt (1990) argues that regardless of the model used in organizational units, a common way to describe the "how" of decision making will be to describe a productive way to find solutions to an organization's problems. Chait (1979) would offer that the process would be enhanced by identifying one's clear objectives and defining goals, a process essential to identifying what the journal cancellation means to both faculty and librarians in a time of retrenchment. When the reasons that librarians find faculty input crucial to the success of the process are identified, faculty may more clearly see why and how librarians are using the information obtained (Lynch, 1990).

While decision sharing exists in libraries, we do not see where faculty are allowed to go beyond the formulated structure of higher education and become fully involved in the process of canceling journals. The chain of usage of the information between faculty's input into the decision and the librarian's use of the input may be at the crux of the disconnect (Kaplan, 1977). Generally, the larger the organization, the more the decisions are allowed to filter through the organization in a decentralized way. Even though faculty are included in decision making, the weight of their input may not be used strategically (Blau, 1970).

Institutional Decision-Making Processes

What institutions do know about their decision-making styles informs us that looking at decisions only as singular, discrete decision events and not viewing decisions as part of a larger process, both socially and organizationally, is a flawed approach (Garvin & Roberto, 2001). In examining decision-making approaches, enhanced institutional effectiveness is argued by several theorists (Baldridge, 1971; Chaffee, 1983; Cohen & March, 1974). Yet, in areas where higher levels of performance are found, decisions are allowed by multiple groups in participative decision processes (Birnbaum, 1992). Lynch (1976), however, indicates disagreement, offering that library decision-making by groups should only be employed when it is seen as a way for the organization to be more effective than when following authoritarian models.

There are indications that faculty relations and institutional effectiveness are associated with such participation in decisions (Cameron, 1985). About faculty involvement in journal cancellation, Walter (1990) specifies that where faculty are involved in the process of canceling journals, the process produces faculty support, which is seen as a further possibility for the journal cancellation project to be considered as a success.

Decision-making studies have demonstrated that differences exist in decision-making models on academic campuses (Giesecke, 1993). However, few have attempted to understand the constraints that cause participation to be low in some decisions on academic campuses, for example, in the decision-making needed for the cancellation of journals.

East (1997) found that participation in decision making in academic units may be affected by outside influences. From these influences, East presents his barrier elements, used in this study to examine if faculty are not included in library decision-making opportunities for other reasons. Raffel (1974) notes that "there is no economic way to resolve differences among alternatives meeting different objectives held by different subgroups; where political conflict exists, a political solution must be found" (p. 415). In working within two groups, such as faculty and librarians, if the problem is exclusively viewed as an economic or library finance problem, we fully ignore the greater organizational decision-making issue that library decision makers must address for this complex issue.

Literature Review Conclusion

What is left unaddressed in the literature is an investigation of how faculty as decision makers consider the process of canceling journals in academic libraries. By examining the factors used to cancel journals, we may find librarians better able to operationalize the input of faculty members for the cancellation of journals.

RESEARCH METHODOLOGY

Overview of Methodology and Research Questions

The deployment of this examination of (1) how faculty participate in decisions on the cancellation of academic journals and (2) how librarians view the factors upon which journal cancellations are based, are closely tied to whether librarians use this information to assist in their decision-making process. First, the study attempts to identify the value and ranking of factors used to cancel journals. Second, the study assesses the level of involvement, participation, and decision-making barriers of faculty in library decision-making in higher education. The data collection used to answer these research questions is classed as descriptive and employs techniques of survey research. Such research is non-experimental and uses a sample of respondents to gain information without a manipulation of the subjects (McMillan & Schumacher, 1997).

Populations
Faculty Population. The sample chosen for this study consisted of faculty from 8 departments within an urban institution (four departments in the health/medical sciences and four departments in the hard sciences). To determine the population to study, the researcher examined large, urban institutions with both health/medical science schools and schools of natural, biological, and physical sciences. The research literature identifies science journals as those that are suffering greater losses in collections from the consequences of journal cancellations; therefore, science faculty were

intentionally selected for this study. After locating an urban institution with four departments of equal and representative size, a university with both types of schools (medical and science), a sample of faculty was drawn for the study. Furthermore, the institution involved was chosen because neither library was in a state of financial retrenchment, which could have skewed the results of the study.

Librarian Population. Librarians were the second sample selected for this study, consisting primarily of those involved in canceling and acquisition issues in libraries, named in the library profession as "collection development librarians." These library practitioners usually work most directly with the faculty in this study in the actual libraries used by the faculty of this study. After locating an urban institution with the aforementioned eight departments of faculty, a group of librarians were identified from which a sample for the study could be drawn. For all librarians involved, the researcher worked with the respective library directors to ensure that the appropriate members of the library staff were included in the study.

Instrumentation

The primary instrument, referred to as the Schoch and Abels (1994) factors, was used in this study and administered in a setting similar to that used by Schoch and Abels, specifically science faculty and academic librarians at a large, urban institution. The purpose of this instrument was to enlist faculty in the difficult task of assisting librarians in making the decision of what to cancel in an academic journal collection. In the early 1990s, the impetus for its design was a third round of journal cancellations in a four-year cycle at an urban institution where the faculty and library were both based in the sciences. The creators of the instrument developed lists of criteria upon which to base journal cancellations and then gave it to faculty users to assess.

As faculty were often asked to participate in the decision-making for canceling journals, the instrument creators wanted to find a tool that would assist faculty in providing input for these decisions. Faculty became a primary source for creating these factors, and the instrument creators assumed they would keep these same faculty involved in future cancellation processes.

The specific question addressed by the instrument was whether factors could be identified that would demonstrate some level of value for a specific journal title within a given library collection. This evaluation of factors and the inclusion of faculty created a group of librarians and faculty members similar to the groups in this study. While the list was created by faculty, self-selecting factors to be chosen for inclusion or exclusion in the previous study, the creators did test for validity and reliability with four faculty liaisons who were cognizant of journal cancellation issues.

The development of this instrument, namely in a science library in a university setting, makes the instrument parallel and applicable to both the population and research questions explored here. Here it was used as a way to illustrate how the examined faculty in this study view the factors upon which journals are canceled in the library they are using.

For this study, the instrument was adapted with permission to address possible factors that were not applicable during the time it was first developed (early 1990s), such as use of the Internet and electronic journals. The list of factors to rank, called *valuative factors* by the creators, was replicated in a web-based survey sent to faculty. The factors examined were costs, citedness, authority, currency, language, physical characteristics, indexing, in-library use, availability elsewhere, and "other." "Other" was a category that looked to examine new or emerging trends, such as whether this material is available in other formats in other libraries you have access to; what is your reliance on this library as your primary library resource; and the importance or seminal nature of a given journal to your current research projects.

A second instrument was developed by the researcher, with a panel of subject experts in the library field, and was sent to librarians to test the second survey for validity. The instrument included open-ended questions related to the library literature on cancellation issues, issues of communication, and organizational decision-making.

The second survey, administered only to the librarian group, asked a series of Likert-scaled questions on their self-assessment of involvement, participation, and barriers for faculty making these decisions. Three open-ended questions were asked to provide an opportunity for librarian participants to provide qualitative data on the decision-making process.

Data Collection Procedures
In the data collection portion of this study, the researcher collected data employing a six-step process designed to execute the research in this study. The first process was selecting the appropriate group for analysis. Faculty and librarians were chosen as the two groups for analysis. In this first step, all full-time faculty in eight select departments and all librarians involved in collection development activities were to be sent the survey information; second process was defining the methodology for analyzing the research

questions. A mixed methodology of quantitative and qualitative methodologies was selected; the third step was selecting the instruments applicable to the research questions; the fourth step was to transform the instruments into a web-based instrument, including the informed consent form to clarify for participants what involvement in the study entailed. Added to the web-based instrument were questions of demography, including department or library affiliation; number of years teaching or researching; time spent researching; degrees held; library job titles; and part- or full-time status. The demographic questions were posed to examine whether participants in the sample would be representative of the populations examined; the fifth step was to collect, analyze, and summarize the data, using graphical explanations of the data when applicable; the sixth and final step of the research design was drawing conclusions, making recommendations, and providing recommendations for future research.

To ensure confidentiality, as promised in the informed consent participants received, the respondents had no direct contact from the researcher. The surveys were posted on an anonymous university site, and only the name of the researcher and survey name were listed on the site. To disseminate the survey, the researcher created a list of individuals who received the survey based on their department or library affiliation, but this list was not connected to the data or survey findings in any way. This ensured that no individuals were connected in any way to specific survey findings. To ensure confidentiality, the findings were reported here in aggregate.

Data Analysis

Data analysis for this research study was conducted on the responses from the web-based survey completed by participants. The collected responses, where applicable, were entered into the statistical software program, Statistical Package for the Social Sciences (SPSS) 10.0. The participant groups for the study are (1) faculty from 140 total possible participants with $N = 18$ responding (13 percent); and (2) librarians from a total possible participants of 23 with $N = 20$ (87 percent) responding. Because the response rate was low for all faculty groups (total $N = 18$), faculty respondents here are an aggregate of all the faculty responding.

In terms of technical issues related to the data analysis, one survey was received as unreadable because of a computer error while the participant was completing the survey. All other returned surveys were deemed complete and usable. There were some surveys that did not take full advantage of the opportunity for open-ended question/explanation, but this was not determined as an incomplete survey and, therefore, not cause for exclusion. Of the remaining $N = 38$ participants, $N = 18$ (faculty) and $N = 20$ (librarian), all data were retained and used.

Since the research seeks both open-ended, qualitative responses and quantitative data, the findings will reflect these differences. For the quantitative questions, percentage responses are presented. For the qualitative questions related to research question two, posed only to the librarians, the researcher developed a list of canceling and journal collection themes for analyzing and tabulating the data from the open-ended survey questions posed to librarian participants.

The content analysis of responses included creating lists of responses from librarians and identifying themes of similar responses that the researcher could group together for each question. All of the qualitative questions posed to librarians were collected and analyzed in the same manner. After analysis, these responses were grouped by question, coded, checked by an independent researcher/practitioner for validity of coding, and presented in the findings section of this study.

Research Assumptions and Limitations

Assumptions

For this study, the following assumptions were made:

1. All members of each of the departments studied with any rank of faculty, including such appointments as assistant, associate, visiting, or adjunct professor, are involved in some level of teaching, service, and research. Therefore, their individual needs for professional literature can be assumed to be similar, although they may vary by the volume of research materials needed.
2. Neither library included was currently undergoing an intensive cancellation project at the present time, so bias should not relate to this issue.
3. Faculty members involved in the study will accurately self-identify their status within their department and within the school.
4. While publishing channels may inevitably shift, traditional academic journals still have a firm standing in academic libraries.
5. Research will not be available universally in online formats for a considerable amount of time, and, therefore, journal cancellations will most likely continue to be made by academic librarians. Insights on the process are intrinsically valuable.

Limitations

For this study, the following limitations are acknowledged. Certain limitations may affect the ability to generalize to other populations.

1. The study was to be conducted at one urban university, containing both medical sciences and hard sciences.
2. Faculty from eight departments were selected from both hard sciences and health/medical sciences; librarians were selected from both campus libraries, one health/medical science library and one general library with a hard science collection.
3. The low response rate from faculty should be taken into consideration when comparing the faculty (low) and librarian (high) participant results.
4. Participants in this study needed some level of technological ability to participate. These included the ability: to use email, to open an HTML web link and to open a PDF file attachment. Response rates could have been affected by how the survey was created, disseminated, and completed.
5. Adjunct faculty members were not necessarily under the same requirement to perform research, which possibly could reduce their needs for journals.
6. Data collection was limited to members of the university during one semester only.
7. Since this study was being conducted at one institution, the findings cannot be generalized.
8. Content analysis of the qualitative results was designed by the researcher.

RESEARCH FINDINGS

The findings presented are reported from data collected from the two surveys described previously. Both the descriptive and qualitative data sets were received from the faculty and librarians, and a third section of findings summarizes the information from librarians. This provides a basis for the discussion, conclusions, and recommendations drawn at the conclusion.

Faculty Findings

The sample chosen for this study consisted of faculty from eight departments within an urban institution. Faculty participants were asked to rank factors upon which journals should be canceled, from 1 (LEAST

Table 4. Ranking of the Factors by Faculty.

Factors	Percentage Value (%)
In-library use	83
Citedness	82
Authority	82
Other	80
Language	76
Indexing	72
Currency	66
Physical characteristics	66
Availability elsewhere	56
Costs	44

Note: Percentages represent the ranking of factors showing a preference for the factor by a ranking of 5 or higher ($N = 18$).

IMPORTANT) to 9 (MOST IMPORTANT), or to 10 (where appropriate) (Table 4).

The faculty here show by percentage, that their cumulative percentages given, a mid-range or higher (5 and higher) rank, that their preferences are: In-Library Usage (83 percent), Citedness (82 percent), and Authority (82 percent). Faculty participants were offered the option to provide comments on the factor noted as *other* in the survey. No respondents clarified what their individual response of *other* may have meant. Examples provided in the survey are listed below. Since there were no explanations offered by participants, it cannot be determined which reason participants using *other* attempted to indicate by this response.

- Other (please specify) (Include other factors, such as whether this material is available in other formats in other libraries you have access to; what is your reliance on this library as your primary library resource; importance or seminal nature of a given journal to your current research projects, etc.).

Faculty were then asked: what do you think are the three most important factors your library should consider in canceling journals?

In the discussion of the implications of this research, there is a clear match between faculty factors and what librarians list as how librarians believe they should proceed in making these tough, cancellation decisions (Table 5).

Table 5.   Factors Faculty Believe as Important for Librarians to
Consider.

Factor Groups	Percentage
	$N = 18$, 54 possible responses, 53 provided responses
	47%
• Reputation of the journal • Authority in the field • Publish in the journal	25 responses fit into this grouping of responses related to authority of the journal to the field. The comments were related to factors to evaluate, such as the reputation of the journal, the known career of the author/colleagues published, editorial board or columnist commitments, and whether on-campus colleagues were related to the journal in any capacity
	33%
• Access issues • Interlibrary loan availability • Consortium access • Personal copies of journal • Electronic database access	18 responses named access to the journal articles elsewhere as being a factor to evaluate, including access in another library on campus or in town, in other's offices on campus, or at home
	20%
• Relevant to current role	11 responses from faculty named relevancy to their current role either as an educator or researcher on campus, courses taught, whether they were advising students to read the journal, etc.

Librarian Findings

Librarian participants in this study were librarians from two academic libraries within an urban institution. As with the faculty participants, librarians were first asked to rank these factors from 1 (LEAST IMPORTANT) to 9 (MOST IMPORTANT), or to 10 (where appropriate) when considering making a recommendation regarding the cancellation of journals.

These findings show the responses by percentage for the librarian group. Examining the cumulative percentages given, a mid-range or higher (5 and higher) rank, it is found for librarians the three highest percentage rankings for factors are: Authority (100 percent), In-Library Usage (100 percent), and Costs (95 percent) (Table 6). As with faculty, librarian participants were also offered the option to provide comments on the factor noted as *other* in the survey. No respondents clarified what their individual response of *other* may

Table 6. Ranking of the Factors by Librarians.

Factors	Percentage Value (%)
Authority	100
In-library use	100
Costs	95
Indexing	85
Citedness	85
Language	70
Availability elsewhere	65
Currency	55
Physical characteristics	30
Other	35

Note: Percentages represent the ranking of factors showing a preference for the factor by a ranking of 5 or higher (*N* = 20).

have meant. Since there were no explanations offered by participants, it cannot be determined which reason participants using *other* attempted to indicate by this response (Table 7).

Librarians were asked eight questions to address the second research question of this study.

(1) What do you think *your faculty* consider as the three most important factors your library should consider in canceling journals?

(2) How would you rate your involvement in selection and cancellation of journal titles? Of the librarian participants, 70 percent of respondents in the librarian survey were individuals truly involved in these issues, seen either as their primary responsibility or that they are involved in journal concerns. Therefore, these librarians self-evaluated their involvement at 69 percent in these two categories, with a breakdown of 32 percent reporting that issues of journal cancellations were their primary responsibility and 37 percent naming themselves fully involved in journal cancellation. Librarians with positions in management and technology, such as directors or the systems librarian, may fall into categories such as "not involved" reported here, yet their inclusion is of assistance in the study, because they may have more direct access with faculty in other venues. The perceptions of what the faculty should consider as important from the librarians are reported in Table 8.

(3) How often do you discuss journal selection and cancellation concerns with faculty members? (Table 9)

Discussions with faculty on the topic of journal selection or cancellation, report that conversations with faculty regarding new journal selections were

308 JAMES H. WALTHER

Table 7. Factors Librarians Choose as the Best Factors by which to Cancel Journals.

Factor Groups	Percentage
	$N = 20$, 60 possible responses, 50 provided responses
• In-library usage	30%
	15 responses from librarians focused on library usage, such as amount of use, lack of use, and cost-relative use. Several commented that unused journals should be more closely examined as to why they are still purchased
• Reputation of the journal	26%
• Authority in the field	13 responses fit into this grouping of responses related
• Overall importance of journal title	to authority of the journal to the field. Librarians reported that the evaluation should be made on such factors as reputation of the journal, authority of the publisher and authors, importance of the articles and authors
• Cost	16%
• Cost per usage ratio	8 responses from librarians named cost a factor to closely evaluate. Amount of use in relationship to cost was reported as a representative evaluation factor for librarians
• Access issues	14%
• Interlibrary loan availability	7 responses named access to the journal articles
• Consortium access	elsewhere as a factor to consider when canceling, such as using interlibrary loan relationships, consortium access as an option after canceling a journal title
• Citation ranking	14%
• Indexing	7 responses from librarians named auxiliary factors often cited in the library literature worthy of examination. These factors included where the journal was indexed, how often the articles were cited by others; each indicating possible importance to the field

ongoing or frequent discussions for librarians (several times a year (69 percent)), whereas journal cancellation discussions were seen as more procedural, such as in an annual cancellation project or after a budget shortfall in the library. In the question asking about personal involvement in selection and cancellation of journals, librarians with positions in management and

Table 8. Assumed Factors of Faculty by Librarians.

Factor Groups	Percentage
	$N = 20$, 60 possible responses, 50 provided responses
• Reputation of the journal • Authority in the field • Publish in the journal	50% 25 responses fit into this grouping of responses related to authority of the journal to the field. The comments related to factors to evaluate, such as the reputation of the journal, the respect of the authors published, and whether the editorial board members of the journal were known on campus
• Access issues • Interlibrary loan availability • Consortium access • Personal copies of journal • Electronic database access	34% 17 responses named access to the journal articles elsewhere as being a factor that faculty members would see as a relevant reason to cancel a journal
• Relevant to current role	16% 8 responses from librarians named relevancy to the faculty member's current role either as an educator or researcher on campus, courses taught, whether they were advising students to read the journal, etc.

Table 9. Self-Evaluation of Discussions of Journal Selection and Cancellation with Faculty.

	1 or 2 Times a Week	Several Times a Month	Once in a Month (%)	Several Times a Year (%)	Once in a Year (%)	Only for Projects (%)	Never (%)
Selection			5	63		16	16
Cancellation				32	16	37	16

Note: Librarian sample size $N = 20$.

technology, such as directors or the systems librarian, may fall into categories such as "not involved" reported here, yet their inclusion is relevant here, because they may have close ties with faculty in other venues on campus.

(4) How do you incorporate the use of faculty comments and/or decisions when considering journal cancellations? (Table 10)

(5) How satisfied are you with the level of participation of the faculty in assisting in establishing the journal collection in your library? (Table 11)

As for satisfaction with faculty participation on these issues, librarians are divided in their satisfaction with levels of faculty participation. The category

Table 10.   Librarian Incorporation of Faculty Discussion Comments for
Journal Cancellations.

Representative Comments

- I incorporate their recommendations very carefully. I will only cancel a journal title if a faculty member agrees with the cancellation
- I would pass along any comments I receive from faculty to those librarians involved in decision-making
- While [I'm] not involved in cancellations, I do believe the faculty comments and usage statistics are carefully looked at when considering journal cancellations
- Faculty comments play an important part of the cancellations of journals, but cost and usage play greater roles
- I generally try to abide by the faculty wishes, budget permitting
- [I] work to achieve faculty buy-in. Sometimes [I] move money from book budgets to serials
- Their views are highly considered, but I try to balance them with the needs of the students. I have the final say on which journals are purchased and which are canceled
- I give [the faculty] dollar amounts on how much needs to be cancelled and they give me suggestions for cancellation
- Precancellation lists are routed to faculty for comment
- We generally solicit comments, ask for connections in what they are teaching; and then prioritize them in categories

Note: Librarian sample size $N = 20$.

Table 11.   Satisfaction with Participation Levels of Faculty Involvement
in Selection and Cancellation of Journals.

	Very Satisfied (%)	Somewhat Satisfied (%)	Somewhat Dissatisfied (%)	Very Dissatisfied (%)	No Opinion (%)	Do Not Know (%)
Selection	20	20	25		10	25
Cancellation	16	26	21	5	11	21

Note: Librarian sample size $N = 20$.

somewhat satisfied (26 percent) shows the highest representation for librarians by percentage. The *dissatisfied* categories (26 percent) are the same percentage of librarians participants. With these results, librarians seem more positive with how the process of selecting and purchasing new materials for the library with faculty proceeds than with the level of participation faculty are willing to dedicate to canceling journals. Librarians were offered the opportunity to offer comments on their responses (Table 12).

(6) Do you see any of the following as barriers for more participation from the faculty for journal cancellation projects in your library? (Table 13)

Table 12. Librarian Comments on Faculty Involvement in Journal Cancellations.

Representative Comments
• Participation varies by department. Some [faculty] are very involved and others barely give you the time of day, no matter how much you try and get them involved. Library contacts for the faculty departments are the low men on the totem in departments, and usually the newest professors get the job. These faculty are busily trying to get tenure and do not have the time to devote to library journal cancellations
• Generally, the faculty are OK to work with on journal cancellations, but one department fights my efforts
• Publication costs are aggravating the cancellation process, making the decision process almost an annual event. We sometimes wonder if faculty recognize the rising costs [of journals] and [the] insufficient raises to the library budget to keep tempo with publication
• Faculty often do not accept the realities of library funding, so they want to keep journals even when we show them that the budget can't sustain all the titles. In science and engineering, nearly all faculty put their own needs for titles in narrow research fields above the needs of undergrads and master's students. If the decision is either a general science title over a research title, they always want the more expensive science title to be retained
• While some faculty are interested in the "serials crisis," most faculty decline our attempts to give them the broader picture of what we are considering

Note: Librarian sample size $N = 20$.

Table 13. Librarian Perceptions of Barriers to Faculty Involvement in Decision Making.

Decision-Making Barriers	Librarian Perceptions of Faculty's Barriers (%)
Time (temporal proximity), i.e., do you believe faculty consider themselves too busy to be involved?	$N = 15$ (42)
Text (information), i.e., do you believe faculty do not have information on the depth of journal costs?	$N = 13$ (36)
Constituents (stakeholders), i.e., do you believe faculty consider others on campus should be lobbying for a larger library budget to alleviate financial problems associated with journal costs?	$N = 5$ (14)
Context (environment), i.e., do you believe faculty consider they should not be involved in library decisions?	$N = 3$ (8)

Source: Developed from East (1997).
Note: Librarian Sample Size, $N = 20$, total response possible $= 80$, since participants were allowed to "check all that applied." Of the 80 possible, 36 responses are demonstrated above in percentages and response size.

Table 14.   Faculty Familiarity with Trends in Scholarly Communication Pricing.

Level of Familiarity		Percentages
Very familiar	$N = 0$	(0%)
Somewhat familiar	$N = 8$	(42%)
Somewhat unfamiliar	$N = 7$	(37%)
Very unfamiliar	$N = 4$	(21%)

Note: Librarian sample size, $N = 20$, Size (Responding), $N = 19$.

The findings from this question highlight that librarians perceive that the constraints of non-participation from faculty for involvement in journal cancellation decisions are either because of time (42 percent) or of information (36 percent). Both of these issues were assumed by librarians as the reasons for which faculty may hold low-participation with them on journal cancellation decisions. This finding correlates well with the level of dissatisfaction that librarians generally feel regarding the amount of time faculty will dedicate to assisting in canceling journals.

(7) In your library, how familiar would you say faculty are with the trends in scholarly communication pricing, better known as "the serials crisis," throughout higher education and publishing?

As with faculty participation, librarians see in the faculty a lack of familiarity and knowledge about the actual pricing of journals (Table 14). Librarians indicate that faculty are either *somewhat unfamiliar* or *very unfamiliar* (58 percent) with how journals are actually priced. If this representation is true throughout other faculty groups, librarians must take time to increase participation in journal cancellations and selection, including discussions of journal prices. If faculty are not cognizant of the problems which librarians face in this area, it is questionable whether they will choose to work for a solution.

(8) Are there other ways you would involve faculty in your library decision-making for cancellations, if you could easily obtain participation? (Table 15)

Summary of the Findings

With the dual purpose of examining how faculty and librarians view the factors used in journal cancellations, the results of these groups indicate factor preferences that are highly similar between faculty and librarian groups. The analysis of the similarity shows faculty and librarians selecting

Table 15. Other Ways Librarians Would Involve Faculty in Decision Making for Journal Cancellations.

Representative Comments

- For me, the most helpful thing would be if the deans, university administrators, and possibly the department chairs would allow more focus in disciplines covered and taught at the university. A faculty member can evaluate what journals are important to him/her, but usually we are looking for a range of journals across a whole discipline. It gets tricky to decide to cancel a journal in a specialty field, because each faculty member has their own interest
- I would like an organized annual review of the titles supporting their department/program to determine if some titles should be canceled and others added
- Perhaps in sending a list of the journals we are considering canceling to interested faculty and soliciting their comments
- It is very important to show faculty the entire list of the library subscriptions for their department. This makes it easier for them to consider cancellations. Faculty sometimes have no idea of the expense, especially individual subscriptions are generally far lower than institutional prices
- Perhaps a committee or small group of professors in specific areas who met only 1 or 2 times a year to discuss various journal factors, specific and general. [Faculty should be] better aware of electronic alternatives
- It would be very useful to use the faculty's network of contacts to identify key publications to add to the continuing value of existing publications
- We have been trying to educate faculty on the serials crisis, but it does not seem to make much of an impact here. Any effort to change the model needs to come from the faculty, as they control the tenure process
- [We could] hold a special meeting; invite the librarians to present suggested cancellations; group discussions may help professors hear other's needs
- We work actively to educate faculty about journal pricing and e-publishing issues. I do not believe that they have a very clear understanding of the issues involved and think we make decisions arbitrarily

Note: Librarian sample size $N = 20$.

2 of the 10 factors, namely in-library usage and authority, within close ranking as the most important factor to use in cancellation decisions.

In the examination of librarian inclusion of faculty's involvement in decisions related to journal cancellation, librarians act with strategy and actually use faculty input in their decision making rather than acting arbitrarily. There is much opportunity for further examination of the inclusion of faculty in the area of library decision-making. Since the primary purpose of this research was to study the factors used to cancel journals, if it is found that journal cancellations are inevitable and faculty are in agreement on the factors by which to cancel, this study would indicate that faculty should be further considered and included in future cancellation programs. This is especially true given the similarity in the ranking of the factors.

The strength of the study is the inclusion of the qualitative open-ended questions answered by librarians regarding the process of journal cancellations. The findings of the study demonstrate how faculty and librarians both view the factors of similar importance and how this information is incorporated into cancellation decisions.

Beyond the value of the ranking of factors and the self-assessment of the process for librarians, the included qualitative data results presented here on faculty involvement may indicate examples of how to more fully include faculty in future cancellation projects in today's academic libraries, such as (1) by asking faculty for suggestions for cancellation and (2) identifying which factors faculty believe are important elements by which to evaluate journal titles.

SUMMARY OF FINDINGS, CONCLUSIONS, AND RECOMMENDATIONS

This study attempts to provide a bridge between previous research studies that had only looked at librarian or faculty groups individually, without comparing each group's assessment of the factors used to cancel journals, and their insights into the process. The study describes how faculty and librarians view the factors used to make journal cancellation decisions and how librarians use faculty input.

Conclusions of the Findings

* Faculty and librarians indicate highly similar factor preferences upon which to cancel journals; namely two of ten factors, in-library usage and authority, were named important factors by both groups.

With an assessment of the factors seen through both a faculty and librarian lens, this study descriptively documents how commonly these factors are viewed by both the users and collectors of information. Future collaborative decision-making opportunities between librarians and faculty will further determine whether other groups of librarians and faculty agree upon the use of these factors, and to what degree.

These two factors are especially relevant to examine in the process of cancellation. Librarians and faculty clearly wanted to know if purchased journals are being used (in-library usage) and if these materials are of contextual, subjective value (authority) to library users. The decision to cancel journals grounded on these two factors call librarians into an important place in the canceling of journals with faculty and assert that an open dialogue between these two groups is needed to retain and cancel journals. Because these two factors must be evaluated in different ways, librarians must make decisions with strategic, in-library use of information and discuss with faculty as which journals represent the authoritative research in their area.

• While similarity and agreement existed in the results for these two factors, costs held a different ranking from the faculty and librarian perspectives. These differences present a crucial disconnect between librarians and others in higher education that must be resolved for working on journal cancellations as group decision.

Beyond the findings of the similarity between these two groups in this one decision-making process in higher education, this study could present issues and ideas for other decision-making opportunities in the academy. This study identified the librarians' interest in further faculty participation in decision making and in examining new ways of involving faculty. Surveying users, including faculty in an organized annual review of journal titles and educational seminars for faculty on scholarly communication issues are just a few of the ways librarians suggested to start involving faculty more deeply in library decision-making.

Librarians must work to develop ways to further inform faculty of the annual escalation of journal costs and why these issues must be continually re-examined. Further participation and interest in examining new ways of involving faculty in decision-making were identified in this study from the librarians. Due to this divergence in the interest of examining cost as a factor for faculty, librarians offer that they would like to explore other ways of involving faculty in an organized annual review of journal titles via educational seminars for faculty on scholarly communication issues.

• Librarians are using information solicited from users, in this case faculty, with strategy.

Even if more active participation is not fully achieved, librarians demonstrated they use the current faculty input they are receiving and seem somewhat receptive to expanding the process of faculty inclusion even further. The findings of this study portray a type of institution worthy of engaged inquiry of relationships among decision makers in higher education, especially in light of the similarity of the factors used to assess and make decisions in this setting.

Research Question One

- The preconceived notions of canceling journals only due to cost is not held in agreement by either groups, yet authority of the journal and in-library usage are two highly important factors for both groups.

To examine research question one, whether the factors used by librarians to cancel journals are sufficient enough to inform librarians in the decision-making process, one must look at the demonstrative results given by both groups. The similarity in what each group designates as relevant to assess includes the faculty's naming (1) in-library usage, (2) citedness, and (3) authority; and the librarian's naming (1) authority, (2) in-library usage, and (3) costs.

Important to note is the finding that cost is one of the top three factors for librarians, but one of the lowest factors for faculty. Since costs drive the need for cancellations, librarians must continue to communicate to faculty the depth of the cost problem more fully and forcefully. Annual, journal cancellation reviews could become one of the many ways librarians could work to further educate faculty on the cost aspects of these problems.

Also, it is worthwhile to point out other lowest factors of concern for each group, including faculty reporting costs (44 percent), calculating the mid-range and higher rankings, and librarians naming the physical characteristics (30 percent), using the same mid-range and higher calculation. With these findings, it can be understood in the context of the terms and instrument ranking procedures where the interest of both groups lie.

In the second assessment of participant's preferences, respondents were allowed to examine factors in their own terms. The comments in this section give rich insight as a verification of how important the factors of in-library usage, authority, citedness, cost, and access elsewhere are to both groups.

- The perceptions of the faculty ranking by librarians were similar to their actual responses.

The similarities between what librarians assumed faculty would name as their top factors are almost a mirror representation of how faculty actually reported and ranked their key issues for decision making. An essential difference in these findings is that librarians examine more closely the issue of indexing and citation ranking, a common valuative factor for the information profession.

- Indexing, impact, or citation rankings are not highly ranked by faculty.

Indexing, as a factor, can be seen as essential to the profession of librarianship and tied to assisting in access to journals. Faculty and librarians both named their broad factors of concern about journals, specifically where their use of journal is relevant to (1) courses currently taught on campus, (2) journals directly related to research currently being conducted on campus, (3) materials faculty were either referring to students in class, or (4) materials that librarians were assisting students to locate, as a result of faculty comments and referrals.

Overall and with striking similarity, the findings of the survey questions tied to research question one demonstrate measurable similarity in how faculty use and rank factors to consider when canceling journals and how librarians use and rank these same factors.

Research Question Two

The discussion of research question two is best placed in the context of the research literature previously examining these issues. This study works to confirm and illuminate past research, and also to use the results to inform librarian practitioners in new ways.

- Due to similarity in understanding the decisions to be made by librarians, faculty should be included despite perceived barriers.

On the issue of decision making, this study confirmed what others in the literature have previously reported. In examining librarian perceptions of barriers to faculty involvement in decision making, this study highlights the perceived constraints of non-participation from faculty in journal cancellation decisions. The two highest percentages, time (42 percent) and information (36 percent), were seen by librarians as the reasons faculty would have non- or low-participation with librarians on journal cancellation decisions.

- Faculty participation must be increased in academic library decisions to find a common ground in reaching decisions.

The reported satisfaction with faculty participation levels of involvement in selection and/or cancellation of journals shows that faculty involvement in the process of selection and cancellation could always be enhanced. Past organizational assessments have focused on participation and decision-making failures, such as those defined by the organizational characteristics of a "garbage-can decision-making process," including the high energy used on the decision process, the lengthy time needed to make a decision, and the fluidity or randomness of participation (Cohen, March, & Olsen, 1972).

The literature does not offer this model as a highly productive model for libraries or institutions of higher education (Bell, 1999). In this study, time and information were seen as perceived issues for faculty. If librarians think faculty members are too busy or do not have enough information, such as information on costs, they might not include faculty in their decision processes. This study worked to show the possibilities for the integration of their decision interests based on the similarities in their rankings of the factors supplied.

Librarians report that most faculty are somewhat uninformed on the issues of journal costs. Faculty are asked to provide input for a decision on an issue they do not have much information on. Faculty familiarity on the issues of cost is perceived by librarians to be low, but essential to decision making. Librarians reported in their experience that faculty are either somewhat unfamiliar (37 percent) or very unfamiliar (21 percent) with actual journal costs. To enhance the decision-making value and input, faculty must be better informed on the issues of costs and the need for journal cancellations.

- Similarity in ranking these factors could represent an environment that could encourage other group decision-making opportunities.

This study finds librarians and faculty working in a situation in which decision makers are presented with a variety of decision options. Having an infinite variation of decisions, without prescriptions or set guidelines to follow, a more optimal decision process is provided (Allison, 1971). Especially in this unique setting of academic libraries, where libraries are the conceptual ground floor upon which a research university is built, libraries are responsible to both administration and research user groups (Budd, 1998). Any opportunity for flexibility in the methods to reach decisions may improve strategic decision-making. The findings here on the similarity in value of the factors should encourage library practitioners and faculty to continue examining the value of working together.

- Librarians are not arbitrary in how they use information from faculty, especially in the incorporation of comments on canceling journals.

A final finding highlights the effective usage of faculty input in journal cancellations decisions. Comments from participants demonstrate that librarians are not arbitrary in their incorporation or usage of faculty comments in given decisions on journal cancellation. Representative comments from librarians on how they incorporate faculty input in journal cancellation decisions include:

- "abide by faculty wishes as much as the budget permits"
- "...achieve faculty buy-in"
- "solicit comments (and) prioritize them."

Librarians examined here were taking careful consideration of this information. The comments on faculty involvement, both current and ideal levels, show considerable interest in more fully involving faculty in library decisions. Each of the comments connects to previous research in this area, underscoring the importance of canceling journals as an opportunity to discuss and market these concerns with faculty (Barstow, 1993; Madison, 1999). Even studies in the early stages of the serials crisis point to the need for faculty buy-in and the continual development of faculty–librarian relationships (Stenstrom & McBride, 1979; White, 1980). This study reconfirms this need. In the context of how much worse the situation of journal costs has become in recent years, it is only more fitting that these partnerships be held in higher regard today.

RECOMMENDATIONS TO LIBRARIANS

Librarian Usage of Cancellation Factors

- Understand and utilize the possible similarity of faculty and librarians in evaluating journal cancellation factors.

An essential finding of the study is the matched assessment of faculty and librarians in their evaluation of the factors. In the findings of this study, the similarities of the top rankings of both groups show the opportunity for further assistance with these difficult decisions in academic libraries. What librarians working with journal cancellations can learn from these findings is what researchers have theorized and grappled with before.

- Examine closely rankings, such as impact, or citation rankings, since faculty and recent research do not positively rank these factors.

New research in the area of citation value elicits a recommendation for librarians to closely examine how they are using citation values or citation indexing as a factor when considering evaluating a journal for cancellation. Faculty do not highly rank these values as a cancellation factor. Recent research notes caution when relying on citation factors, questioning the possible misuse of this bibliometric application in relationship to how these are rated by clinical practitioners and scientific researchers (Saha, Saint, & Christakis, 2003). Previous research has argued that library practitioners must look to a variety of factors rather than focusing on canceling journals because of one factor (Bader & Thompson, 1989), and, in this study, cost is not even the highest ranked factor by either faculty or librarian participants. Therefore, this study recommends examining a portfolio of factors, such as those used here.

While cost should not be the primary factor evaluated, a journal's "impact factor," which measures the frequency with which an article was cited by others (Garfield, 1972), would not be the seemingly automatic application of relevancy or gauge of relevancy for selecting journals for purchase, cancellation, research, or even article submission for faculty that it may be used as (Hecht, Hecht, & Sandberg, 1998).

- Realize that other factors exist and that a series of factors must be examined before canceling journals.

Cost, shelf-use, faculty need, and connection with curriculum were all additional essential factors named in this study as relevant to librarians and faculty. Impact factors are only bibliometric indicators that demonstrate the half-life citation value of a journal or article (Garfield & Sher, 1963). In the digital library environments, online usage will skew online articles with a higher measurement, implying something that the measurement was never intended to accomplish: measure scientific quality (Frank, 2003). By design, the factor was not intended to be used as a cancellation indicator. This study should further call into question their usage and recommend that other factors be evaluated by faculty and librarians.

RECOMMENDATIONS TO FUTURE RESEARCHERS

Faculty Involvement in Library Decision-Making

- Allow for institutional growth and advancement by involving faculty throughout the canceling process because of their need for academic research collections.

In concluding this study, it is worthwhile to look at the theoretical undercurrents of this research, the ties to organizational decision-making. As an example of organizational learning, the decision-making opportunities found in academic libraries present themselves as an example of worker-created *intelligence*, which Carnevale (1991) offers as approximately 60 percent of today's competitive advantages in organizations. If such examples of best practices are being developed in academic libraries, and more broadly in higher education, these lessons learned should be more closely examined in the future. Carnevale (2003) presents that this inwardly focused learning of our organizations is found in organizations in which (1) real problems are present; (2) people examine the issues; (3) people learn from an existing problem; and (4) individuals report back to the group with problem-solving strategies. This study attempts to illuminate all four of these elements found in academic libraries that are confronted with the journal problem, and presents a model for dealing with other current or future problems occurring in the academy.

- Assume that organizations can learn from self-examination and work for solutions to problems within the organization.

Robson (1993) and Argyris (1993) examine the practical approaches to learning within organizations and the role that action research can play in allowing solutions to real problems to be found. In the seemingly simplistic model of action research: action (new behavior), data gathering, discussion/feedback, (more) action, and the repetition of cycles until problems are resolved, Burke (1994) presents the model that is commonly used to explain how librarians approach the journal cancellation process effectively with the use of faculty. While Carnevale (2003) points out that action research is applied research, bound by the organizations in which it is found, the search for solutions is a true opportunity to look within to resolve difficult problems in higher education today.

Faculty Input in Academic Library Decision-Making

- More directly provide for opportunities for faculty to become more fully involved in the academic library and the internal decision-making process.

Recommendations from librarian participants in this study offer a rich dialogue that could be opened on the topic of journal costs and cancellations in higher education. Recommendations for suggestions of how librarians could strategically include faculty in the future are:

- Create an annual review of journal titles by title, including cost of the journal and disseminate the information to departmental groups on campus.
- Show faculty members the entire list of journal subscriptions, both of their department and the overall campus, so they can see the various range in expenditures.

- Introduce faculty members to electronic alternatives in publishing opportunities on the Internet, which will further become an issue for tenure and promotion in higher education.
- Communicate with faculty members through multiple venues, such as meetings, group discussions, seminars, library newsletters, and web pages that librarians are working to maintain productive journal collections for faculty members, and are not acting randomly when canceling titles in the library.

In examining the use of information for decision making, Browne (1993) points out how decisions makers, such as the librarians and faculty in this study, may have ample opportunity for the best of intentions, yet in practice, when making final decisions, present and use different information from what is expected. These differences may include the following:

- Decision makers might not use the information collected as a basis for choosing the alternative that is implemented, although they may have intended to.
- Decision makers use information for general enlightenment and to gain a background understanding of the context in which the decision is being made.
- Decision makers are aware of the potential for using information politically to establish a case for additional resources.
- Decision makers use information as a symbol of rationality and, by extension, as an indicator of quality in decision making.

In terms of policy implementation for the decisions related to canceling journals, several of these hold true for how librarians may proceed in practice, rather than in theory. Several of the open-ended responses from librarians in this study found the gathering of faculty comments as essentially worthwhile, but the final decision in collections and journal cancellations were essentially seen as librarian decisions. As librarians continue to search for faculty input in decision making, they must also strive to indicate how much this information is needed and used.

Communication and Information in Higher Education

- Encourage researchers and librarians to further explore the implications for theory and practice of this study.

As the questions posed to librarians were to gain data on how often and how useful faculty/librarian communication was in the process of canceling journals, the issue of communication and decision making of multiple groups in higher education must be further examined. The similarity in ranking the decision factors as an example of decision making in higher education was a worthwhile pursuit; one worthy of having the findings communicated. The opportunities for collaboration in decision making and the ability to create best practices in higher education seem worthy of the endeavor.

In examining higher education's ability to communicate knowledge and information within an organization, it is found that communication may be good within some groups, while assumed powerlessness or "blame cultures" may exist in other units in the university (Dhillon, 2001). As in this current study, information provided to groups to assist in decision making is suggested as a means to confront the differences in groups within a campus. Foster (1998) offers specific ways to provide information, and also notes the preferred use of all types of media in which to communicate information:

- Face to face (verbal communication)
- Print-based material
- Electronic forms (Intranet and E-mail).

The examples of faculty and librarians working together matches well with the open-ended comments from the librarians in this study, who are looking for avenues of better communication and ways to provide relevant information to faculty on the serials crisis.

Electronic Journals

- Consider the constant change of scholarly communication and the rise of electronic communication, as new models of publishing.

As librarians examine other opportunities for access to academic journals, a growing viability is the option of searchable databases from commercial document delivery services, increased and different applications to interlibrary loan, and full-text online databases (Everett, 1993; Gessesse, 1994; Hughes, 1997). While not yet seen as a perfect solution to the reductions of journal collections, Besemer (1993) offers suggestions for the implementation of electronic journals that can be seen as a prescriptive model for success in some libraries. In their evaluation, librarians should:

- Evaluate the political model of their institution. Is the library seen as an arm of administration or is it seen as more directly tied to academic departments and the curriculum?
- Gather support of the university administration for new cost-saving initiatives to provide research content.

- Provide online journal-use workshops to develop the technical ability for usage.
- Assess usage levels and costs of these new journal services.

As the finances of the journal market continue to be of prime concern to administrators, frontline managers, and library users, the situation of journal cancellations may remain constant for quite some time. However, this study presents the interesting finding of a similarity of thought between librarians and faculty and how they approach the factors chosen upon which to make cancel decisions. It is assumed at the conclusion of this study that such decisions will become increasingly more difficult to approach. It is hoped that the study assists in informing librarians how to proceed.

However, one factor that may prove to change or shift the interrelated issues discussed here is that of electronic journals. Could electronic journals, with their desktop and cover-to-cover access, shift this entire situation? Librarians point out that technical capabilities are better than ever and present new options to dealing with the problems of providing scholarly communication at predictable cost (Albanese, 2001). A closer examination is worthwhile. Whether or not these publication channels become solutions or just other options for materials to use and purchase remains to be seen.

At present, the scholarly journal market looks like a bleak and grim reality that few would wish to involve themselves in; yet, scholarly communication is constantly shifting and reshaping itself into new models of providing information to the world's scholars. Several opportunities for other channels of publishing and research now exist with emerging electronic publishing venues. The mix of scholarly communication opportunities today presents a new reality for scholars, similar to the way scholarly societies first started networking and publishing with the first science journal, *Royal Society*, founded in London in 1660 and chartered in 1662 (Birch, 1968). But as librarians struggle to find solutions to budget shortfalls and journal cost increases, these materials present current realities of providing research-level materials to users.

Suggestions on Research Procedures

As a note on the research procedures and recommendations for additional research, future researchers need not alter the Schoch and Abels (1994) instrument as used in this study. As mentioned, participants were offered the opportunity to select an additional comment during the ranking of the factors, noted as *other* in Survey Question I in both surveys. Even though the factor was used, the researcher could in no way examine why the participants would have selected this *other* factor, beyond the suggested examples of:

- whether this material is available in other formats in other libraries to which you have access;
- what is your reliance on this library as your primary library resource; and
- importance or seminal nature of a given journal to your current research projects.

Since respondents using this factor did not clarify what their response should be associated with, it was not seen as an additional factor. However, naming an additional factor, such as these above examples or capturing the issue of electronic journals in the marketplace would be a worthwhile pursuit, as this study made no attempt to consider the decision-making element of canceling a print journal for an online journal.

FINAL THOUGHTS

A review of past studies examining the procedural aspects of canceling journals identifies a gap in the agreement between librarians and faculty in specific factors used for canceling journals. This research study examined the factors found to be most commonly used as factors upon which to evaluate journals for cancellation.

Using a previously developed factor-ranking instrument, this study surveyed faculty and librarian groups to identify whether factors used in journal cancellations are, from the perspective of faculty and librarians, of equal importance in informing librarians for their decision-making process for canceling journals. The study also examined whether faculty input gathered in the decision-making process is used by librarians in their decision making for journal cancellations.

The study expanded previous research in this area by including two libraries and two library user groups (faculty). The study included qualitative questions answered by librarians regarding the process of journal cancellation, offering an opportunity for librarian participants to examine their own process of journal cancellation in their given library settings. The study descriptively describes how faculty and librarians both view the factors of similar importance. In addition to the ranking of factors and the general self-assessment of the process for librarians, the study presents how faculty involvement may be further expanded in future journal cancellation projects

or in other decision-making processes. This exploration into the relationships of how these cancellation factors are viewed by both groups is an
examination that is worthy of further study.

REFERENCES

Albanese, A. R. (2001). Revolution or evolution. *Library Journal, 126*(18), 48–51.
Allison, G. T. (1971). *Essence of decision.* Boston, MA: Little, Brown.
Argyris, C. (1993). *Knowledge for action: A guide to overcoming barriers to organizational
    change.* A Joint Publication in the Jossey-Bass Management Series and the Jossey-Bass
    Social and Behavior Science Series. San Francisco, CA: Jossey-Bass.
Association of Research Libraries. (1989). *Report of the ARL serials pricing.* Washington, DC:
    Association of Research Libraries.
Association of Research Libraries, the Association of American Universities, & the Pew Higher
    Education Roundtable. (1998). To publish and perish. *Policy Perspectives, 7*, Retrieved
    June 19, 2002 from http://www.arl.org/scomm/pew/pewrept.html
Astle, D. L. (1993). Libraries and the use of price studies. *Serials Librarian, 23*(3/4), 129–136.
Astle, D., & Hamaker, C. (1988). Journal publishing: Pricing and structural issues in the 1930s
    and the 1980s. *Advances in Serials Management: A Research Annual, 2*, 1–36.
Atkinson, R. (1993). Crisis and opportunity: Reevaluating acquisitions budgeting in an age of
    transition. *Journal of Library Administration, 19*(2), 33–55.
Atkinson, R. (1995). The academic library collection in an on-line environment. In: B. P. Lynch
    (Ed.), *Information technology and the remaking of the university library. New directions
    for higher education* (Vol. 90, pp. 43–62). San Francisco, CA: Jossey-Bass.
Bader, S. A., & Thompson, L. L. (1989). Analyzing in-house journal utilization: An added
    dimension in decision making. *Bulletin of the Medical Library Association, 77*, 216–218.
Baldridge, J. V. (1971). *Power and conflict in the university.* New Haven, CT: Wiley.
Barstow, S. (1993). Quickly selecting serials for cancellation. *Technical Services Quarterly,
    10*(4), 29–42.
Bell, S. J. (1999). Acquiring a library automation system: An analysis of a strategic decision
    event. *Advances in Library Administration and Organization, 16*, 263–299.
Bennion, B. C. (1994). Why the science journal crisis? *Bulletin of the American Society for
    Information Science, 20*(3), 25–26.
Bentley, R. J., & Blackburn, R. T. (1990). Changes in academic research performance over time:
    A study of institutional accumulative advantage. *Research in Higher Education, 31*,
    327–345.
Berberet, J., & McMillin, L. (2002). The American professoriate in transition. *ACB Priorities,
    18*, 8–15.
Besemer, S. P. (1993). Addressing the serials problem with simple online searching and docu-
    ment delivery: Making lemonade from lemons. *Proceedings of the Sixth International
    Conference on New Information Technology, 6*, 9–16.
Bieber, J. P., & Blackburn, R. T. (1993). Faculty research productivity 1972–1988: Develop-
    ment and application of constant units of measure. *Research in Higher Education, 34*,
    551–567.
Birch, T. (1968). *The history of the Royal Society of London.* New York: Royal Society.

Birnbaum, R. (1992). *How academic leadership works.* San Francisco, CA: Jossey-Bass.

Blackburn, R. T., & Lawrence, J. H. (1996). *Faculty at work.* Baltimore, MD: Johns Hopkins University.

Blau, P. (1970). A formal theory of differentiation in organizations. *American Sociological Review, 35*(2), 201–218.

Born, K., & Van Orsdel, L. (2001). Searching for serials utopia: Periodical price survey 2001. *Library Journal, 126*(7), 53–58.

Bourne, C. P., & Gregor, D. (1975). Planning serials cancellations and cooperative collection development in the health sciences: Methodology and background information. *Bulletin of the Medical Library Association, 63*(4), 366–377.

Branin, J. J., & Case, M. (1998). Reforming scholarly publishing in the sciences: A librarian perspective. *Notices of the AMS, 45*(4), 475–486.

Broadus, R. N. (1985). A proposed method for eliminating titles from periodical subscription lists. *College and Research Libraries, 46*(1), 30–35.

Broude, J. (1978). Journal deselection in an academic environment: A comparison of faculty and librarian choices. *The Serials Librarian, 3*(2), 147–166.

Browne, M. (1993). *Organizational decision-making and information.* Norwood, NJ: Ablex.

Budd, J. M. (1998). *The academic library: Its context, its purpose, and its operation.* Littleton, CO: Libraries Unlimited.

Burke, W. W. (1994). *Organizational development: A process of learning and change* (2nd ed.). Upper Saddle River, NJ: Pearson, Addison-Wesley.

Cameron, K. S. (1985). Investigating the casual association between unionism and organizational effectiveness. *Research in Higher Education, 23*, 387–411.

Carnevale, A. P. (1991). *America and the new economy: How new competitive standards are radically changing American workplaces.* Jossey-Bass Management Series. San Francisco, CA: Jossey-Bass.

Carnevale, D. G. (2003). *Organizational development in the public sector.* Cambridge, MA: Westview.

Case, M. (1998). Views of the current marketplace for scholarly journals. *ARL Bimonthly Newsletter of Research Library Issues, 200*, Washington, DC: Association of Research Libraries, Office of Scholarly Communication. Retrieved July 13, 2002 from http://www.arl.org/newsltr/200/200toc.html

Case, M. (2001). The impact of serials costs on library collections. *ARL Bimonthly Newsletter of Research Library Issues, 218*, Washington, DC: Association of Research Libraries, Office of Scholarly Communication. Retrieved October 13, 2001 from http://www.arl.org/newsltr/218/218toc.html

Chaffee, E. E. (1983). *Rational decision-making in higher education.* Boulder, CO: National Center for Higher Education Management Systems.

Chait, R. (1979). College mission statements. *Science, 205*, 957.

Chrzastowski, T. E., & Schmidt, K. A. (1993). Surveying the damage: Academic library serials cancellations. *College and Research Libraries, 54*(2), 93–102.

Chrzastowski, T. E., & Schmidt, K. A. (1997). The serials cancellation crisis: National trends in academic library serials cancellations. *Library Acquisitions: Practice and Theory, 21*(4), 431–443.

Clark, L. (1987). Material costs and collection development in academic libraries. *Journal of Library Administration, Pricing and Costs of Monographs and Serials: National and International Issues, 8*, 97–109.

Cohen, M. D., & March, J. G. (1974). *Leadership and ambiguity: The American college president*. New York: McGraw-Hill.

Cohen, M. D., March, J. G., & Olsen, J. P. (1972). Garbage can model of organizational choice. *Administrative Science Quarterly, 7*(1), 1–25.

Cox, J. E. (1998). The changing economic model of scholarly publishing: Uncertainty, complexity, multimedia serials. *Library Acquisitions: Practice and Theory, 22*(2), 161–166.

Create change. (2000). Retrieved July 20, 2001 from http://db.arl.org/journals

Creswell, J. W. (1986). Concluding thoughts: Observing, promoting, evaluating and reviewing research performance. In: J. W. Creswell (Ed.), *Measuring faculty research performance. New Directions for Institutional Research* (Vol. 50, pp. 87–102). San Francisco, CA: Jossey-Bass.

Cummings, A. M., Witte, M. L., Bowen, W. G., Lazarus, L. O., & Ekman, R. H. (1992). University libraries and scholarly communication: A study prepared for The Andrew W. Mellon Foundation. Washington, DC: Association of Research Libraries for The Andrew W. Mellon Foundation.

Dain, P. (1990). Scholarship, higher education, and libraries in the United States: Historical questions and quests. In: P. Dain & J. Y. Cole (Eds), *Libraries and scholarly communication in the United States: The historical dimension* (pp. 1–44). Westport, CT: Greenwood.

Dhillon, J. K. (2001). Challenges and strategies for improving the quality of information in a university setting: A case study. *Total Quality Management, 12*(2), 167–177.

Dow, R. F., Meringolo, S., & St. Clair, G. (1995). Academic collections in a changing environment. In: G. B. McCabe & R. J. Person (Eds), *Academic libraries: Their rationale and role in American higher education* (pp. 103–123). Westport, CT: Greenwood.

Drucker, P. (1966). *The effective executive*. Boston, MA: Harper & Row.

Durey, P. (1976). Weeding serials subscriptions in a university library. *Collection Management, 1*(3–4), 91–94.

East, W. B. C. (1997). Decision-making strategies in educational organizations. *The Journal of Physical Education, Recreation and Dance, 68*(4), 39–45.

Everett, D. (1993). Full-text online databases and document delivery in an academic library: Too little, too late. *Online, 17*(2), 22–25.

Fallon, M., & Young, L. L. (1983). Evaluating a periodicals collection. *Community and Junior College Libraries, 2*, 3–8.

Farrell, D. (1981). Why is there a crisis in collection management? *Foundations in Library and Information Science, 17*, 279–286.

Foster, A. (1998). Grasping the tacit knowledge nettle. *Knowledge Management, 1*(April), 32.

Francq, C. (1994). Bottoming out the bottomless pit with journal usage/cost relational index. *Technical Services Quarterly, 11*(4), 13–26.

Frank, M. (2003). Impact factors: Arbiter of excellence. *Journal of the Medical Library Association, 91*(1), 4–6.

Fry, B. M., & White, H. S. (1976). *Publishers and libraries: A study of scholarly and research journals*. Lexington, MA: D.C. Heath.

Fry, B. M., & White, H. S. (1979). Impact on economic pressures on American libraries and their decisions concerning scholarly and research journal acquisition and retention. *Library Acquisitions, 3*, 153–237.

Fussler, H. H., & Simon, J. L. (1961). *Patterns in the use of books in large research libraries*. Chicago, IL: University of Chicago Press.

Gardner, J. (1991). The challenge of maintaining research collections in the 1990s. *Journal of Library Administration, 14*(3), 17–25.

Garfield, E. (1972). Citation analysis as a tool in journal evaluation. *Science, 178,* 471–479.

Garfield, E., & Sher, I. H. (1963). New factors in the evaluation of scientific literature through citation indexing. *American Document, 14*(3), 195–201.

Garvin, D. A., & Roberto, M. A. (2001). What you don't know about making decisions. *Harvard Business Review, 79*(8), 108–119.

Gessesse, K. (1994). Scientific communication, electronic access and document delivery: The new challenge to the science engineering reference librarian. *International Information and Library Review, 26*(4), 341–349.

Giesecke, J. (1993). Recognizing multiple decision-making models: A guide for managers. *College and Research Libraries, 54*(2), 102–114.

Grefsheim, S., Bader, S., & Meredith, P. (1983). User involvement in journal de-selection. *Collection Management, 5*(1/2), 43–52.

Hamaker, C. (1993). Toward a calculus of collection development. *Journal of Library Administration, 19*(2), 101–123.

Hanson, R. K. (1981). Serials deselection: A dreadful dilemma. In: S. H. Lee (Ed.), *Serials collection development: Choices and strategies* (pp. 43–59). Ann Arbor, MI: Pierian.

Harrington, S. A., & Grice, I. M. (1992). Serials cancellation: A continuing saga. *The Serials Librarian, 23*(1/2), 99–112.

Hawkins, B. L. (1998). The unsustainability of the traditional library and the threat to higher education. In: B. L. Hawkins & P. Battin (Eds), *The Mirage of continuity: Reconfiguring academic resources for the 21st century* (pp. 129–153). Washington, DC: Council on Library and Information Resources and the Association of American Universities.

Hawthorn, M. (1991). Serials selection and deselection: A survey of North American academic libraries. *The Serials Librarian, 21*(1), 29–46.

Hecht, F., Hecht, B. K., & Sandberg, A. A. (1998). The journal "impact factor": A misnamed, misleading, misused measure. *Cancer Genet Cytogenet, 104,* 77–81.

Hubbard, J., & Williams, B. W. (1989). Basing journal cancellation decisions on usage data: The Wichita State University Libraries' experience. In: *Enter Save Delete...: Libraries Pioneering Into the Next Century, Proceedings of the Mountain Plains Library Association, Academic Library Section Research Forum Joint Conference* (pp. 60–81).

Hughes, J. (1997). Can document delivery compensate for reduced serials holdings? A life sciences library perspective. *College and Research Libraries, 58*(5), 421–431.

Johnson, S. (1983). Serial deselection in university libraries: The next step. *Library Acquisitions: Practice and Theory, 7,* 239–246.

Kaplan, L. (1977). On decision sharing in libraries: How much do we know? *College and Research Libraries, 38*(1), 25–31.

Kaser, R. T. (1995). Secondary information services—mirrors of scholarly communication: Forces and trends. *Publishing Research Quarterly, 11*(3), 10–24.

Kohl, D. (2001). *Scholarly communication today: What's wrong and what together can we do about it.* Washington, DC: Association of Research Libraries. Retrieved July 10, 2002 from http://www.arl.org/sparc

Kotter, W. R. (1999). Bridging the great divide: Improving relations between librarians and classroom faculty. *Journal of Academic Librarianship, 25*(4), 294–303.

Kovacs, B. (1989). The impact of weeding on collection development: Sci-tech collections vs. general collections. *Collection Management in Sci-Tech Libraries, 9*(3), 25–36.

Kyrillidou, M. (2000). Journal costs: Current trends & future scenarios for 2020. *ARL Bimonthly Report, 210,* Retrieved June 20, 2001 from http://www.arl.org/newsltr/210/costs.html

Lawal, I. O. (2002). Science resources: Does the Internet make them cheaper, better? *The Bottom Line: Managing Library Finances, 15*(3), 116–124.

Lynch, B. (1976). The role of middle managers in libraries. *Advances in Librarianship, 6,* 253–277.

Lynch, B. P. (1990). Management theory and organizational structure. In: M. J. Lynch (Ed.), *Academic libraries: Research perspectives* (pp. 215–233). Chicago, IL: American Library Association.

Madison, O. M. A. (1999). From journal cancellation to library strategic visioning faculty leadership. *Journal of Library Administration, 28*(4), 57–70.

Marks, K. E., Nielsen, S. P., Petersen, H. C., & Wagner, P. E. (1991). Longitudinal study of scientific journal prices in a research library. *College and Research Libraries, 52,* 125–138.

Mattlage, A. (1999). Perspectives on: Networked scholarly communication. *Journal of Academic Librarianship, 25*(4), 313–321.

McCabe, M. J. (2001). The impact of publisher mergers on journal prices: Theory and evidence. *The Serials Librarian, 40*(1/2), 157–166.

McCarthy, P. (1994). Serial killers: Academic libraries respond to soaring costs. *Library Journal, 119,* 41–44.

McMillan, J. H., & Schumacher, S. (1997). *Research in education: A conceptual introduction* (4th ed.). New York: Longman.

Metz, P. (1992). Thirteen steps to avoiding bad luck in a serials collection project. *Journal of Academic Librarianship, 18*(2), 76–82.

Metz, P., & Cosgriff, J. (2000). Building a comprehensive serials decision database at Virginia Tech. *College and Research Libraries, 61*(1), 324–334.

Milne, S. J. (1990). Periodicals and space constraints. *Indiana Libraries, 9*(2), 55–58.

National Enquiry into Scholarly Communication (1979). *Scholarly Communication.* The Report. Baltimore: Johns Hopkins University Press.

Neame, L. (1986). Periodicals cancellation: Making a virtue out of necessity. *The Serials Librarian, 10*(3), 33–42.

Nisonger, T. E. (1998). *Management of serials in libraries.* Littleton, CO: Libraries Unlimited.

Nisonger, T. E. (2000). Use of the *Journal Citation Reports* for serials management in research libraries: An investigation of the effect of self-citation on journal rankings in library and information science and genetics. *College and Research Libraries, 61*(3), 263–275.

Nutt, P. C. (1990). Preventing decision debacles. *Technological Forecasting and Social Change, 38,* 159–194.

Odiorne, G. S. (1969). *Management decisions by objectives.* Englewood Cliffs, NJ: Prentice-Hall.

Okerson, A. (1986). Periodical prices: A history and discussion. *Advances in Serials Management: A Research Annual, 1,* 101–134.

Okerson, A., & Stubbs, K. (1991). The library "doomsday machine". *Publishers Weekly, 238,* 36–37.

Paul, H. (1984). Serials: Higher prices vs. shrinking budgets. *The Serials Librarian, 9*(2), 3–12.

Perkins, D. L. (1990). Weed it and reap. *The Serials Librarian, 18*(1/2), 131–140.

Raffel, J. A. (1974). From economic to political analysis of library decision-making. *College and Research Libraries, 35,* 412–423.

Richards, D. T. (1991). Monographic collections in scientific libraries: Sacrificial lambs in the library lea? *Journal of Library Administration, 14*(3), 27–47.

Robson, C. (1993). *Real world research: A resource for social scientists and practitioner-researchers* (2nd ed.). Oxford, UK: Blackwell.

Saha, S., Saint, S., & Christakis, D. A. (2003). Impact factor: A valid measure of journal quality? *Journal of the Medical Library Association, 91*(1), 42–46.

Sapp, G., & Watson, P. G. (1989). Librarian-faculty relations during a period of journals cancellations. *Journal of Academic Librarianship, 15*, 285–289.

Schoch, N. (1994). Relationship between citation frequency and journal costs: A comparison between pure and applied science disciplines. *Proceedings of the American Society for Information Science (ASIS), 31*, 34–40.

Schoch, N., & Abels, E. G. (1994). Using a valuative instrument for decision-making in the cancellation of science journals in a university setting. *Proceedings of the American Society for Information Science (ASIS), 31*, 41–50.

Schwartz, C. A. (1998). Restructuring serials management to generate new resources and services with commentaries on restructurings at three institutions. *College and Research Libraries, 59*(2), 115–128.

Segal, J. (1986). Journal deselection: A literature review and application. *Science and Technology Libraries, 6*(3), 25–42.

Slote, S. J. (1982). *Weeding library collections II* (2nd ed.). Littleton, CO: Libraries Unlimited.

Stankus, T. (1985). New specialized journals, mature scientists, and shifting loyalties. *Library Acquisitions: Practice and Theory, 9*, 99–104.

Stenstrom, P., & McBride, R. B. (1979). Serial use by social science faculty: A survey. *College and Research Libraries, 40*, 426–431.

Stephens, J. M. (1993). Keeping the serials beast at bay: A case study of collaborative serials review. *The Serials Librarian, 24*(3/4), 241–244.

Tallman, K. D., & Leach, J. T. (1989). Serials review and the three-year cancellation project at the University of Arizona Library. *Serials Review, 15*(3), 51–60.

Tenopir, C., & King, D. W. (1997). Trends in scientific scholarly journal publishing in the United States. *Journal of Scholarly Publishing, 28*, 135–170.

Tenopir, C., & King, D. W. (2000). *Towards electronic journals: Realities for scientists, librarians and publishers.* Washington, DC: Special Library Association.

Tierney, W. G. (1999). *Building the responsive campus: Creating high performance colleges and universities.* Thousand Oaks, CA: Sage.

Tucker, B. E. (1995). The journal deselection project: The LSUMC-S experience. *Library Acquisitions: Practice and Theory, 19*(3), 313–320.

University of Virginia. (1999). *Issues in Scholarly Communication,* Retrieved June 20, 2002 from http://www.lib.virginia.edu/scholcomm.html

Walker, T. J. (1998). Free Internet access to traditional journals. *American Scientist, 86*(3), 463–471.

Walter, P. L. (1990). Doing the unthinkable: Canceling journals at a research library. *The Serials Librarian, 18*(1/2), 141–153.

White, H. S. (1980). Factors in the decision by individuals and libraries to place or cancel subscriptions to scholarly and research journals. *The Library Quarterly, 50*(3), 287–309.

White, H. S. (1988). The journal that ate the library. *Library Journal, 113*, 62–63.

Williamson, H. (1977). Journal growth by division. *IEEE Transactions on Professional Communication, 20*, 89–92.

Williamson, M. L. (1985). Seven years of cancellations at Georgia Tech. *The Serials Librarian, 9*(3), 103–114.

Yocum, P. B. (1989). The precarious state of academic science library collections. *Science and Technology Libraries, 9*(3), 37–46.

Ziman, J. M. (1980). The proliferation of scientific literatures: A natural process. *Science, 208*, 369–371.

SENIOR UK MANAGERS' IDENTIFICATION OF ATTRIBUTES OF INFORMATION ASSETS

Joan Stenson

INTRODUCTION

This paper presents the major findings of recently completed research in the UK concerning the attributes of information as an asset and its impact on organisational performance. The research study employed an automated information asset- and attribute-scoring grid exercise and semi-structured open-ended interviews with 45 senior UK managers in four case study organisations. The information asset-scoring grid was developed to provide a simple visual representation of information assets and attributes using Excel charts. The semi-structured open-ended interviews aimed to identify the attributes of information assets considered significant by 45 senior UK managers and to explore relevant issues such as the value of information and organisational effectiveness.

CONTEXT

The definition of information as an asset has its origins in a resource-based view of information. Black and Marchand (1982, p. 205) trace the rise of this view of information from the mid-1970s when the US Government realised

Advances in Library Administration and Organization, Volume 23, 333–414
Copyright © 2006 by Elsevier Ltd.
All rights of reproduction in any form reserved
ISSN: 0732-0671/doi:10.1016/S0732-0671(05)23009-2

that it was in danger of drowning under paperwork and doing so at an unsustainable cost. It set up a Commission on Federal Paperwork, which stated that:

> ...as a resource, data and information can and must be managed just as we manage human, physical and financial resources. Data and information must be subject to the same budgetary, managerial and audit disciplines as any other resource.
>
> (Black & Marchand, 1982, p. 207)

Burk and Horton (1988) epitomised the resource-based view of information in their work on identifying key corporate information resources. These were the information resources vital for organisational activities. Burk and Horton's (1988) approach concentrated on harnessing information resources already present in organisations and identifying uses of these resources. Values were assigned to information resources based on strategic weightings (where the organisation's overall business strategy provides criteria for weighting individual information resources in terms of their usefulness for particular strategies). Only when weightings had been assigned were costs considered. An information audit then periodically ensured that "best value" was attained for costs expended. The approach concentrated on the productivity of information resources in relation to their costs (Black & Marchand, 1982, p. 206). The link between business strategy and information resources identified by Burk and Horton (1988) was a critical one.

The resource-based approach to information was adapted in the 1990s by two highly regarded and well-publicised reports, the Hawley Report (KPMG/IMPACT, 1994) and Reuter's *Information as an asset: The invisible goldmine* (Reuters, 1995), both of which attempted to identify information as an "asset". The Hawley Report (KPMG/IMPACT, 1994) was produced by KPMG with the backing of the Confederation of British Industry (CBI). It argued that information is a vital resource and proposed that someone at board level should be responsible for its management. The key finding of this report was that:

> ... all significant information in an organisation, regardless of its purpose, should be properly identified, even if not in an accounting sense, for consideration as an asset of the business. The board of directors should address its responsibilities for information assets in the same way as for other assets, e.g. property, plant.
>
> (KPMG/IMPACT, 1994, p. 23)

The Hawley Report (KPMG/IMPACT, 1994) recommended that information assets should be identified and classified by value and importance, and that skilled resources were needed to manage information assets and harness them. This was to ensure information assets were providing the maximum business benefit. Dr. Robert Hawley (1995, p. 237), the chairman of the committee that produced the Report, pointed out that many intangibles (like brands, people and intellectual property) had received attention in the business literature. This meant that boards of directors were at least aware of most of them – and aware that attention should be paid to them. In contrast, very few organisations recognised the value of information. The Hawley Report (KPMG/IMPACT, 1994) positioned this recognition of the importance of information as being pivotal. If boards of directors were not paying attention to information, then there was, at best:

> ...a lack of consistency in strategic understanding, planning, budgeting, management and control, and at worst, the very existence of the organisation can be under threat.
>
> (Hawley, 1995, p. 237)

The Hawley Committee (KPMG/IMPACT, 1994) argued that the first step in benefiting from the information held and used by organisations was a formal process of identification. They found that a number of information types or assets were consistently identified across organisations. Information assets were defined as "...information that is or should be documented and which has value or potential value" (KPMG/IMPACT, 1994, p. 23). The eight categories of information assets identified by the Hawley Committee were:

- *Market and customer information*, e.g., regional utilities have large amounts of data on every household in their regions; trade names and trade marks.
- *Product information*, e.g., the depth of knowledge in particular technologies that support particular products such as fluid and thermal dynamics in the aerospace industry. This includes both registered and non-registered intellectual property rights (IPR).
- *Specialist knowledge* and information for operating in a particular area, which is often in people's heads (e.g., retailing know-how among managers of grocery supermarkets who find even associated areas of retailing difficult to move into. Since the publication of the Hawley Report, retailers (e.g., the supermarket Tesco) in the UK have become very successful in expanding their markets into associated consumer durables. This type of knowledge is also now addressed in part by knowledge management techniques but, at the time of the Hawley Report, knowledge management was not a well-established activity).
- *Business process information* that underpins the workings of the business within the broader context, e.g., economic, political, share price and other information that financial markets use.

- *Management information*, particularly that on which major policy, competitive decisions or strategic plans will be based, e.g., economic statistics or cost base information.
- *Human resource information*, e.g., skills databases, particularly in project-based organisations such as consultants in a technology company who need to be brought together to support a client project. Again, these days knowledge management attempts to address this area.
- *Supplier information*, e.g., trading agreements or networks of contacts for services or product development.
- *Accountability information*, e.g., legally required information including shareholder information, health and safety information or environmental pollution evidence (KPMG/IMPACT, 1994, pp. 9–10).

The identification of information as a vital asset for business was further developed by the publication of *Information as an asset: The invisible gold-mine* (Reuters, 1995), which reported the results of 500 telephone interviews with senior managers in UK companies. The main conclusions of this report were that one in four UK companies said that information was its most important asset; half thought it was more important than trade names and registered trade marks; and one in 10 valued its information more than its staff. However, more than 40% of respondents said their companies had not awakened to the value of the information they had.

The results showed that companies wanted to capitalise their expenditure on information, yet some 25% of the respondents said they could not capitalise information assets because they found it too hard to identify what the value of the assets were (Reuters, 1995). These reports seemed to indicate that organisations would benefit financially from defining information as an asset and that new ways of identifying, measuring and managing information would eventually emerge. Despite the wide publicity and high regard with which both the Hawley Committee and Reuters reports were received they had in fact little impact on the ways in which organisations addressed the management of their information resources. In a study of 12 high-performing organisations by Owens and Wilson (1997), it was found that traditional information roles were being taken over by Information Technology (IT) personnel. This puts an emphasis on the effective storage and retrieval of information rather than the quality of the information itself (Owens & Wilson, 1997, p. 26). The traditional information specialist was playing a diminishing role in the organisations surveyed. The IRM approach, though not widely applied, was significant, however, because it not only identified the cost of information but also sought to identify its value. It remained focused on cost and productivity and this led to criticism of the approach. In particular, Eaton and Bawden (1991, p. 156) summarised the views of many when they pointed out that "if information is a resource, it is different in kind from most others". The "value of information" debate is central to this criticism and is discussed in the following section.

The Value of Information

Some attempts to calculate the value of information assets are outlined next with reasons suggested for their lack of success.

Value

The definition of value itself is problematic and provides little basis for a value of information. Boisot (1998, p. 72) states that there is no settled definition of value and traces the development of the concept of value in economic theory from before the 1870s when physiocrats (who believed land was the main generator of value) opposed mercantilists (who believed mineral wealth such as gold and silver were the ultimate source of value).

Others argued that value resided in the transformation that humans wrought upon nature rather than nature itself. Some viewed human or animal labour as the source of all value. This view was shared by classical economists such as Adam Smith and David Ricardo. Physiocrats, mercantilists and classical economists all took value to be energy-based. In no case did information play any significant role. In the second half of the nineteenth century, value became relational and contingent, being established through the interplay of the supply and demand conditions for goods. Information was never treated as the central focus in a transaction and hence as an object of exchange in its own right (Boisot, 1998, p. 72). As a result, attempts to place a financial value on information were not rooted in sound foundations.

Attempts at Information Valuation

Badenoch, Reid, Burton, Gibb, and Oppenheim (1994, pp. 23–62) attempt at finding information value into four categories:

1. Econometric approaches (e.g., economic value-added).
2. Organisational management and resource management perspectives (e.g., IRM).
3. Costing, pricing and evaluation of library and information services (e.g., performance measurement).
4. The social value of information (e.g., contribution to social good).

The value of information depends on its context and use (Eaton & Bawden, 1991, p. 163), and its value to users is impossible to determine in advance. Eaton and Bawden (1991) argued that identifying information as a resource had become shorthand for "information is important." In other words, concentration on quantifying information detracted from the dynamic role information played in organisations. Attempts to measure value limited the dynamic nature of information and ultimately destroyed innovation in organisations.

None of the methods gained widespread acceptance and Badenoch et al. (1994, p. 62) conclude that this is because "we cannot consider the value of information out of context of the activity or decision it supports".

Valuation Methods

The following examples of attempts to place a value on information demonstrate some of the difficulties that are often encountered when trying to place an objective value on information.

Griffiths and King (1991, p. 109) focused on estimates of the cost of information to users of in-house information services (e.g., desk research, online searching). Their approach saw the main factor in valuing information not as the value of the resource itself but the value of the time and effort spent by users in obtaining information elsewhere when these resources were not available. This seems an objective measure of the cost of information. However, if we consider that any one user's time may be worth more or less than that of other users and that many users in practice would not be interested in obtaining information from elsewhere, then the measure appears less than objective. It also assumes that the user will apply the information to create value for the organisation. The information found may be of no use at all, i.e., it may have a cost but no value.

Glazer (1993) attempted to value transaction-based information and identified two levels of value: the value of information as it is currently being used and potential ways in which information could be used: $V(a)$ is the current actual value and $V(p)$ potential value of information.

Glazer (1993) undertook a valuation exercise in an electronics company using the above categories of value. This resulted in a figure of $25 million for the value of information that could be generated from potential uses of transaction-based information. Glazer's method assumed that all the information held by the organisation was valuable. This was by no means certain since, as Orna (1996, p. 20) points out, "information has no inherent value in itself".

An Objective Value for Information?

Arriving at a value of information is not an objective exercise. Different stakeholders (e.g., customers, employees, managers, suppliers, society, owners and investors) will employ different methods depending on their various perspectives. Their evaluations will be subjective. Attempts to value information and place it on the balance sheet of organisations does have benefits in that it positions information within an area of financial management with which all senior managers are concerned. However, an objective value of information (and indeed of traditional and non-traditional intangible assets) is not possible. Information value by its very nature is subjective, and is dependant on the interpretation of the individual or team members who employ information in particular situations for particular purposes. In any case, objective measures are often far less reliable than they at first appear. Accounting has been highlighted as an area where organisations such as Enron and Worldcom can present seemingly objective and audited financial statements, which have in fact little to do with their real underlying financial position.

If information assets themselves cannot be valued or recognised as intangible assets, then perhaps their attributes can provide a mechanism whereby users can attempt to gain a more complete picture of them. Capturing these attributes is a tall order and has a long and varied treatment in the literature.

Repo (1986, p. 374) lists the unique attributes that information possesses:

1. Information is human. It exists only through human perception.
2. Information is expandable. The free flow of information maximises its use.
3. Information is compressible.
4. Information is substitutable. It may save money by substituting the use of other resources.
5. Information is easily transportable by using applications of new IT.
6. Information is diffusible. It tends to "leak" even if we try to contain it.
7. Information is shareable; giving it away does not mean losing it.

Burk and Horton (1988) argue that it is the role which information plays that defines it as an organisational resource, not its similarities to other resources. Information has value in encouraging innovation and change. Information has identifiable and measurable characteristics (Burk &

Horton, 1988, p. 18). These measurable characteristics can help to define its value and include:

1. *Quality of the information itself.* Degree of accuracy, comprehensiveness, credibility, relevance, simplicity and validity.
2. *Utility of information holdings.* Degree of intellectual and physical accessibility, ease of use, flexibility and presentation.
3. *Impact on productivity of organisation.* Contribution to improvement in decision-making, product quality, efficiency of operation or working conditions, time-saving and promotion of timely action.
4. *Impact on effectiveness of organisation.* Contribution to new markets, improved customer satisfaction, meeting targets and objectives and promoting more harmonious relationships.
5. *Impact on financial position.* Contribution to cost reduction or cost saving, substitution for more expensive resource inputs, increased profits and return on investment (Burk & Horton, 1988, p. 93).

Many of the attributes identified by Repo (1986) and Burk and Horton (1988) are revisited by Orna (1996, p. 20). In her view information must be transformed by human cognition.

1. Where inflows of information necessary to maintain knowledge and support appropriate action are blocked, disaster can follow, either quickly (as in aircraft disasters) or in the form of a gradual run down of competence and chaos.
2. Where information is hoarded for the exclusive use of a limited number of people, it can actually fail to achieve its full potential value for those who hoard it. If it is exchanged and traded the value resulting from its use increases for all parties to the transaction.
3. Information has no inherent value in itself.
4. Information is a diffused resource that enters into all activities of businesses and forms a component of all products and services that are sold.

The elements identified by Repo (1986) and Burk and Horton (1988) and revisited by Orna (1996) cover three distinct types of attributes. These are attributes inherent to information, attributes concerned with the impact of information and economic attributes of information.

Inherent Attributes
The first two characteristics identified by Burk and Horton (1988), quality and utility, can be seen to be inherent to information as an entity in itself. They can be identified and measured according to a set criterion within a

particular context or organisational setting. Attributes such as expandable, compressible, storable, transportable and substitutable (Repo, 1986) also fall into this category.

Impact Attributes
Impact attributes include productivity and effectiveness. These are not so readily identifiable or measurable. The main difficulty is that information, although useful, is in all likelihood only a tiny factor in any productivity or effectiveness improvements. While information underpins improved productivity and effectiveness, it cannot be easily separated from all the other elements that impact on these areas. To have this impact information must be "transformed by humans"(Orna, 1996; Repo, 1986). Information also has an impact in encouraging innovation and change (Burk & Horton, 1988, p. 93).

Economic Attributes
The economic attributes of information are their most interesting. Burk and Horton (1988) include an economic category of financial impact. However, it is very difficult to show any financial impact from information, other than cost (which reduces rather than increasing profit).

Economic attributes identified by Arrow (1984, p. 142), which emphasise the inappropriability of information, actually exclude it from the definition as an economic good. This is because information once transferred becomes the possession of both buyer and seller – "…information is inappropriable because an individual who has some can never lose it by transmitting it" (Arrow, 1984, p. 142). This means that the same information can benefit both the giver and receiver. Unlike a traditional economic good, for example a car, information can never really become the sole possession of the receiver. If I have an idea and I share it with another person, not only does that person benefit, but I can still retain and benefit from the idea. Value is added by the sharing of information (Orna, 1996) since both parties are able to use it to enhance their activities. The attributes of "exchanged" and "traded" identified by Orna (1996) are also economic attributes and there is evidence, for example, the selling of customer information data, to support their inclusion as economic attributes. Inherent, impact and economic attributes of information assets are summarised in Exhibit 1.

All three categories of attributes of information assets may be under-recognised by senior managers because they underpin everyday organisational activities rather than appearing as revenue generators. Indeed the attributes described in the literature may not be those relevant to senior managers. While it is very difficult to identify the value of individual attributes, their

Exhibit 1.   Attributes of Information Assets.

Inherent Attributes	Impact Attributes	Economic Attributes
Utility/quality (Burk & Horton, 1988)	Productivity/effectiveness (Burk & Horton, 1988)	Financial position (Burk & Horton, 1988) No inherent value (Orna, 1996)
Expandable/compressible/ storable (Repo, 1986) Transportable/substitutable (Repo, 1986)	Transformed by humans (Orna, 1996; Repo, 1986) Encouraging innovation and change (Burk & Horton, 1988)	Exchanged and traded (Orna, 1996) Shareable (Arrow, 1984; Orna, 1996; Repo, 1986)

effects on the strategic activities of organisations, on their competitiveness and decision-making processes, can be more readily shown. In other words, they can be shown to enhance the performance of organisations.

Organisational Performance and Information Assets
The proposal for a link between organisational performance and information is a tentative one. Such a link has long been discussed in the information science literature (Allen, 1966) but until recently there has been little progress made in establishing a coherent link (Marchand, 2000; Marchand et al., 2001a, b; Orna, 2004).

Allen (1966), in his famous study of the use of scientific and technical information by research teams, found that better performers (information gatekeepers) used internal sources of information more while poorer performers used outside sources which they tended to overrate. Better performance of research teams was not linked by Allen to improved organisational performance. We still know very little about the connection between information and organisational performance. Similarly, attributes of information, such as quality and utility, are well documented but their impact on organisational performance is unclear. This may be because information cannot be easily separated from other factors, which influence organisational performance, such as the information-seeking behaviours of research teams.

Progress has been made in recent years, particularly by a team of researchers at the Institute of Management Development (IMD), working with the support of Accenture, the management consultancy firm, and led by Donald Marchand. A 28-month research project entitled "Navigating Business Success" was conducted by the team at the IMD between September 1997 and December 1999. The project involved over 1200 senior managers in 103 companies across 26 industries and 37 countries (Marchand, Kettinger, & Rollins, 2001b, p. xv). The research study sought to discover how people, information and IT interact to affect business performance (Marchand, Kettinger, & Rollins, 2001a, p. 9). The research provides a context for the development of information strategies through the interaction of three information capabilities. "Information strategy is the detailed expression of information policy (an information policy is founded on an organisation's overall business objectives and the priorities within them) in terms of objectives, targets and actions to achieve them for a defined period ahead" (Orna, 2004, p. 8). The three information capabilities described by Marchand et al. (2001a) are:

1. The IT practices (ITP) capability
2. The information management practices (IMP) capability
3. The information behaviours and values (IBV) capability.

Together, these three capabilities interact to form an integrated "information orientation" (IO) measure. This measure provides senior managers with an integrated new business metric to help build business capabilities and behaviours for effectively using information in their companies to achieve better business performance (Marchand et al., 2001b, p. 48).

Marchand et al. (2001b) found that senior managers had a complex and comprehensive view of effective information use that integrated dimensions of behavioural, information management and IT thinking. This integrated view is, according to Marchand et al. (2001b, p. 7), a much better predictor of organisational performance than any single view.

IT Practices
The senior managers' perception of ITPs is concerned with the practical outcomes of applications of IT in supporting organisational operations, processes, innovation and managerial decision-making (Marchand et al., 2001b, p. 49). Marchand et al. (2001b, p. 72) conclude that, while IT strategies may work well to achieve intended strategies, ITPs alone will not lead to superior organisational performance.

Information Management Practices
IMPs are seen as a process or life cycle (see Exhibit 2) that involves sensing, collecting, organising, processing and monitoring information to enhance its use for decision-making.

Sensing is an important element of the life-cycle process, but it is often ignored in traditional definitions of information life cycles (Best, 1996, p. 4).

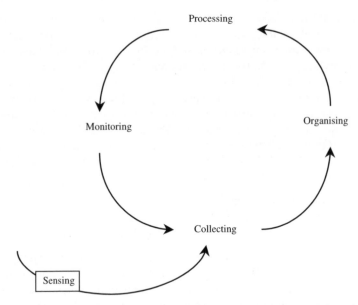

Exhibit 2.   Life-Cycle of Information Management. *Source*: Marchand et al. 2001a,
p. 76.

Sensing involves the active seeking and scanning of new information in
external environments. Information sensed about the external environment
helps define information needs and drives changes to what information
would be collected within an organisation. Marchand et al. (2001b, p. 98)
found that senior managers perceive all of the five separate stages of the
information life cycle as being "distinct and valued ideas". However, it was
found that while "the sensing phase does exist as a discrete dimension in the
minds of senior managers the concept is not as well formulated as other
information management practices". In particular, sensing information on
economic, social and political changes affecting the business seems to be
least developed in formal information practice. The practices associated
with sensing information are less structured than the other life-cycle stages
(Marchand et al., 2001b, p. 93).

It is interesting to note that the senior managers interviewed for the
Marchand et al. study were also less concerned with monitoring information
than with using it. Monitoring information was perceived slightly less
clearly than processing, collecting and organising information. Managers
perceived updating and refreshing information for future use as being more

significant than the reuse of existing information (Marchand et al., 2001b, p. 91). Marchand et al. concluded that managers do recognise the time and financial resources expended in collecting quality information will be wasted if it is not maintained. However, reusing information is a lesser priority than having information available when it is needed.

Information Behaviours and Values
Marchand et al. (2001b, p. 94) identified a linkage between positive information usage behaviours and good IMPs, which is most evident in sensing practices. The argument is that "those people who actively use cognitive skills to sense for information will also make better evaluative judgments about the applicability of certain information to decision contexts" (Marchand et al., 2001b, p. 94). The information behaviours recognised by senior managers include:

- Integrity – guarantee the information is truthful.
- Formality – formal information resources are perceived to have higher reliability and quality.
- Information control – provision of trustworthy and formal information related to individual and organisational performance.
- Transparency – treating errors, mistakes, failures and surprises as constructive learning opportunities accelerates the feedback loop between a company's intended strategy, its actions to implement the strategy and the ability to correct or change course along the way (Marchand et al., 2001b, pp. 102–103). (Openness and transparency in relation to single- and double-loop learning have been discussed in the learning organisation literature (Senge, 1990; Argyris & Schön, 1996)).
- Sharing – managers' willingness to share the most important information in the organisation about their own and the company's performance with employees.
- Proactive information use – active concern to think about how to use information, obtain new information and the desire to put useful information into practice (Marchand et al., 2001b, pp. 125–126).

Senior managers did recognise that people should use information to respond quickly in the competitive environment of the company (Marchand et al., 2001b, p. 126). Senior managers do not believe that improvements in information behaviours alone, without the support of solid IT practices or competent information practices, will result in substantial improvements in business performance. It is the interaction of the three capabilities, the IO, which is the significant indicator.

The IO Measure

The IO measure developed is intended as a business measure of effective information use. IO is not a measure of overall organisational performance, but it is a powerful measure of how senior managers perceive their companies possess the capabilities associated with effective information use to achieve enhanced organisational effectiveness. There are several key characteristics of IO:

- IO incorporates a people-centric view of information use.
- IO is causally linked to business performance.
- IO is an organisation-wide metric, not limited to the IT department or other information management support functions.
- IO applies universally across international borders.
- IO can be used as a key performance indicator over time to assess the effectiveness of management actions to improve information behaviour and values, IMPs and IT practices (Marchand et al., 2001a, pp. 11–12).

While the IO is a significant advance in the linking of information and organisational performance, a caveat to the research is given by Orna (2004) when she looks back over a career in information consultancy which spans over 50 years. Orna (2004, pp. 115–116) states that her long experience of information consultancy in organisations points to a much more limited practice by senior managers of the IBVs quoted by Marchand et al. Orna (2004, p. 116) points to information integrity in particular:

> The sorry trail of corporate wrongdoing, based on deliberate flouting of information integrity, and ultimate exposure initiated by the Enron case should act as an awful warning.

CASE STUDY RESEARCH

Four case studies formed the central part of the research study and were undertaken between November 2001 and March 2002. The case studies comprised open-ended, guided interviews with 45 senior managers and an information asset-scoring grid exercise, which was used to familiarise the senior managers with a range of information assets and attributes. The senior managers who participated in this research were those in long-term careers whose views have been developed over many years and who will continue to have influence in their organisations. Within information-intensive organisations, such senior managers form a high-level group or an elite, which represents the most influential people in the organisation. Targeting such groups is termed elite interviewing (Marshall & Rossman, 1989, p. 54). Elite interviewing focuses on the influential, the prominent, and the well-informed people in an organisation or community. These are the people who have both the will and the means to enact change in their organisations. The numbers of senior managers interviewed for each case study were

Case Study	Number of Senior Managers Interviewed
1	14
2	9
3	10
4	12

Two of the organisations were based in the South of England (Case studies 1 and 4) and one in the Midlands (Case study 2). Case study 3 was based in East Anglia. With Case studies 2 and 4, the majority of interviews were conducted at head office but a small number of interviews were also conducted at one of the regional offices. Regional senior managers were far more critical of the organisations' information management than those located at head offices. A major concern of regional senior managers was access to information assets. Case study 3 was a public sector organisation whereas Case studies 1, 2 and 4 were public limited or limited companies.

Developing the Information Asset- and Attribute-Scoring Grid

The grid was developed using a number of sources. These included a review of the literature. Burk and Horton's (1988) attribute categories were used to form the vertical rows of the grid while the information assets which formed the horizontal categories were based on the revised Hawley Committee identification of information assets (KPMG/IMPACT, 1994). One small change was made to the information asset "organisational information." The word "culture" was added to provide immediate context for this asset.

The development of the information asset-scoring grid attributes row involved a detailed listing of attributes identified by Burk and Horton (1988, pp. 91–99) together with an open category of "Other". Senior managers could see that the attribute quality was concerned with, for example, accuracy and relevance but they were also free to create their own attributes under the "Other" category. (Only two of the managers used the "Other" category.)

The grid was primarily used to introduce senior managers to a range of attributes and assets and to help discriminate among them. The grid developed is shown in Exhibit 3.

The information asset- and attribute-scoring grid was designed to collect a large amount of data. An Excel spreadsheet was written to allow easy entry and access to this information and for ease of later analysis. The spreadsheet featured a white grid in the middle with information assets heading the columns and their attributes shown against the rows. Ratings were added, in the form of stars shown as most significant (gold), next most significant (silver) and least significant (blue). Blue was chosen because the bronze colour available was rather dark and unappealing. (Significance was used in an "importance" rather than statistical sense.)

The interviewees completed their own grids by adding stars to cells by simply selecting a cell and clicking on one of the three stars. Each case study organisation had its own sheets, which contained the individual grids elicited from individual senior managers. The grids provided a good introduction to the concepts of information assets and their attributes. Some senior

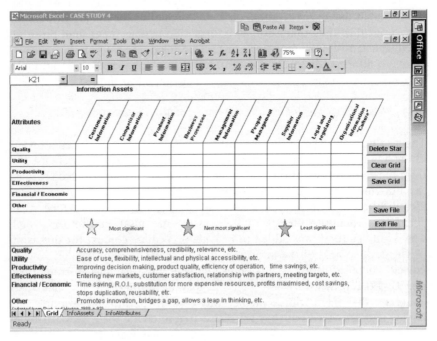

Exhibit 3.   Information Asset and Attribute-Scoring Grid.

managers reported that they found it difficult to discriminate between attributes, arguing that different attributes became important for different information assets at different times. At the time, adding a situational dimension to the grid would have over-complicated the exercise. However, on reflection this would have added a useful context to the information asset-scoring grid and might be an area for future development.

Developing the Case Study Interview Schedule

The development of the case study interview schedule (see the appendix) was undertaken over nine months from January to September 2001 and reflected the results of the earlier repertory grid interviews with senior executives and the interviews with internationally active information professionals.

The case studies focused on five major themes as shown in Exhibit 4. They are represented by bricks, which together build understanding. Themes 1 and 2 are general areas of interest while Themes 3, 4 and 5 focus on specific issues, namely the identification, use and measurement of the effects of information assets.

1. The organisation and information strategy (O + IS).
2. The organisation and its effectiveness (O + E).
3. Identifying information assets (IIA).
4. Using information assets (UIA).
5. Measuring the effects of information assets (M).

Approaches to Analysis of Case Study Data

Information Asset-Scoring Grid
The information asset-scoring grid was used to provide a simple visual representation of assets and attributes using Excel charts. Charts for individual senior managers were produced. A simple visual count of gold stars (yellow bars) was taken to show the most significant assets and attributes scored.

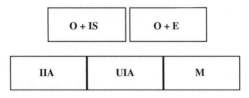

Exhibit 4. Five Major Themes.

Open-Ended Guided Interviews

Analysis was conducted using a grounded theory approach. Strauss and Corbin (1990, p. 10) define the grounded theory approach as "a qualitative research method that uses a systematic set of procedures to develop an inductively derived grounded theory about a phenomenon" (p. 26).

Two levels of analysis were employed: qualitative using a specialist qualitative data analysis (QDA) software package and quantitative using Excel.

Excel Analysis

Questions such as "do information assets feature on the management agenda?" were analysed using Excel to give a simple count of yes, no and do not know answers. Exhibit 5 shows a view of the Excel data. The job title of the senior managers interviewed, case study number and coding for Theme 1 Question 1 are also shown.

Theme 1 Question 1 comprised seven statements based on the five guiding principles of strategic information management suggested by Horton (1993, p. 2). This theme was suitable for analysis at either qualitative or

Position	Case s	1a	1b	1c	1d	1e	1f	1g	2a	2b
Finance Director	4	4	5	5	4	4	4	3		0
Managing Director - Business Development	4	4	4	5	5	5	2	1		1
Director of Transportation Software	4	4	4	5	4	2	2	1		0
Director - Highways	4	4	4	3	4	5	4	3		1
Director - Corporate Services	4	4	5	5	3	4	2	4		1
Human Resources Manager	4	4	4	2	4	4	3	4		0
Marketing Information Systems Manager	4	3	4	3	2	2	3	4		0
Manager - Information Resources	4	4	4	2	2	2	2	2		1
Divisional Director	4	4	4	4	4	4	2	2		1
Senior Manager - Transportation and Highways	4	4	4	4	3	4	3	4		1
Senior Manager - Transportation and Highways	4	4	4	2	2	4	4	2		0
Senior Engineer	4	3	4	4	5	5	3	2		1
Process Control Manager	2	5	5	4	4	4	4	3		1
Programme Manager	2	5	5	3	5	5	4	1		1
Engineering Director	2	5	5	1	5	5	3	2		0
Commercial Director	2	5	5	4	4	5	2	3		0
IT Director	2	5	5	4	4	4	3	4		0
Technical Manager	2	5	5	4	4	3	2	1		0
Marketing Manager	2	4	4	5	4	3	4	3		0
Financial Controller	2	5	5	1	5	4	4	1		0
Executive Director	2	4	3	4	4	4	5	5		0
Director of Technical Consulting	1	4	4	3	4	4	4	2		0
Lead Consultant	1	5	5	4	3	3	4	2		0
Human Resources Manager	1	5	5	4	2	2	2	2		1
Lead Consultant 1	1	4	4	4	3	2	2	2		0
Lead Consultant 2	1	5	4	2	4	2	4	1		0
Computing Services Manager	1	4	5	2	2	2	3	4		0
Director	1	5	2	3	4	5	4	2		0
Financial Controller	1	2	2	2	2	3	2	2		1
Managing Director	1	4	2	4	4	2	4	2		0
Principal Consultant	1	3	2	2	4	2	4	2		0
Business Manager	1	3	3	4	2	4	4	2		2
Defence Business Manager	1	5	5	4	3	5	2	2		0

Exhibit 5. Excel Data.

quantitative levels or at a combination of both as supporting statements were made to provide context for the numeric ratings given. The key factor in deciding which level of analysis to use was that the supporting statements were of more interest. It was decided to focus on the statements made although initial analysis was performed using Excel to give prompt feedback to case study facilitators.

Selection of QDA Software

The QDA package selected for the analysis of the interview data was ATLAS/Ti. ATLAS/Ti is an acronym, which stands for "Archiv fuer Technik, Lebenswelt und Altagssprache" translated as "archive for technology, the life world and everyday language". The extension "Ti" stands for text interpretation. It was developed by Project ATLAS (1989–1992) at the Technical University of Berlin and is based on grounded theory. The other well-known QDA package which was considered for use was NUD*IST (version 4). NUD*IST uses trees to structure concepts in an index but lacks the conceptual graphs which ATLAS/Ti offers. NUD*IST does have benefits in that it imposes a hierarchy so that specific concepts can become subsets of a number of more general ones. However, a major drawback of the package is the lack of a printing facility for code trees. This drawback has been addressed by a new version of the software (version 5). A comparison of the features of ATLAS/Ti and NUD*IST is shown in Exhibit 6.

Getting started with analysis using ATLAS/Ti is relatively easy. The package is accessible and flexible, if somewhat slow and prone to falling over at intervals. NUD*IST, on the other hand, is less accessible and flexible, making it much slower to get started. The researcher had the benefit of access to an ATLAS/Ti practitioner, Mr. Ralph Godau, through a contact

Exhibit 6. Comparison of ATLAS/Ti and NUD*IST.

ATLAS/Ti	NUD*IST
User-friendly interface	Rougher interface
Hypertext links between data, codes and documents	Fewer links between data, codes and documents
No limits on coding	Coding has to be decided in advance and used throughout
Networks can be printed/exported	No option to print tree display of codes
Creative/visual – but unstructured	Hierarchical – limited

Source: Barry, 1998, p. 8.

known to Ms Henczel, Manager, CAVAL Collaborative Solutions, which
also influenced the choice of software.

Loading and Organising the Case Study Interview Data

A project file, termed a Hermeneutic Unit (HU) in the ATLAS/Ti programme, was created. This was used to store all of the interview files associated with the case studies. The file was named Case study 4.hpr. Exhibit 7
shows a screenshot of the HU with the transcript of the interview with Lead
Consultant 2 displayed. The coding area is shown in the margin to the right.

The Analysis Approach

Familiarisation/Coding
The first step in analysis is free and open coding, which involves the first
coding of concepts and themes (see Exhibit 9). This stage was primarily used
to organise the data and to initially code concepts and can be seen as the

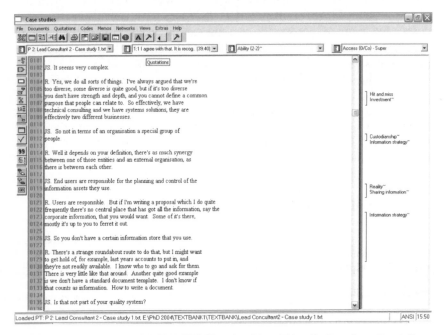

Exhibit 7. Screenshot of ATLAS/Ti Showing User-Friendly Interface (Lead Consultant 2, Case Study 1).

Familiarisation step in the grounded theory process. Open coding was also used to code yes/no and do not know answers, providing a simple output of numbers of occurrences which could be checked with the Excel count. This double counting increased the reliability of the data. Once the initial coding has been performed, it is important to review codes and merge or rename codes that have been duplicated or which have very similar meanings. This is the *Recoding step* in grounded theory. For example, both the words accurate and accuracy were coded in different documents as attributes of information assets. These codes were merged to form a single-code accuracy. The software retains a record of the merged code in a comment box linked to the new or over-riding code.

Reflection/Memoing

The second step of the grounded theory process, reflection, is not adequately covered by ATLAS/Ti but can be approximated by re-reading literature and noting important issues as memos. Importantly, there is an opportunity to create memos at any stage of the analysis so that ideas and important breakthroughs can be written down and revisited as the analysis progresses. Memos provide the opportunity for theory building with unlimited text space.

Conceptualisation/Category Building and Axial Coding

The conceptualisation step of grounded theory is mirrored by the building of categories in ATLAS/Ti. The first step in this process involves placing each issue in context so that its causes and results can be related. This is the most time-consuming stage of the coding as it requires extensive mapping of relationships across themes and concepts. This building of relationships and linkages is termed Axial coding in ATLAS/Ti and is located within the network function. Networks are, basically, conceptual graphs, which help to explore ideas using intuitive graphical representations. They provide a visual representation of the data, which helps to reduce cognitive load when handling complex relationships.

Linking/Networks

Networks consist of nodes (nodes can be codes, memos or quotations) and are connected by arcs which can be directed or undirected. Codes are the most commonly used form (http://www.atlasti.com/glossconcepts.shtml). Focused networks can be generated very easily from codes with associated text (by importing an object and its neighbours) or can be independently created by importing into a blank network. Arcs can be given one of a built-in set of relation names such as "causes" (Richards & Richards, 1994, p. 459). These relations are role indicators for concepts and can be seen in Exhibit 8.

In Exhibit 8, a broken leg is shown as the cause of pain. (The broken leg could also be shown as the consequence.) Its properties are multiple fractures, sensation present, and a fall on an icy street. Strategies employed to deal with the issue of pain are taking pills, reading a book and placing a splint on the leg. The consequence of these strategies is temporary relief. The contexts in which they occur involve obtaining prompt help and a visit to hospital. The intervening condition, the untrained first aider, shows the different unexpected conditions such as an untrained first aider that impacted on the issue of pain.

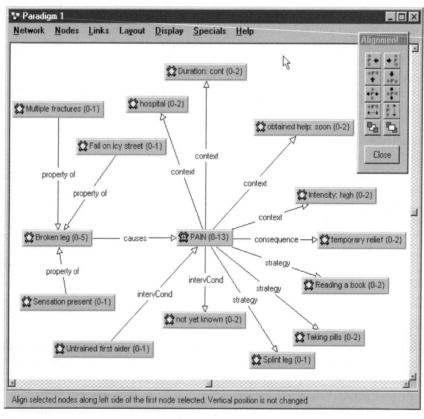

Exhibit 8.   Showing Linkages for Broken Leg.

Some default relations are pre-loaded at start up of ATLAS/Ti, for example:

<isa> Links specific concepts to general concepts – dog <isa> Mammal
<is-cause-of> Links cause and effect–broken leg <is-cause-of> Pain

These can be supplemented by user-defined relations as in Exhibit 8, where "strategy" is a user-defined relation. The default relations are useful for building networks that represent situations rather than the abstract concepts that are the focus of this research. As a result, user-defined relations were created to represent linkages in the data.

Nine user-defined relations were defined as follows:

- Asset – an information asset.
- Attribute – a characteristic of a concept or of an information asset.
- Context – to signify the conditions in which the issue is raised.
- Determine – the impact of one factor on another.
- Feedback – the suggestion made by an interviewee for addressing the issue raised.
- Issue – the concept/problem under investigation.
- Part – a partial connection between concepts and sub-concepts.
- Relate – a relationship between concepts.
- Result – the outcome of the issue raised.

Re-evaluation/Selective Coding

The final stage is "selective coding" which involves the integration of the categorised material into a theory (see Exhibit 9). This integration is achieved by selecting a category as a "core category" around which the rest of the categories can be organised. Memo writing helps to provide insights into the theory as the grounded theory process and coding stages come together.

Conclusions on the Use of Case Studies

The data collection methods employed, subjects, data collected and analysis approach are shown in Exhibit 10.

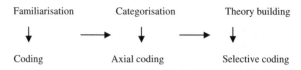

Familiarisation		Categorisation		Theory building
↓	→	↓	→	↓
Coding		Axial coding		Selective coding

Exhibit 9. The Grounded Theory Process and Coding Stages.

Exhibit 10.   Case Study Summary Table.

Data Collection Method	Subjects	Data Collected	Analysis Approach
Information asset scoring grid	45 senior managers	Information asset scoring grid charts	Excel
Open-ended guided interviews	45 senior managers	Interviews	Excel and ATLAS/Ti

The case studies conducted involved two major stages of data collection.

- An information asset-scoring grid was used to introduce senior managers to a range of information assets and attributes.
- Open-ended guided interviews conducted with 45 senior managers collected rich qualitative data.

The case study method itself provided an opportunity to discuss issues concerning senior managers and information within the setting of their own organisations. The method provided access to a range of views so that a deeper understanding of the issues could be gained. Case studies also provided an opportunity to gather contextual background information to the issues raised by the interviewees since the researcher was on site for several days and had access to company Intranets, sales and marketing information, company websites and electronic libraries. This provided a much more detailed picture of the organisations and their members so that the issues raised could be placed in context.

The case study organisations were both large and small, geographically dispersed and located on one site, private and public sector, consultancy and manufacturing based. Senior managers interviewed ranged from board directors to marketing managers, all high-level users and contributors of information assets. The multiple case study design allows for cross-sites analysis and adds confidence to the findings and so helps increase the external validity of the data. However, the organisations which participated in this research were seen as primarily individual case studies. The extent to which they could be usefully compared was limited.

FINDINGS OF CASE STUDY DATA

In this section, findings of the case study research are presented. Four case studies were conducted in information-intensive UK organisations during late-2001 and early-2002. A total of 45 senior managers were interviewed. The organisations were drawn from both the private and public sectors. The case study interviews commenced with the completion of an information asset-scoring grid by the senior managers. Interviews were then conducted using an open-ended guided interview schedule.

Findings of the information asset- and attribute-scoring grids. Findings are shown individually for each grid completed, with senior managers identified by their job title. Senior managers scored information assets and attributes using a gold, silver and blue star system. These were then outputted as Excel Charts, and the most significant assets and attributes scored (gold) were counted for each manager. Where the senior manager gave all the information assets and attributes a gold star, the word "All" is used to describe this approach. Excel Charts were generated for information assets and attributes. The information asset and attributes scored as most significant for each case study organisation are shown in Exhibits 11–14. The term "significant" is not used in a statistical sense but rather it denotes the importance of the information asset or attribute to the senior manager. In all, 44 information asset- and attribute-scoring grids out of a possible 45 were completed. An Executive Director, Case study 2, did not complete the grid saying that he preferred to concentrate on issues concerning his own organisation. Exhibit 15 provides a summary of the most important information assets and attributes scored by the senior managers for all the case study organisations.

As shown in Exhibit 11, quality was identified as the most important attribute by senior managers in Case study 1. (A count of the number of occurrences of each attribute scored gives this result.) Product, customer, organisational information and "culture" information assets were also rated.

A focus on the quality of information assets and on product and customer information assets shows an awareness of the wealth of internal knowledge and experience in the organisation in dealing with commercial imperatives. The scoring of organisational information "culture" may indicate that the senior managers recognise substantial cultural barriers exist in the organisation to exploiting information assets.

The organisation had undertaken a major restructuring programme. Some of the senior managers interviewed saw restructuring as a positive step. The new business groupings were clearly defined and reporting structures visible. The restructuring was identified, however, by several senior managers as hindering information sharing and information management capabilities. Business groupings encouraged a focus on making one's own

Exhibit 11.   Case Study 1 – Most Significant Information Assets and
Attributes by Manager.

Job Title	Information Assets	Attributes
Lead Consultant	Business processes	Quality
	Product information	Utility
	Management information	
Business Area Manager	Customer information	Effectiveness
	Product information	Quality
Quality Manager	Organisational information "culture"	Quality
		Utility
Director of Technical Consulting	Customer information	Quality
	Business processes	
Lead Consultant 1	Product information	Quality
		Effectiveness
Lead Consultant 2	Organisational information "culture"	Quality
Computer Services Manager	Organisational information "culture"	Effectiveness
	Customer information	
	Competitor information	
	Product information	
Director	Product information	Productivity
	Business processes	Financial/economic
		Other
Financial Controller	Competitor information	Quality
	Management information	Utility
Managing Director	Product information	Utility
	Management information	Financial/economic
	Legal and regulatory	
Principal Consultant	Customer information	Quality
	Product information	Utility
Lead Consultant 3	All	Quality
		Utility
Business Area Manager	Organisational information "culture"	Quality
	Management information	Productivity
Human Resources Manager	All	Quality
		Utility

group successful rather than contributing to the success of the organisation
as a whole. This was referred to as "siloing" by some senior managers:

> There's internal tension to make the best of your business unit and use your resources
> best before perhaps you think about other resources in the company but that's inevitable
> by setting up separate profit and loss areas. I wouldn't say competition as such but the
> restructuring creates that. The geography from the point of view of creating a better
> bottom line is a good thing, but from the point of managing information it's possibly
> something we need to stand back and look at.
>
> Lead Consultant 3, Case study 1

Exhibit 12. Case Study 2 – Most Significant Information Assets and Attributes by Manager.

Job Title	Information Assets	Attributes
Process Control Manager	Customer information Competitor information Product information	Quality Effectiveness Other
Programme Manager	Customer information People management	Productivity Utility
Engineering Director	Business processes Management information	Quality Utility
Commercial Manager	Customer information Business processes	Effectiveness
IT Director	Customer information Supplier information Organisational information "culture"	Utility Effectiveness Financial/economic
Technical Manager	Customer information	Quality Utility
Marketing Manager	Competitor information	Financial/Economic
Financial Controller	All	Productivity

Exhibit 13. Case Study 3 – Most significant Information Assets and Attributes by Manager.

Job Title	Information Assets	Attributes
Head of Internal Audit	Product information Management information	Quality Utility
Head of Information Systems	All	Utility Quality
Director of Training Strategy	All	Quality
Director of Finance and Support	All	Utility Quality
Head of Human Resources	Business processes Management information Legal and regulatory Organisational information "culture"	Financial/Economic
Legal Officer	Business processes Management information	Quality
Head of Policy	Supplier information	Effectiveness
Board Secretary	Supplier information	Quality Utility
Area Manager	Business processes People management Organisational information "culture"	Quality Utility
Training Manager	Customer information	Productivity

Exhibit 14.   Case Study 4 – Most significant Information Assets and
Attributes by Manager.

Job title	Information Assets	Attributes
Finance Director	People management	Utility
	Organisational information "culture"	Productivity
Managing Director – Business Development	Customer information	Effectiveness
	Organisational information "culture"	Quality
Director of Transportation Software	Customer information	Quality
	Product information	Productivity
Director – Business Unit	All	Quality
		Effectiveness
Director – Corporate Services	Customer information	Quality
	Competitor information	Utility
Human Resources Manager	All	Quality
		Financial/ Economic
Marketing Information Systems Manager	Customer information	Quality
	Organisational information "culture"	Utility
Manager – Information Resources	Customer information	Quality
	Organisational information "culture"	Effectiveness
Divisional Director	All	Productivity
		Financial/economic
Senior Manager	Product information	Quality
	Management information	Productivity
		Financial/economic
Senior Engineer	Product information	Quality
	Supplier information	Utility
Board Director	Product information	All
	Legal and regulatory	

As seen in Exhibit 12, the eight grids completed showed a strong identification of customer information as the most important asset. Competitor information and business processes were also scored. Attributes such as quality and utility were identified as being important. The identification of customer information as an important asset reflects the organisation's customer-oriented approach. The Managing Director's commitment to engendering a customer service ethos among all staff is apparent. The Managing Director of this organisation said that difficulty was encountered in his organisation, not, for example, in managing internally generated customer

Exhibit 15. Summary Table of Most Significant Information Asset and Attribute-Scoring Grids.

	Information Assets	Information Attributes
Case study 1	Product information	Quality
	Customer information	
	Organisational information "culture"	
Case study 2	Customer information	Quality
	Competitor information	Utility
	Business processes	
Case study 3	Management information	Quality
	Business processes	Utility
Case study 4	Customer information	Quality
	Organisational information "culture"	Utility
	Product information	Productivity

information, but in acquiring such information from customers in the first instance. Customers often relied on his organisation to provide their order and sales information. The identification of financial and economic attributes of information assets as important by the IT Director and Marketing Manager is interesting in an organisation with a traditional product base operating in a static market. The organisation had experienced exceptional growth (by taking market share from a bigger but less flexible competitor) over the previous few years, and many of the senior managers saw future growth and efficiency as being dependant on the continued development of an IT infrastructure that was "world class". The organisation had carefully cultivated technological leadership in its sector and, although it was competing on price and efficiency, its main competitive advantage arose from its innovative use of the Internet and Information and Communications Technology (ICT).

As can be seen from Exhibit 13, the marginally more important assets were management information and business processes. Quality was the most highly scored attribute followed by utility. This public sector organisation (Case study 3) did not score customer information as frequently as the three other organisations in the information asset-scoring grid. The organisation was in the mid stages of implementing a five-year ICT strategy. The strategy had highlighted the commercial possibilities of internally generated information that the organisation had built up over a number of years and this had led to a clear focus on improving the exploitation of information assets.

As can be seen from Exhibit 14, of the nine information assets scored, customer information was of most importance to the senior managers in

Case study 4. It was followed by organisational information "culture", reflecting a concern with internal communication structures. Product information was also scored highly. Quality was the most highly scored attribute followed by utility and productivity. The organisation was described by the senior managers as very large, diverse and geographically dispersed around the UK where 80% of its offices are based. Rapid growth of the organisation had resulted in frequent restructuring and management changes. The more recent of these had resulted in its current structure of 15 strategic business units that were "customer facing". Strategy was high on the agenda, with a great deal of senior management effort expended on developing a common vocabulary so that common goals could be met from a shared starting point. As in Case study 1, individual business units were in internal competition, and this was seen by some managers as a barrier to information sharing:

> Not so much custodians as hoarders! And that's just the culture. One of the reasons for that is that during the recession of the 90's, late 80's, early 90's, we were only about 2000 strong, we went into the recession and were split up into different units. People were told that if they made a profit they would survive, if they made a loss they would be cut, and everyone learned to do exactly as they wanted in order to achieve that. They came out of the recession with something like 8000 strong. They'd taken over other companies that had gone to the wall and added value and then they were trying to bring them back centrally which is a hard job when they've been divided. The fact that they'd be controlled from somewhere, that's one of the reasons for hoarding, fragmented units and constant re-structuring, there's been three since I've been here.
>
> Manager, Information Resources, Case study 3

As shown in Exhibit 15, customer information was scored most highly by the managers in Case studies 1, 2 and 4. Management information was scored most highly by managers in Case study 3. Attributes of quality were scored as important by senior managers in all four case study organisations. The information asset and attribute-scoring grids provided a focused overview of a range of information assets and attributes. The grids encouraged managers to discriminate between different information assets and attributes using a simple scoring system. This provided a useful introduction to the open-ended guided interviews which formed the major component of the case study research.

Open-Ended Guided Interviews – Case Studies

Findings are presented for the open-ended guide interviews conducted with 45 senior managers in four case study organisations. Five major themes were covered in the open-ended guided interviews.

Theme 1: The organisation and information strategy
Theme 1 Question 1: The organisation and information strategy. Theme 1 Question 1 asked participants to rate their organisation against seven statements relating to information management in their organisation on a one to five scale, with one being strongly agree and five being strongly disagree. Participants then were asked to explain their scores, and these comments were used for textual analysis. Textual analysis, using ATLAS/Ti, provided insight into the strategic vision of the case study organisations. Analysis of scores in Excel provided prompt feedback reports to case study participants at the conclusion of the case study visit, since analysis could be performed quickly.

Case study 1. The senior managers interviewed generally saw their organisation's information strategy as being poor. There was a good awareness of the issues involved in managing information and in creating usable and accessible information assets, which were protected and managed adequately. However, this was hampered by a lack of information systems and infrastructure according to interviewees.

Case study 2. Many of the senior managers interviewed said that the management and application of IT to their business, especially through the use of the Internet, was exceptional. There was a great deal of emphasis on creating structured databases and information systems to help in achieving competitive advantage in a technically demanding product area. Emphasis was on providing access to customers and suppliers over an international global network. The building of knowledge bases through contributions from employees was less successful; this was especially apparent in the introduction of an electronic library. Overall the scores were high, but this may have been as a result of an exceptional IT department rather than the existence of good information management strategies.

Case study 3. Many of the senior managers scored the organisation highly on information strategy. This was due, in the main, to a recent information audit that had been carried out by an independent consultant. The senior managers cited the information audit as an example of the organisation's awareness of the importance of information. The results of the audit had yet to be implemented within the organisation's overall strategy.

Case study 4. Senior managers said the organisation was actively addressing information strategy. However, there were reservations. In particular, there was concern about the management of information life cycles. There seemed to be no policy in place for evaluating the relevance of historical and current information resources across this large organisation or their value to the organisation. In particular, many of the senior managers were concerned about project information which, in their view, was not being captured in a reusable or knowledge-creating format.

There was no formal information strategy in any of the four case study organisations. Rather, the area was included within ICT.

Theme 1 Question 2 (a): Information assets and the management agenda. Of the 45 senior managers who participated in interviews, 33 said that information assets featured on the management agenda for their organisations. Twelve said that they did not. By case study (see Exhibit 16), these were:

Many senior managers gave examples of concrete information assets such as new accounting systems and customer databases as evidence that information assets featured on the management agenda. When asked later what information assets their organisation had identified as being important, these concrete information assets also featured. Less concrete assets, especially those that related to people management were, however, also strongly identified.

Theme 1 Question 2 (b): Discuss the value of information assets. As can be seen in Exhibit 17, some 38 senior managers said that the value of information assets was discussed in management meetings, whereas seven senior managers said it was not discussed.

The senior managers (38) who said they discussed the value of information assets were asked to describe what kinds of issues were raised in these

Exhibit 16.   Information Assets and the Management Agenda.

	No. of Managers	Yes	No	Total
Case study 1	14	12	2	14
Case study 2	9	6	3	9
Case study 3	10	10	0	10
Case study 4	12	5	7	12
Total	45	33	12	45

Exhibit 17.   Discuss the Value of Information Assets.

	No. of Managers	Yes	No	Total
Case study 1	14	10	4	14
Case study 2	9	9	0	9
Case study 3	10	9	1	10
Case study 4	12	10	2	12
Total	45	38	7	45

discussions (see Theme 1 Question 2 (c)). Those who said the value of information assets were not discussed (7) were asked why they thought this issue did not feature on the management agenda (see Theme 1 Question 2 (d)).

The recognition of the value of information was a central issue. A senior manager, Case study 2, stated that his position as a board director in the organisation was "implicit recognition" of the value placed on information in his organisation.

> Strongly agree. IT is a board position which is implicit recognition of the value.
>
> IT Director, Case study 2

Theme 1 Question 2 (c): Discuss the value of information assets – issues raise. When asked what issues were raised when the value of information assets was discussed, comments included reusing information, customer relationship management, communication, the value of people, implementing electronic information systems and duplication of resources. Reusing project-based information was of major concern to the two project-based organisations studied, Case studies 1 and 4.

The reuse of project-based information is of increasing concern, since new accounting treatments (Roberts & Felsted, 2002, p. 12) have meant that the costs of putting together bids and tendering for contracts can no longer be written off. This makes the bidding process far more expensive as many contracts are not, in fact, won. Case studies 1 and 4 were using their Intranets and, in the case of Case study 4, knowledge management systems to optimise project planning and bidding processes. Much effort was directed towards improving communication among staff so that lessons from previous projects could be used to speed the contract bidding process. Similarly, publicising skill sets of key staff involved in and available for project-based work meant that bids with named participants could be put together quickly.

Case study 1 encountered difficulties in implementing its Intranet, a lack of use was identified as an issue of concern. The organisation planned a document management system to give the Intranet "critical mass" which it believed would improve usage by employees throughout the organisation. This would then lead to more re-use of existing project-based information in the organisation.

> I think a lot of the work we do can be repeated. I don't think that we necessarily make as much use of the knowledge that we've gained in doing a piece of work in the next job.
>
> Director of Technical Consulting, Case study 1

The reuse of information was also an important issue for Case study 4:

> How do you replicate and extract value time and time again? We use our knowledge to try and reinvent a solution instead of sitting back and saying if we have a real set of processes here we don't just fish the solution out of the filing cabinet, and modify it a little bit. We tend to say we've got a lot of knowledge, let's create the solution and then we find out right, well that's a very similar solution to one we created five years ago, and all that time and effort, and I think that shows that we haven't yet got the process that means hang on, haven't we seen that issue, that problem before? Yes, we have, well, go and look at that, and what was the solution? It was this, we can modify the same solution, we could save thousands of man hours and boost our profits.
>
> Board Director, Case study 4

Theme 1 Question 2 (d): Value of information not discussed.

Of those who said the value of information was not discussed (7), the reasons given for not discussing the value were well thought out. Information value was not discussed because it had an automatic role in the "higher level" management of the business:

> We don't discuss the value of the information as such, rather we discuss it because it has a role in the management of the higher level stuff.
>
> Area Manager, Case study 3

Difficulties involved in quantifying the value of information, as identified in the literature review (Reuters, 1995, p. 5), were also raised by the Managing Director of Case study 1, who said:

> Because I think we find it difficult to quantify. Our clients don't, if you like, buy my knowledge generally in a sort of a nice quantified way. They tend to buy effort and therefore it's actually quite difficult to get to. If we put that much effort in and had better deployment of knowledge, how much more would our customers pay? It's not an easy sum to do.
>
> Managing Director, Case study 1

There appeared to be little incentive to value information assets. Customer demands were for value-added services rather than quantifiable goods.

Theme 1 Question 2 (e): Monetary value.

Some 12 senior managers said they placed a monetary value on information assets whereas 33 said they did not (as shown in Exhibit 18).

Traditional measures such as cost and time saving featured as the most often used monetary measures:

> Yes, we do put monetary value on them. We have just introduced a new financial system into the company which actually will make productivity savings over the course of the next financial year, and that's an information asset, so yes we do. Saving overheads, manpower and time.
>
> Lead Consultant, Case study 1

Exhibit 18. Monetary Value of Information Assets.

	No. of Managers	Yes	No	Total
Case study 1	14	5	9	14
Case study 2	9	3	6	9
Case study 3	10	2	8	10
Case study 4	12	2	10	12
Total	45	12	33	45

There was recognition that monetary measures were limited – especially in terms of knowledge value:

> I think we had difficulty understanding how to do that. We were looking at the cost of recruitment and therefore the cost of not managing retention and that has been identified as an issue but what we haven't looked at is the loss of particular key skills or key knowledge bearers really. And that is difficult then to put a monetary value on. We haven't gone down the line to management and said...what would be the loss of that person or that person, what is their knowledge value?
>
> Human Resource Manager, Case study 4

For those who said they did not place a monetary value on information assets, the subjective nature of information value appeared to be the major factor. There was an awareness also that value resided in less tangible areas such as people management. There was concern that, since different information assets became important at different times and for different purposes, values were constantly changing. Quality of information was again important, the idea that up-to-date information was of more value than outdated information was an important issue:

> No, I don't think we consider information assets as having a value, we obviously know which bits of information are valuable at a given time. Yesterday's bid, which might have been a winning bid, has a lot more value than one we did two years ago.
>
> Senior Manager, Case study 4

Theme 1 Question 2 (f): Rank the value. The idea of ranking information assets was used as a way of identifying whether senior managers were discriminating between information assets in terms of their value. This would not necessarily involve placing a monetary value on information assets. However, even fewer senior managers (10) said that they ranked the value of information assets compared to those who placed a monetary value on information assets (12). A total of 35 senior managers said they did not rank the value of information assets, as shown in Exhibit 19.

Exhibit 19.   Rank the Value of Information Assets.

	No. of Managers	Yes	No	Total
Case study 1	14	2	12	14
Case study 2	9	3	6	9
Case study 3	10	2	8	10
Case study 4	12	3	9	12
Total	45	10	35	45

Of the senior managers (10) who did rank the value of information assets. Examples of ranking include:

> It'll be ranked on whether it's good for the people, good for the clients, good for the profitability of the business and efficiency of the business.
>
> Director of Technical Consulting, Case study 1

And,

> Yes, definitely, Health & Safety information, for example, is more important than other types of information.
>
> Training Manager, Case study 3

ATLAS/TI analysis Theme 1. Information strategy.

A central view of the data for Theme 1: information strategy was created using ATLAS/Ti. In Exhibit 20, the issue of information strategy is seen within the context of management attention. Associated issues are the management agenda and information assets. Business Manager, Case study 1, says that the value of information is not discussed but that information assets such as the contact management system and corporate picture are discussed. Attributes of information assets identified are maintenance, recognition and delivery. Maintenance of information assets is identified as part of the risk analysis strategy of the organisation with an added caveat that maintenance should be appropriate. The recognition of information assets is seen as part of management attention, which is also an attribute of information assets. In addition, delivery, for example, delivery of products on time to customers, is related to appropriate management attention being given.

In Exhibit 21, the issue of information strategy is seen within the context of management attention with an attribute of Investment. Associated issues are the management agenda and information assets. Human Resources Manager, Case study 2, identifies competitive advantage as an information asset with an attribute of monetary value. Information assets and their

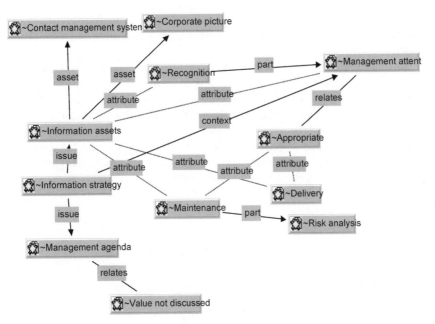

Exhibit 20. Information Strategy – Business Manager – Case Study 1.

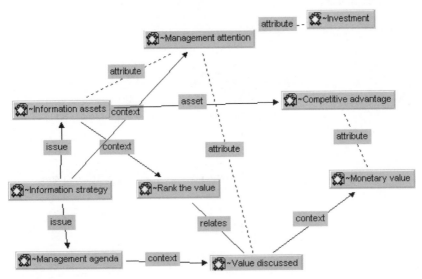

Exhibit 21. Information Strategy – Human Resources Manager – Case Study 2.

ranking in terms of value is discussed within the context of the management agenda. Management attention is an attribute of the value of information assets.

In Exhibit 22, the issue of information strategy is seen within the context of management attention. Associated issues are the management agenda and information assets, which for the Board Director are seen within the context of business information. Competitive advantage is given as an information asset and the issue associated with this is the organisation's databases. The existence of business information determines the management attention given to information assets. An attribute of management attention is Investment, and there is also a part relationship between management attention and responsibility as Investment decisions require responsibility to

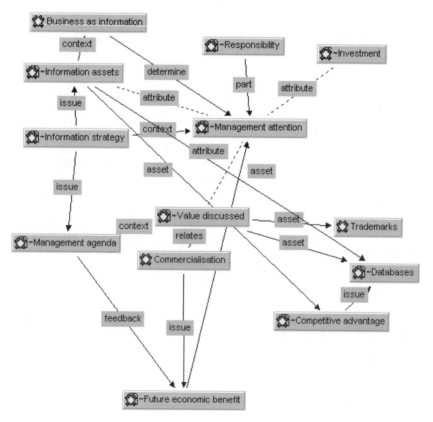

Exhibit 22.   Information Strategy – Board Secretary – Case Study 3.

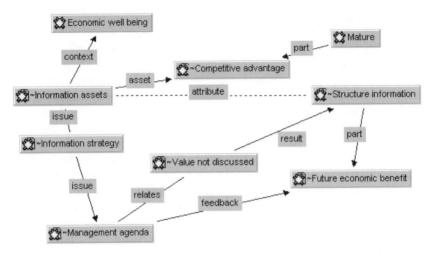

Exhibit 23.   Information Strategy – Finance Director – Case Study 4.

be taken. The value of information is discussed, in particular, in relation to the commercialisation of information assets such as trade marks and databases. The issue associated with commercialisation is future economic benefit, which results in competitive advantage for the organisation and feeds back into management attention.

In Exhibit 23, the issue of information strategy is not seen within the context of management attention. Associated issues are the management agenda and information assets which are seen within the context of the economic well being of the organisation. Competitive advantage is an information asset, which is partly related to the maturity of the organisation's information. The attribute identified as important is the structuring of information assets which has a part relationship to future economic benefit for the organisation. Failure to structure information effectively is seen as the result of the value of information not being discussed.

Commonalities between Exhibits 20–23

Competitive advantage was identified by three senior managers (Exhibits 21–23) as a factor when considering their organisation's information strategy. Management attention was also identified as a factor by three senior managers (Exhibits 20–22).

Theme 2: The organisation and effectiveness

Theme 2 Questions 3 (a) and (c): Is your organisation effective? Is it becoming more or less effective over time? Senior managers were first asked to describe whether they considered their organisations to be effective. They were then asked to give a definition of organisational effectiveness for themselves and for their team. The order of the questions may seem inappropriate but it was hoped that, by not asking for an early definition of organisational effectiveness, more thought would be given to the impact of organisational effectiveness. The effectiveness or ineffectiveness of the organisation provided a clear starting-off point, which situated the interviewee within the theme. Senior managers were then asked to describe whether their organisations were becoming more effective, less effective or remaining the same over time. Effectiveness is seen as a long-term proposition.

Some 38 senior managers described their organisations as effective, as shown in Exhibit 24. Of these, 31 said their organisations were effective and becoming more effective. Three said their organisations were effective but becoming less effective, and four said their organisations were effective and remaining the same. Seven senior managers described their organisations as ineffective. Of these, four said their organisations were ineffective but becoming more effective, two said their organisations were ineffective and becoming less effective and one said his organisation was ineffective and remaining the same.

Becoming more effective was seen in terms of access to both individual and corporate experience and the leveraging of that experience:

> I think we could be substantially more effective if we were able to rapidly access the best individual experience and the best corporate experience and deploy it onto each project.
> Managing Director, Case study 1

Exhibit 24. Effectiveness, Becoming More or Less Effective or Remaining the Same.

	No. of Managers	E	I	E + M	E + L	E + S	I + M	I + L	I + S
Case study 1	14	9	5	7	1	1	3	1	1
Case study 2	9	9		6	1	2			
Case study 3	10	10		9		1			
Case study 4	12	10	2	9	1		1	1	
Total	45	38	7	31	3	4	4	2	1

Note: Key: E = Effective, I = Ineffective, E + M = Effective and becoming more effective, E + L = Effective and becoming less effective, E + S = Effective and remaining the same, I + M = Ineffective and becoming more effective, I + L = Ineffective and becoming less effective, I + S = Ineffective and remaining the same.

Becoming less effective was identified by senior managers in Case study 1 with the restructuring of the business, which was seen as creating barriers to information sharing:

> I think less, it's because we have restructured which has had various positive aspects for the business in the sense that it compartmentalises profit and loss areas, but what it also does is create to a certain degree some barriers about information assets, less knowledge in one group about what the other group is doing.
>
> Lead Consultant 3, Case study 1

Becoming less effective was also identified with being unable to keep up with the pace of change in information and resulted in competitive disadvantage.

> No, it is not effective and I worry that it's going to become less effective than it was – it's going back to the point about the pace of change of information, it's becoming greater and greater and my concerns are that large companies such as us are unable to respond to that increasing pace whereas smaller companies are and will be. My concern is that we will become less competitive as a result of that.
>
> Senior Engineer, Case study 4

Theme 2 Question 3 (b): Define organisational effectiveness. Senior managers were asked to define organisational effectiveness for themselves and their team. Definitions of organisational effectiveness varied from specifics such as meeting clients' expectations to more general definitions such as achieving objectives.

> Well, organisational effectiveness is really the ability to meet client expectations and therefore generate continuing work.
>
> Director of Software Development, Case study 4

And,

> For the corporate body it's achieving its objectives and all these subsidiary bits. It's whatever its objectives are, and the extent to which we achieve those is, I think, organisational effectiveness.
>
> Board Secretary, Case study 3

A disparity between internal and external effectiveness was illustrated by a Senior Manager (Case study 3). In his organisation, customer complaints were going down, making the organisation more effective externally, but employee satisfaction was also going down making it less effective internally:

> I suppose its customer satisfaction. The levels of complaint for customers are getting lower, but internally the employee satisfaction level is falling.
>
> Area Manager, Case Study 3

The effectiveness of people was also an important aspect of organisational effectiveness:

> I think as the business changes over time from very much a small business to medium to a larger business, the effectiveness of new employees is important. The time in which they can become effective is dependent on us managing information better. The same knowledge management system, allows quite inexperienced people to specify a product. They probably still need an underlying engineering knowledge but we are doing all we can in order to make the new employees more effective. I think that is one of our biggest challenges as we grow over time. Getting new people of the right standard and giving them the information. It's very easy when you have got a small organisation to manage knowledge. You can't have one expert at the end of the 'phone anymore when you have got a large business.
>
> IT Director, Case study 2

Definitions of organisational effectiveness given are summarised in Exhibit 25.

As can be seen in Exhibit 25, the most common definition of organisational effectiveness across the four case study organisations concerned achieving customer satisfaction, the delivery of products and services and quality of those products and services focusing on external effectiveness. Senior managers in Case studies 1 and 2 gave definitions related to internal effectiveness such as improved decision-making and optimum working but the overall emphasis was on external effectiveness in relation to meeting clients' expectations and needs.

Theme 2 Question 3 (d): Information assets and organisational effectiveness. The role of information assets in enhancing organisational effectiveness was described in terms of improving communication:

> Communication at the moment. Until recently there was no real construct apart from word of mouth to deliver operational, I mean corporate information and operational

Exhibit 25. Summary of Definitions of Organisational Effectiveness.

	Customer Satisfaction/ Delivery/ Quality of Product	Achieving Objectives/ Strategy	Cost Effectiveness/ Profit/Market Share	People/ Culture/ Decision-Making/ Optimum Working	Survival
Case study 1	√	√		√	
Case study 2	√	√	√	√	√
Case study 3	√		√		√
Case study 4	√	√	√		√

information apart from going and telling someone which is fine, but that's not being methodically pre-designed in terms of communication strategy, message audience and delivery method.

Principal Consultant, Case study 1

And, identifying hoarders of information assets:

I think it's central, there are a lot of people issues. There are a lot of pressures on meeting financial targets which are area driven, therefore people are holding on to that information. On the basis we have the right information we can perhaps do a job more effectively and therefore make more money out of it, yes.

Business Manager, Case study 1

Information assets were also seen to have a role in enhancing the effectiveness of decision-making, which required good quality information assets:

Their role is very important because a lot of the decision-making, certainly more detailed decision-making analysis, will stem from good quality information assets and if we get that right then the more high-level decision-making, more conceptual decision-making probably would be more accurate, more relevant. Thinking of the bottom-up approach, to get to the higher level, if you've got good quality information assets that will feed into the pyramid and should ensure that when it comes to the crunch decisions, all the right factors have been considered and that's how I see it. Management need to check their strategy and to check their strategy again they need good quality information assets to test the strategy and confirm its relevance or otherwise. Either way you look at it, information assets are very important.

Head of internal audit, Case study 3

ATLAS/Ti analysis. Theme 2: The organisation and effectiveness.
In Exhibit 26, the definition of organisational effectiveness given by Managing Director, Case study 1, is based on securing competitive advantage based on price and production. The organisation is effective and making improvements in his view. Information assets provide context for his definition of organisational effectiveness but only in as far as they are related to competitive advantage and production. Organisational effectiveness feeds back into competitive advantage so that these two concepts are linked.

In Exhibit 27, Commercial Manager, Case study 2, sees his organisation as effective but becoming less effective. His definition of organisational effectiveness is phrased in terms of rapid response to customers and accuracy. Information assets provide context for the definition of organisational effectiveness. Time constraints and a "just-in-time" approach to information assets means that the organisation is becoming less effective. Commercial Manager, Case study 2, ascribes this loss in effectiveness to the rapid growth of the organisation, saying it is a "victim of its own success."

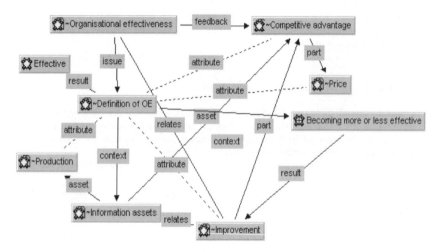

Exhibit 26. Organisation and Effectiveness – Managing Director – Case Study 1.

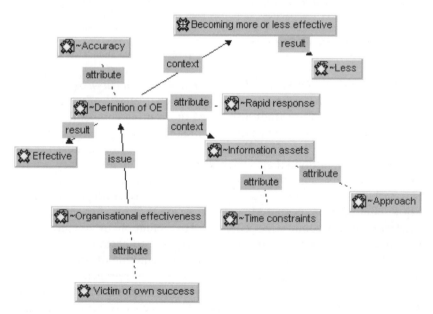

Exhibit 27. Organisation and Effectiveness – Commercial Manager – Case Study 2.

In Exhibit 28, Head of Policy, Case study 3, sees his organisation as effective and becoming more effective. The definition of organisational effectiveness given focuses on cost and quality and people management. People management is defined as an information asset within the context of organisational effectiveness. Understanding in the context of people management is also an attribute of the definition of organisational effectiveness and is identified as an information asset.

In Exhibit 29, Senior Manager, Case study 4, provides a definition of information assets with attributes of development and "trying to be better." The organisation is becoming more effective. "Trying to be better" is part of management attention which has related issues of people management and communication. People management is defined as an information asset and communication is seen as an attribute of information assets. Information assets are seen in the context of organisational effectiveness, particularly in promoting development, people management and communication.

Commonalities between Exhibits 26–29

Information assets were identified by all four senior managers when considering their organisations and effectiveness.

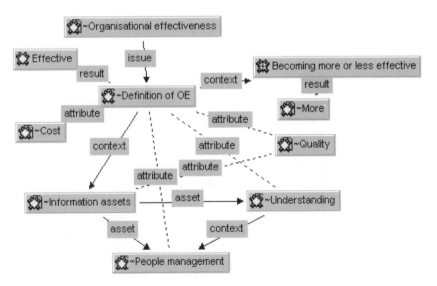

Exhibit 28. Organisation and Effectiveness – Head of Policy – Case Study 3.

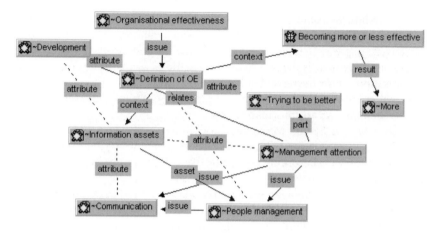

Exhibit 29. Organisation and Effectiveness – Senior Manager – Case study 4.

Exhibit 30. Organisation and Manager Identified (MI) Information Assets.

	No. of Managers	Yes	No	MI	Total
Case study 1	14	12	1	1	14
Case study 2	9	9	0	0	9
Case study 3	10	9	1	0	10
Case study 4	12	9	1	2	12
Total	45	39	3	3	45

Theme 3 Question 4(a): Identifying information assets. A total of 39 senior managers said their organisations had identified information assets considered important for the business. Six said their organisation had not identified any such information assets. As can be seen in Exhibit 30, three of these six senior managers then went on to identify information assets which they themselves considered were important (manager identified (MI) information assets).

Theme 3 Questions 4 (b) and (c): What are the information assets and what are their attributes?. A wide range of information assets was identified. The senior managers were also asked to describe attributes of the information assets they identified. Customer information was identified by the senior managers as an information asset in all the case study organisations. Attributes concerned with the quality and utility of information assets (e.g., up to date, accessible, accurate) were identified as important attributes.

Quality of information was a major concern, for example:

> The problem I've got is that it's taking me 12 hours at least to gather information and that should be at the press of a button and where I want to go for the future it needs to be a press of a button. But we need to make sure that the system, the information in the system is good quality so we can use reports because at the moment we're having to do it long hand.
>
> Engineering Director, Case study 2

The wide range of information assets and attributes identified by the senior managers demonstrate that "one size does not fit all". The different business environments of the four case study companies produced a variety of information assets and attributes, which are individualistic but reflect dynamic business environments.

Exhibits 31–34 show the range of information assets and attributes that the senior managers said their organisations had identified. Some senior managers also identified assets, which they said their organisations had not recognised but which they saw as being critical for the organisation. As shown in Exhibit 30, these are identified as MI assets (Case studies 1 and 4 and Exhibits 31 and 34 have extended titles to include these). Senior managers were asked to describe attributes of the information assets they or their organisations had identified. Where they do not describe any attributes, this is shown by the term "none given". Senior managers tended to list a number of assets and then list attributes for only one or two of those assets.

Theme 3 Question 4 (d): Identification mechanisms. Senior managers were asked to describe mechanisms used in their organisations to identify information assets. Identification mechanisms for information assets included Intranets, customer reviews, management meetings, quality systems, staff management, information audits and brainstorming. Identification mechanisms were both formal (databases and management information) and informal (brainstorming and meetings). Customers also drove the identification and exploitation of information assets with customers' needs, demands and increasing involvement with organisations as long-term partners being important factors. Examples of identification mechanisms include:

> Brainstorming. There will be occasions when we just sit down and try and sort out what we have got, so yes, that sort of thing. But probably not more formal than that. From very, very cut and dried management information through to all sorts of things. So, trying to identify those sorts of information I think a lot of it's implicit, you know you've got these fairly structured or very structured information systems in place and the rest of it just tends to happen and there's probably a lot just stuck in the middle as well. The spectrum goes right across. And also we mustn't forget I meet my management team on a monthly basis. The executive meets once a fortnight, so it does value the fact that it does need to structure the organisation across mutually shared information.
>
> Director of Training Strategy, Case study 3

Exhibit 31. Case Study 1 – Organisation and Manager Identified (MI)
Assets and Attributes.

Job Title	Information Assets	Attributes
Human Resources Manager	Company policies	Accuracy
Business Area Manager (MI)	Contact information	Quality up to date
Lead Consultant 1		
Quality Manager		
Business Area Manager (MI)	Contract management	Accessibility
Principal Consultant	Corporate and financial	Quality
		Timeliness
Lead Consultant 3	Corporate track record	Appropriate level
		Concise
		Usability
Managing Director	Customer information	Customer satisfaction
Quality Manager		Quality
Principal Consultant	Customer related	None given
Computer Services Manager	Customers	Acted upon
Financial Controller		Not time consuming
		Purpose
		Usability
Director	Domain knowledge	None given
Computer Services Manager	Employees	Time saving
Director Quality Manager	Financial information	Accuracy
		Judgment
Business Area Manager (MI)	Focused on customers	Accuracy
		Timeliness
Human Resources Manager	Recruitment information	Accuracy
Director	Information systems	Accuracy
		Clarity of presentation
		Timeliness
Lead Consultant 1	Internet	Non given
Lead Consultant 2	Management information	Future planning
		Management decisions
Director of Technical	Marketing material	None given
Consulting		
Managing Director	Measurement and	None given
	quantification	
Principal Consultant Quality	Operational performance	None given
Manager		
Managing Director	Past outputs	None given
Principal Consultant	People appraisals	None given
Computer Services Manager	Planned document	None given
	management system	
Director of Technical	Processes	Efficiency
Consulting		
Lead Consultant 2	Project cycles	Quality assurance

Exhibit 31. (*Continued*)

Job Title	Information Assets	Attributes
Managing Director	Regulatory information	None given
Managing Director	Relevant experience	Accessibility
		Transferable
Director of Technical Consulting	Reuse knowledge	None given
Director of Technical Consulting	Sales support material	None given
Lead Consultant	Series of databases	Accuracy
		Cohesiveness
		In time
		Market relevance
		Transport electronically
Human Resources Manager	Training	Ease of access
Lead Consultant 1	Yellow pages	None given

Barriers to identification also existed:

> No. We have the quality system, but that is a very blunt instrument, that tells you that everything has to be archived for a very long time, but that's just like taking everything in a project and sticking it in a vault somewhere.
>
> Lead Consultant 2, Case study 1

Senior managers in Case study 3 had recognised a lack of identification of information assets as a strategic issue. The organisation had substantial, but organically grown, information assets, and this had resulted in duplication. To address this, an information audit consultant was contracted to interview staff and create a database of the resources available and being used in the organisation. The thinking behind the decision to conduct an information audit is illustrated by a Senior Manager, Case study 3. The information audit is seen as a starting point rather than a solution showing that identification is seen as not an end in itself:

> I think we're back into the grown organically arena again. Hopefully the information audit will give us a line in the sand that we can build on.
>
> Head of Information Systems, Case study 3

Theme 3 Question 4 (e): Manage and protect. Many of the managers mentioned IT security policies and user policies. The management and protection of information assets was seen primarily in terms of IT policies with security issues such as virus protection and data protection of concern. User policies

Exhibit 32. Case Study 2 – Organisation Identified Assets and Attributes.

Job Title	Information Assets	Attributes
IT Director	Business processes	None given
Engineering Director	Business system	None given
Process Control Manager	CAD (Computer-aided design) system	None given
IT Director	Commercial information	None given
Marketing Manager	Customer database	Accuracy
		Efficiency
		Time saving
Commercial	Customer Databases	Empowerment
Manager		Control and monitor
Technical Manager		Speed of reaction
Technical Manager	Design	None given
Engineering	Electronic library	Centralised information
Director		Lost information
Commercial		Repetitive cycle
Manager		Access
Programme Manager	Electronic systems	Quality
Engineering Director	Internet	Contact with customers
Technical Manager		Empowerment
Engineering	Intranet	Communication tool
Director Technical		Manage procedures
Manager		
Process Control		
Manager		
Process Control Manager	Manufacturing database	Delivery
Financial Controller	Nominal ledger	Compliance
Executive Director	Operational information	Position against competitors
		Profit
Engineering	Product Database	Control Data
Director		Easy to Use
IT Director Financial		Time Saving
Controller		Access
Process Control		
Manager		
IT Director	Product information	None given
Programme Manager	Quarterly action plans	Effectiveness
Financial Controller	Salary database	Accuracy confidentiality
Financial Controller	Sales order history	Retrievability
IT Director	Software	None given
Technical Manager	Training	Access
IT Director	Training database	None given

Exhibit 33. Case Study 3 – Organisation Identified Assets and Attributes.

Job Title	Information Assets	Attributes
Director of Finance and Support	Background information	Improves relationships
Head of Information Systems	Booking system	None given
Director of Finance and Support	Customer databases	Concise
		Personalisation
		Relevant information
Area Manager	Customer information	Accuracy
Head of Information		Currency
Systems		Legal costs
Legal Officer		Source of information
Head of Policy	Customers needs	None given
Head of Internal	Databases	Accuracy
Audit		Ease of access
Head of Information		Easy to use
Systems		Flexibility
		Openness
Legal Officer	Electronic information	None given
Head of Policy	Financial information	None given
Board Secretary	Know-how	None given
Director of Training Strategy	Labour market information	Accuracy
		Comprehensiveness
		Credible
Director of Training Strategy	Networking intelligence	Reality checks
Board Secretary	Publications	None given
Training Manager	People management	Communication
Director of Training Strategy	Skill demand data	Currency
Board Secretary	Web sites	None given

were also frequently reported as mechanisms to protect information assets. Internal security measures surrounding IT usage predominated:

> We certainly have security policies, in place, around IT. Every employee signs a network usage policy and security policy. We have quality assurance around what we do. So, for example, things like password changes, deletion of users from systems when they leave the business, other things you would expect.
>
> IT Director, Case study 2

The major concerns of senior managers in relation to the protection of information assets was focused not on external risks to the business but on internal risks such as employee abuse. Protection mechanisms were primarily people based with only a few managers mentioning IPRs or patent protection.

Exhibit 34.   Case Study 4 – Organisation and Manager Identified (MI)
                Assets and Attributes.

Job Title	Information Assets	Attributes
Senior Engineer (MI)	As built information	Intuitive
Managing Director – Business Development	Business development	None given
Director – Business Unit	Business intelligence	Indicator
Human Resources Manager	Client information	Access Consistency
Managing Director – Business Development	Commercial information	None given
Finance Director	Competitive advantage	Expertise
Finance Director	Customer information	Accessibility
Director – Corporate Services		
Marketing Information Systems Manager (MI)	Enquiry system	Group wide
Board Director	Experience	None given
Director – Corporate Services	Financial information	None given
Managing Director – Business Development	Health and safety information	Currency
Senior Manager		
Managing Director – Business Development	Intranet	Communication Intuitive
Senior Manager		Key tool
Director of Software Development		Reliable information Targeted Up to date
Divisional Director	Intranet areas	Accessibility Coding Structure information

Two senior managers in Case studies 2 and 3 did show concern about IPRs
and patent protection:

> Again that's the other thing that's important, it is our intellectual property, we do have
> patents, we do have copyrights, on software and all the drawings on all the designs.
> > Technical Manager, Case study 2

And,

> We are bringing into place a .... . e-learning portal and the whole issue of intellectual
> property rights comes up. Internally the IT systems are very well protected because
> obviously they are our lifeline to funds.
> > Director of Training Strategy, Case study 3

Exhibit 35. Replacement Cost.

	No. of Managers	Low	Medium	High	Do not Know	Total
Case study 1	14	3	1	1	9	14
Case study 2	9	1	2	0	6	9
Case study 3	10	1	0	0	9	10
Case study 4	12	0	0	1	11	12
Total	45	5	3	2	35	45

Theme 3 Question 4 (f): Replacement cost. As shown in Exhibit 35, five managers said that the replacement cost of information assets was low, three said it was medium, and two said it was high. The replacement cost was described in terms of man hours needed to replace information. A Senior Manager in Case study 2 highlighted the speed with which information could become obsolete by saying that only the previous six months information should be replaced.

However, some 35 senior managers said they did not know the replacement cost.

The "do not know" group, which was by far the largest, did give a wide range of reasons why they did not feel comfortable assigning a replacement cost to the information assets which their organisations or they themselves had identified. These reasons illustrate the difficulties faced in assigning a replacement cost to information assets.

Many of the senior managers, who said they did not know the replacement cost, described information assets as irreplaceable because information assets were people based and employees rather than their organisation retained ownership of them:

Actually replacing some of the information would be very difficult because it's in people's heads so lose a person particularly when you know it's senior people and you automatically will lose a lot of information because it will not be recorded anywhere else within the organisation. The organisation in that sense doesn't own all the information because it's never been handed over. The barrier is information is power and status and position and protection. Perhaps if you run into more difficult times the fact that you have this information that is very valuable to the company and people have to come to you for it means that you think, some people might think they are less likely to be considered for say redundancy or something. So, there are a lot of issues associated with owning that information in your head. We are all positively individual.

Lead Consultant 3, Case study 1

And,

> They are all our people, basically because we are very much, I would describe us as a black book organisation. If we lost that person we would lose our business and we have seen that happen. So you know you can translate that to loss of business, a lack of knowledge dissemination equals cost of business unless we have got a solid culture.
>
> Principal Consultant, Case study 1

And,

> The problem is you couldn't replace it because, well, you'd have to throw people at it, because where we are now in the stage in our development we couldn't ... it's alright spending 10 years to develop something when you're moving from being a 20 man organisation to a 200 one. When you get to 500 you would have to compress it into a very, very short period of time and it would be incredibly difficult.
>
> Executive Director, Case study 2

The senior managers' awareness of employees as holders and owners of information assets was interesting. Management attention was focused on the structuring of information assets and sharing using IT but individual employees were recognised as creators, exploiters and owners of important information assets.

Theme 3 Question 4 (f): Level of investment in information assets. Some 14 senior managers said investment in information assets was low, two said it was medium, 25 said it was high and four said they did not know the level of investment (see Exhibit 36).

Of the 25 senior managers who said that investment was high, investment in traditional information assets such as databases and information systems predominated. Managers were aware that information was more than IT:

> High, in terms of IT yes, but there is more to information than IT.
>
> Programme Manager, Case study 2

However, when it came to investment, concrete and tangible information assets based in IT systems and strategies were funded rather than less tangible

Exhibit 36. Level of Investment.

	No. of Managers	Low	Medium	High	Do not Know	Total
Case study 1	14	10	0	2	2	14
Case study 2	9	1	0	8	0	9
Case study 3	10	0	1	7	2	10
Case study 4	12	3	1	8	0	12
Total	45	14	2	25	4	45

investments such as employee training. In particular, creating customer databases and implementing new financial reporting systems were highlighted as an area for additional investment:

> The information systems is top. Information systems that are key to the company. We invest a lot of money into those products and information systems. Massive investment in information systems.
>
> Engineering Director, Case study 2

The Engineering Director, Case study 2, also estimated that management were investing 8–10% of his organisation's turnover in information systems.

The funding of infrastructure to deploy information assets was a concern for senior managers in Case study 1, where 10 out of 14 senior managers said that investment in information assets was low:

> The infrastructure to actually use the information effectively is insufficient. The infrastructure to deploy repeatedly that's the problem, we just use it once and throw it away. It's closer to that end than having the information readily stored and then re-managed and re-used, and a lot of what we do could be re-used I believe.
>
> Managing Director, Case study 1

Financial constraints were reported as a barrier to investment. Although a long-term view of investment in information assets was apparent, financial commitments meant that a balance had to be found:

> The level of investment is what we can afford. It's as simple as that, it's just a fact of life. We would not make the decision to invest in order to increase our profitability in the short-term, we would take a long-term view of this, but you always have to balance these things against shareholders' needs.
>
> Director, Case study 1

Theme 3 Question 4 (g): Why not identify information assets?. Three managers reported that their organisations had not identified information assets. The reasons they gave were lack of communication, understanding and awareness:

> Communication I think. I don't know there are certain things, for example, if you want to start working for a new client, one of the things we do is background checking so that's obviously recognising important information, but that kind of level of information gathering is invisible to most people and all that information is doing is establishing the company will pay us for the job.
>
> Business Manager, Case study 1

And, lack of understanding:

> Before you could do that you'd have to say to people why it's important they do it and I don't think most people would understand, they say, what do you want to do this for? And you'd need to soften people up and position them first. I don't think that's happened.

Yes, winning hearts and minds, it is saying, you need that to do that, and it's also the slightly more reasonable: why it's so important to us. It's easy to talk about intranet and various things but these are only tools at the end of the day or platforms and what do we do with it once we've got it?

Head of Human Resources, Case study 3

Lack of awareness was given as a reason why organisations did not identify information assets even when anecdotal examples suggested that the organisation's members were benefiting from knowledge-sharing initiatives:

I don't think it's crossed its mind that it needs to. It's up to individuals to find out what they need and where they can get it, hence the use of the knowledge base in some instances. Even getting people for jobs is difficult, when we were waiting for the old office to be refurbished I was up on one of the other floors and sitting opposite a man who spent much of his time 'phoning round different offices to find out if a certain type of engineer was available for a certain project at a certain time, without much success. So this gave me an idea for a sort of "body shop" on the intranet pages which has never really come into fruition but the knowledge exchange has been used for that in the past. So that somebody who was with a client up in the north and he worked up in the north they said to him do we have any engineers in this particular field? because they needed some more work done. He didn't really know but he 'phoned up a couple of offices where he knew they had this kind of engineer and drew a blank, and he was one of the first people to use the knowledge exchange saying that he'd got this client and needed somebody and within a couple of hours he had three different people from different parts of the company answering him with different engineers on offer.

Manager, Information Resources, Case study 4

This example shows that providing linkages between people is a key role for this senior manager. The Intranet's role in improving communication is also clear in this particular example.

ATLAS/Ti Analysis

Theme 3: Identifying information assets

In Exhibit 37, Human Resources Manager, Case study 1, identifies three information assets and their associated attributes: company policies and accuracy, recruitment information and accuracy and training and access. Access is also seen as a general attribute of all information assets. The recruitment information asset raises the issue of the organisation's knowledge management strategy for this senior manager with the retention of key staff a central concern. The replacement cost of information assets and level of investment in them is low raising the issue of future economic benefit. Management and protection of information assets has the attribute of basic information showing that this manager believes that only basic provision has been made.

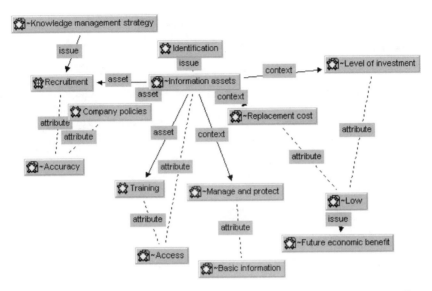

Exhibit 37.   Identifying Information Assets – Human Resources Manager– Case Study 1.

In Exhibit 38, Process Control Manager, Case study 2 identifies four information assets and three attributes: product database and time saving and access, CAD system, Intranet and manufacturing database and delivery. The Intranet is identified as an identification mechanism for information assets and also as a management and protection mechanism. The replacement cost of information assets and level of investment in them is high. The process control manager says that replacement cost cannot equal value recognising that the value is far greater. Physical hardware can be replaced but the lost customers attributable to lost information mean that a replacement cost for information assets is not a measure of its value to the organisation.

In Exhibit 39, Training Manager, Case study 3, identifies people management as an information asset with communication its attribute. The level of investment in information assets and their replacement cost is not known, replacement cost is seen as having attributes of both training costs and recruitment costs connected to an attribute of the learning curve which new employees must undergo to become effective in the organisation. There is a role for information assets in shortening the learning curve of new employees and thereby increasing organisational effectiveness. The learning curve is also, therefore, an attribute of information assets.

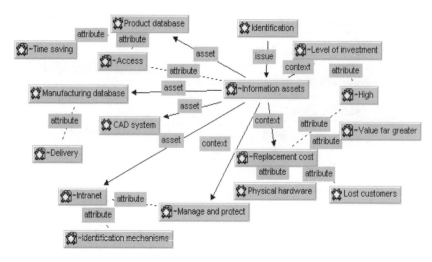

Exhibit 38. Identifying Information Assets – Process Control Manager – Case Study 2.

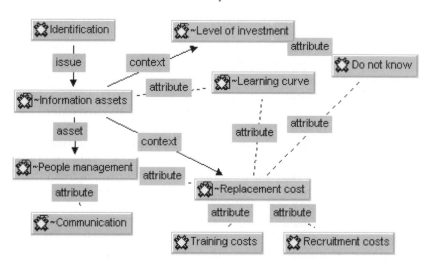

Exhibit 39. Identifying Information Assets – Training Manager – Case Study 3.

In Exhibit 40, Director of Software Development, Case study 4, identifies the information asset Intranet with attributes of targeted, up to date and intuitive, which is also an attribute of information assets generally. The Intranet is also an identification mechanism for information assets and for

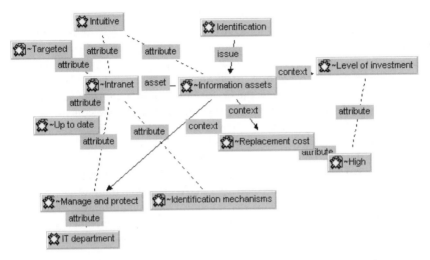

Exhibit 40. Identifying Information Assets – Director of Software Development – Case Study 4.

their management and protection, which is the responsibility of the IT department. The replacement cost and level of investment in information assets is high.

Commonalities between Exhibits 37–40

Senior managers in two of the case study organisations (Exhibits 37 and 38) identified access as an important factor in identifying information assets. Recruitment and recruitment costs (Exhibits 37 and 39) representing unnecessary costs to the organisation were also given as reason for identifying information assets.

Theme 4: Non-routine decision
Senior managers were asked to provide examples of non-routine decisions they had made in the previous few months at work. Non-routine decisions made varied from people management issues to the formulation of company car policies. Some examples of the non-routine decisions made were:

Lead Consultant 1. Case study 1: The non-routine decision taken by Lead Consultant 1 was a marketing decision. A new marketing campaign was not "bearing the fruits that I expected it to be". He concluded that "we were targeting the wrong people" and that there was a need to refocus the campaign.

Engineering Director. Case study 2: The non-routine decision taken by Engineering Director was to look at contract performance. While winning contracts was very much the recognised measure of success for the organisation, the Engineering Director took a pragmatic view "it's very important that we step back and see how profitable that contract is ... it's very important that we actually review the performance of that contract so when we embark on the next contract we learnt from our losses". He concluded that information regarding key areas such as manufacturing times were "poor" and required a refocus on inputs to the business systems in the organisation.

Head of Information Systems. Case study 3: The non-routine decision taken by Head of Information Systems was to discontinue shift working in the IT Department. This affected two staff, reducing their wages by approximately 20%. It also meant that more forward planning was needed so that work that had been carried out overnight could be included within a normal working day. She concluded that "we decided in the end that we wouldn't continue shift working".

Director, Business Unit. Case study 4: The non-routine decision taken by Director, Business Unit involved the opening of a new regional office for a group of people working on a project. The decision involved not only the acquiring of new premises but a commitment to building up a team that could win and carry out further work. The project team could have been accommodated within an existing regional office but the creation of a new office demonstrated a strategic and long-term commitment to both the team and its work. He concluded that it was important to get the "team built up".

Theme 4 Question 5 (a): Categories used and liked. The senior managers were asked to describe the categories of information they used to make their non-routine decisions and to describe any categories they might have found useful had they been available. The term "categories" was used to allow senior managers who did not necessarily view information as an asset to describe important information used for decision-making in their organisations. In the event, no senior managers objected to a definition of information as an asset. The categories of information used and liked do provide an insight into the difficulties faced by senior managers in accessing information assets of a suitable quality for decision-making.

Lead Consultant 1. Case study 1 – marketing decision: The lack of any sales revenue from the marketing initiative was the category of information used by the Lead Consultant:

> It was basically the fact that we hadn't got any sales.

The categories of information that he would have liked to have used were related to the targeting of the marketing initiative, in particular, information on customers' needs.

Engineering Director. Case study 2 – contract performance: The Engineering Director explained that information used for his decision was data collected by means of operatives using swipe cards. This information was not reliable since one man could operate two or three machines but his time would only be allocated to one of them. This made it difficult to identify what costs were involved in discrete contracts.

> So the one job gets all the time allocated to it and the other two get nothing allocated to them so the information going into the business systems is not accurate.

The categories of information he would have liked to have used were information on what products were not being produced "profitably".

Head of Information Systems. Case study 3 – discontinue shift working: The information used by the Head of Information Systems was primarily financial information and human resources information. There was also some research into the technology of automating back-ups so that hands on work was not required. There were no other categories of information that she would have liked to have used.

Director, Business Unit. Case study 4 – open a new regional office: The Director of the Business Unit stated that the decision was "based virtually wholly on staff issues. The knowledge that we could build up a team of people there and, if we didn't have one there, that we could lose the potential".

He identified a range of information assets he would have liked to have had access to including business opportunities in the regional area, access to the wider organisation in order to identify anyone else keen to have a presence in the region. This was described as "market intelligence but also internal market intelligence to make the decision stronger".

The non-routine decisions made also highlighted senior managers' concerns over lack of quality and utility of information assets in their organisations.

> Because it has brought it home to me that we really do need to do it better because it would have made life easier. I'm sure there are other parts of the organisation where information could be better. I think it's well known in the organisation, including my staff, that customer databases are not as good as they ought to be. And they are huge, substantial databases.
>
> Board Secretary, Case study 3

Theme 4 Question 5 (c): Decision success or not. A total of 30 senior managers said that the non-routine decisions they had made were a success justifying their view with comments, such as "We won the competition and the contract has been awarded".

Lead Consultant 2. Case study 1: Sometimes, success brought interest from colleagues:

> It has been a success, it's achieved what I wanted out of it for my particular need and since then two or three other business units have come on board. They've seen it and said, "Ah, I'm interested now", you say, "I thought you weren't interested before". It's the cart before the horse.
>
> Director, Business Unit, Case study 4

Fifteen senior managers said that the outcomes of their decisions were not known. Usually this was related to a non-routine decision, which they had taken very recently. For example, in the "Review Marketing Decision" where a review of a marketing initiative was undertaken when sales revenue failed to materialise, the senior manager commented:

> Too early to tell. We've been going a couple of months. There's a bit of interest, but I wouldn't say it's successful yet.
>
> Lead Consultant 1, Case study 1

Perhaps not surprisingly, none of the senior managers said their decision was not a success, although one manager did say that his team had made the right decision but that it had resulted in the wrong outcome:

> It was the right decision with the wrong outcome. We made the right decisions, it happens the outcome wasn't what we wanted, but it wasn't the fault of our decision-making.
>
> Managing Director, Case study 1

The conclusion to be drawn might be that the senior managers interviewed were experienced enough in their work to make successful non-routine decisions without necessarily using information assets. This has implications for decision-makers with less experience, be they new employees or newly promoted senior managers.

Theme 4 Question 5 (d): Decision and perception. Had information assets been instrumental in making a non-routine decision it was thought that this might impact on the senior managers' perceptions of the value of the information asset used. However, non-routine decisions, even successful ones, did not seem to change the perceptions of the value of information assets for many managers. Senior managers recognised that there were underlying problems in their organisations which information assets and their management could address. However, directing management attention towards these was a matter of priorities. As long as the organisation was effective at the macro level, the micro level was not addressed:

> It's not changed because we know about our problems … the problem in the business is that we've got that many ideas and we know our problems: it's all about prioritising, and up to this last quarter, we've had other priorities, because at the macro level it's working. If it didn't work at the macro level then yes, we'd then sort the micro level out, but because it's working at the macro level then it's pretty much ok, but it can get better.
>
> Engineering Director, Case study 2

ATLAS/Ti Analysis: Theme 4. Non-routine decision.

Exhibit 41 shows a non-routine decision concerning whether to make a bid for a contract taken by Lead Consultant 1, Case study 1.

In Exhibit 41, management attention has a part relationship with bid for contract as this issue engages management in resourcing and decision-making activities, which require their attention. Management attention is a concept that linked across many issues so that it eventually emerged as an important category.

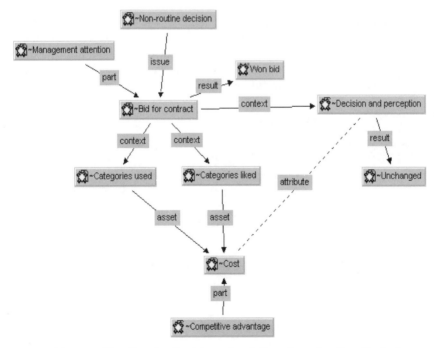

Exhibit 41. Non-Routine Decision – Lead Consultant 2 – Case Study 1.

As can be seen in Exhibit 41, the cost of the bidding process was mentioned in both categories used and categories liked. Cost is therefore identified as an information asset and linked to decision and perception. Assessing whether a bid was cost-effective was seen to be a part of competitive advantage, a concept that again emerged across many issues raised and was identified as an important category. The senior manager's main concern in this example was maintaining competitive advantage by controlling the cost of the contract bid. More cost information was required (especially the cost information of competitors) but this would have been very difficult if not impossible to access. Two results are also shown. The result of the non-routine decision was a winning bid. However, the senior manager's perception of the information he used to make this decision remained unchanged.

In Exhibit 42, the non-routine decision taken by Technical Manager, Case study 2, involved the recruitment of a specialist external contract engineer in a field, which his organisation was considering entering. A recruitment decision attracts management attention shown by a part relationship. The categories of information used were the Internet to check out competitors' current projects to identify suitable candidates and his own specialist knowledge of transferable skills in the industry. The categories of information he would have liked to have used was knowledge of the extent to which contract engineers had access to or could provide copyrighted information. The decision was a success, a suitable candidate was identified and recruited and the success did make a difference to the manager's perception of the

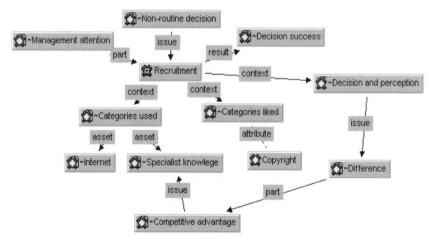

Exhibit 42.   Non-Routine Decision – Technical Manager – Case Study 2.

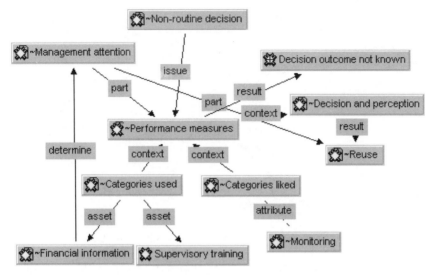

Exhibit 43. Non-Routine Decision – Head of Policy – Case Study 3.

value of the information he used. In particular, he identified competitive advantage as an issue related to specialist knowledge, and this made a difference in his perception of the value of the information used.

In Exhibit 43, the non-routine decision taken by Head of Policy, Case study 3, involves the use of performance measures in his organisation. The categories of information used are financial information and supervisory training. The number of managers in the organisation taking up opportunities for supervisory training has an impact on the financial results of the organisation as these two variables are connected in the business plan. The categories of information he would have liked to have used was monitoring information from local staff of training uptake. Financial information in the organisation determines management attention, which has a part relationship with performance measures and the reuse of information. The outcome of the decision is not known. The decision has changed the perception of the Head of Policy of the value of the information used. He is much more aware of opportunities to reuse information which are being lost.

In Exhibit 44, the non-routine decision taken by Senior Manager, Case study 4, involves choosing an Advertising vehicle for the organisation, which was part of management attention. The categories of information used were basic information on what advertising routes were available. The categories liked would have been much more detailed information on what

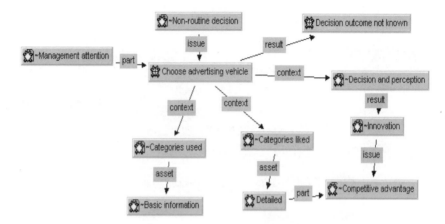

Exhibit 44. Non-Routine Decision – Senior Manager – Case Study 4.

would be eye-catching for particular audiences. He saw this as part of gaining competitive advantage. The outcome of the decision was not known, but the manager did say that the decision had changed his perception of the value of the information used. He saw the use of information as resulting in Innovation raising the issue of Competitive advantage.

Commonalities between Exhibits 41–44

Competitive advantage was identified as an important factor by three senior managers (Exhibits 41, 42 and 44) when making non-routine decisions.

Theme 5: Measuring the effects of information assets

Theme 5 Question 6 (a): Measure the effects of information assets. A total of 11 senior managers said their organisations measured the contribution which information assets made to the business whereas 34 managers said their organisations did not attempt measurement, as shown in Exhibit 45.

Question 6 (b). How is measurement achieved? The measurement of information assets and their attributes was described almost exclusively in terms of cost and time saving. Measures in place were whole business measures, for example:

> I think they do to the extent that the whole investment is being measured but I don't think there is a separate measure for the value of information assets. I think it's a value of the product and that is a combination of a number of things including the hardware, the software and the information itself, so we measure the combination rather than individually.

> Director, Corporate Services, Case study 4

Exhibit 45. Measure the Effects.

	No. of Managers	Yes	No	Total
Case study 1	14	1	13	14
Case study 2	9	3	6	9
Case study 3	10	2	8	10
Case study 4	12	5	7	12
Total	45	11	34	45

And, operational measures:

> The only real measure that's important is, again, the operational performance measures like more business, more sales, better project management, on-time delivery, cost of delivery. Those are the real tangible things that people will be looking for, now there is a million and one ways to measure those.
>
> Principal Consultant, Case study 1

And, accumulation measures:

> Measure how much extra information is put in.
>
> Director of Technical Consulting, Case study 1

Many of the senior managers saw measuring the contribution information made as "pointless". The impact of information on the business in terms of improvement was seen as being of more importance.

> I'm not sure I want to measure it to be honest. I think it needs to be recognised that it needs to be valued, but measuring it, unless it's measuring performance improvement with the use of that information, measuring its value *per se* I think is pointless. Looking for a constant performance improvement, goes back to one of your earlier questions, I think that's important, but I think measuring its value no.
>
> Senior Manager, Case study 4

In their view, measuring the value of information assets would not provide senior managers with any more reassurance that improvements were being made. Rather, information assets and their measurement appeared to be best situated within a holistic and strategic view of the organisation.

Theme 5 Question 6 (c): Suggested measures. Suggested measures for the contribution which information assets made to their business were operational measures such as number of hits into information and team performance measurement:

> Yes, you could do it like a web-site, do hits into certain sets of information.
>
> Director of Technical Consulting, Case study 1

And,

> I think you could measure, thinking about the way, or what I do with contracts, you could maybe correlate what areas are responsible for each management team, team leaders as well. If you look at audits and claw-backs for not doing the job you could maybe do some sort of correlation between where a management team's been in place for a while and they all understand the information that they're working with, how they perform in relation to an area that's had a completely new management team who are still getting to grips with everything and look at the delivery, the claw-backs on the process and audit trails and was that good audits or bad audits? Success rates, and that goes for re-assessed ones too, we have one area that one person had been quite successful with it but the person dealing with it has been around for a while and has a lot of ideas down on paper but you've got other teams that are struggling.
>
> Training Manager, Case study 3

Senior managers in Case study 3 said that there was a long learning curve involved in their joining the organisation and saw good quality information assets and universal access to them as a tool to shorten the learning curve for new employees.

Similarly, the role of people in managing information outweighed the issue of measurement.

> Well, I think there's been an acknowledgement that there is a need for the information now. I don't think there's a measure of the effectiveness of the information except for collecting information and having a strategy of how we do business. The strategy is there and one will look back and be able to see the value has been in being able to get success in those things but I don't think there's anything that measures it but at least we acknowledge it, we realise that it enables different things to occur. Of course, you need a lot more than the information to do it, it's people to harness it then do something with it but I think the acknowledgement of the fact that it's important is there and that we value it.
>
> Managing Director, Business Development, Case study 4

ATLAS/Ti Analysis. Theme 5: Measuring the effects of information assets. In Exhibit 46, Executive Director, Case study 1, identifies development and growth of the organisation as key measures. These measures determine organisational effectiveness, which he sees as part of competitive advantage and growth. Measures also relate to future economic benefit and result in growth and competitive advantage.

In Exhibit 47, Marketing Manager, Case study 2, identifies resource information and growth as key measures for his organisation. These measures determine organisational effectiveness and are related to future economic benefit. Future economic benefit results in growth and in a recognition of the importance of information.

In Exhibit 48, Head of Policy, Case study 3, identifies measures of customer involvement and employee satisfaction survey as key measures. The

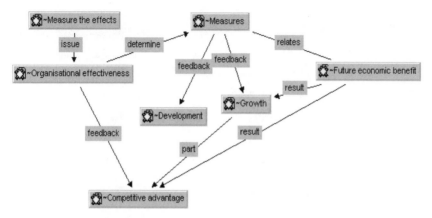

Exhibit 46. Measure the Effects – Executive Director – Case Study 1.

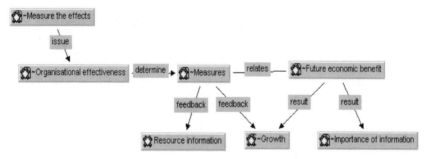

Exhibit 47. Measure the Effects – Marketing Manager – Case Study 2.

employee survey has an impact on organisational effectiveness since employees are involved with customers and their satisfaction with the organisation is related to the effectiveness of the organisation. Customer involvement results from future economic benefit, which relates to the measures identified.

In Exhibit 49, Divisional Director, Case study 4, identifies the overall financial results of the organisation as useful measures. Measures relate to future economic benefit for the organisation, which is seen as having a part relationship with risk analysis, meaning that risks to the business have to be identified to result in success. Organisational effectiveness determines which measures are important and are related to the overall financial results of the organisation.

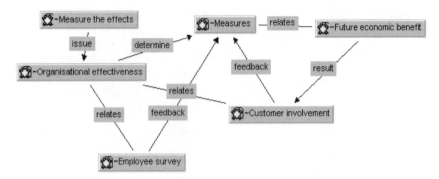

Exhibit 48.   Measure the Effects – Head of Policy – Case Study 3.

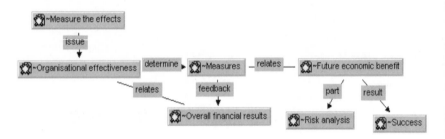

Exhibit 49.   Measure the Effects – Divisional Director – Case Study 4.

Commonalities between Exhibits 46–49

Future economic benefit was identified by all of the four senior managers as an important issue when measuring the effects of information assets. Growth also appeared to be an important factor (Exhibits 46 and 47) and was identified across individual case study organisational boundaries.

Theme 5 Question 6 (d): Importance of information in next five years. Some 44 managers said they thought the identification and management of information assets would become more important over the next five years (as shown in Exhibit 50). One manager (Case study 4) said it would remain unchanged because in his organisation:

> The culture needs to change and I'm not in charge of that. If you want my opinion, I would say it won't change. At worst it might deteriorate because I don't really think the people at the top have got their eye on the ball, if you like, they've got bigger fish to fry, more important things to do. I suppose as I say, if you change the strategy of a company and reorganise the spin offs from that in terms of management, you've got to change

Exhibit 50. Next Five Years.

	No. of Managers	More Important	Less Important	Unchanged	Total
Case study 1	14	14	0	0	14
Case study 2	9	9	0	0	9
Case study 3	10	10	0	0	10
Case study 4	12	11	0	1	12
Total	45	44	0	1	45

> things. Hopefully there's time, they might realise that OK they've made all these changes but people need information to make decisions, to do their jobs.
>
> Marketing Information Systems Manager, Case study 4

Senior managers saw information assets becoming more important in terms of better recognition, competitive advantage and growth leading to increased need for formal communication mechanisms:

> I think it will become more important, it's clearly recognised, we're updating our financials system, we're looking at contact management systems, we're looking at internal communications. Certainly it is recognised and the senior people in the company do recognise the importance of that.
>
> Lead Consultant 1, Case study 1

And,

> It will actually determine who will survive and who will fail commercially, because information gives you competitive advantage.
>
> Lead Consultant, Case study 1

And,

> Growth of the group means that informal systems of communication of information are no longer going to be robust and efficient enough to cope.
>
> Financial Controller, Case study 2

The importance of information assets over the next five years was seen in both positive and negative ways by the senior managers interviewed. On the one hand, information could be harnessed to improve communication and relationships with customers. On the other hand, more information required more management attention to ensure it was maintained and managed well and to avoid information overload:

> And we're all more swamped by information now so the ability to keep your head around everything that comes to you these days is important, it is not possible to manage it all yourself.
>
> Managing Director, Business Development, Case study 4

SUMMARY OF MAJOR FINDINGS

The major findings of the case studies are summarised below:

Information asset-scoring grids

- Findings for the information asset-scoring grid identified customer and management informations as the most important information assets and quality as the most important attribute for the senior managers.
- The restructuring of organisations into separate business groups was identified as a significant barrier to information sharing.

Open-ended guided interviews

- Information strategy was described as poor by senior managers in Case studies 1 and 4 and as good or exceptional by senior managers in Case studies 2 and 3.
- The value of information was discussed at management meetings with the reuse of information, especially project-based information, an important issue.
- Difficulty in quantifying a value for information as identified in the literature (Reuters, 1995, p. 4) was given as a reason for not placing a monetary value on information showing that this remains an issue today.
- Discriminating between different information assets by ranking them did not feature as an alternative to the discussion of information value with only 12 senior managers saying they attempted to rank the value of information assets.
- Senior managers who said their organisations were effective gave reasons such as "improved access to corporate experience" and "leveraging of that experience".
- Senior managers who said their organisations were becoming ineffective gave reasons such as an inability "to keep up with the pace of change".
- Many senior managers in the four case study organisations defined organisational effectiveness in terms of external effectiveness, e.g., customer satisfaction, delivery of product and services and quality of product and services. Senior managers in Case studies 1 and 2 also defined organisational effectiveness in terms of internal effectiveness such as improved decision-making.
- The role of information assets in enhancing organisational effectiveness was described as improving communication, identifying hoarders (non-sharers) of information assets and enhancing decision-making, essentially internally focused roles.

- A wide range of information assets were identified. Customer information was identified as an important information asset by senior managers in all four case study organisations. Quality and utility were identified as important attributes of information assets. Employees were seen as creators, exploiters and owners of information assets.
- Both formal and informal mechanisms for identification of information assets were described.
- Management and protection of information assets was primarily security focused, e.g., preventing misuse of IT by employees. Some recognition of IPRs was demonstrated in Case studies 2 and 3.
- Good awareness of issues surrounding cost of replacing information assets. Only a few senior managers said that information assets could be replaced demonstrating awareness that cost does not equal value.
- Level of investment in information assets was described as high by 25 of 45 senior managers. Investment in IT systems predominated, for example, purchasing financial management systems.
- Reasons given for not identifying information assets were lack of communication, lack of understanding and lack of awareness within the organisation sometimes in the face of strong anecdotal evidence that information assets were adding value.
- Non-routine decisions made using information assets were varied, ranging from people management issues to policy decisions.
- Senior managers used a range of information assets to make non-routine decisions. A range of information assets were identified but many of these were basic information assets that could or should have been available again highlighting issues of quality and access.
- Senior managers either judged their non-routine decision to be a success or said that the outcome was not yet known. The use of information assets to make non-routine decisions did not appear to impact on the senior managers' perceptions of their value.
- Measurement of the effects of attributes of information assets, where it occurred, focused on cost- and time-saving measures. Traditional measures were recognised as limited with a focus on the impact of information, for example, in terms of business improvement seen as a more important indication of value.
- Suggested measures for the effects of attributes of information assets were again focused on cost- and time-saving measures. There was recognition that information had a role in improving organisational effectiveness in, for example, shortening the learning curve of new employees, which outweighed issues of measurement.

- The identification and management of information assets was seen as becoming of more importance over the next five years. A variety of reasons was given, including survival, coping with growth and ensuing communication problems, and coping with information overload.
- Competitive advantage, customer involvement and management attention emerged as central issues.

CONCLUSIONS

The four case studies revealed a practical and focused approach to information assets and their management. Customer information assets were identified by senior managers as critical to their businesses. People management was also an important information asset, reflecting a growing understanding of the role of employees as owners and managers of information. Attributes of information assets identified were again wide and varied, the focus was on practical issues of quality and utility rather than impact or economic benefits of information assets. This was not to say that such benefits were not recognised or indeed sought, rather, the role of information assets and their attributes in underpinning value-creating activities was foremost.

Information Assets

Roslender and Fincham (2003) found that managers are paying significant attention to knowledge-based intangible assets even if they do not recognise the term Intellectual Capital. Information assets were used in decision-making and strategic activities by the senior managers interviewed. A central role for information assets in organisations was identified in the case study research, but this was tempered by recognition that the ownership of information assets remained with the employee rather than the organisation with relatively few senior managers willing to place a monetary value on information assets or state a replacement value for them. This is supported in the literature on organisational learning and communities of practice, which highlights the role of the individual as the enabler of value creation. This led to a focus on external effectiveness with customer information assets being the most frequently identified asset category.

The role of information assets in enhancing competitive advantage emerged as the most common concern of the senior managers interviewed in the case studies for this research. Competitive advantage demanded management's attention. Ensuring competitiveness focused on meeting customers' needs rather than building less traditional but perhaps, in the longer term, more valuable information assets. However, customers represent only one variable involved in achieving competitive advantage and, as new challenges emerge, organisations which rely solely on existing customers may be threatened. Yet, the focus on customers was a necessary determinant of success for the senior managers interviewed and did result in external effectiveness. All the organisations studied were successful businesses, but many of the senior managers also saw their organisations as being internally ineffective with the re-use of information and "lost" information being of concern. The redirection of management attention towards less traditional information assets is not proposed but rather a focusing of the available management attention to less traditional information assets is recommended.

Attributes of Information Assets

Marchand et al. (2001b, p. 91), in a European study involving over 1200 senior managers, found that the quality of information (updating and refreshing) was of greater concern than its reuse. This finding is supported by the research findings. The quality of information was identified as its most important attribute by senior managers in all four case study organisations. However, the reuse of information, especially project-based information, was also of importance to the consultancy-based organisations, Case studies 1 and 4. It would be interesting to investigate whether there is a relationship between the type of business operation (e.g., manufacturing, consultancy) undertaken by the organisations studied by Marchand and the attributes identified as being significant by them. Quality of information was also identified as a source of competitive advantage by Broady-Preston and Williams (2004) in their study of City of London legal firms.

Attributes of information assets described by the 45 senior managers in the case study organisations were also much wider than those identified in the literature. Those identified in the literature fell into three categories: inherent, impact and economic attributes. While all three categories were reflected in the research findings, it was clear that economic attributes were far more rarely recognised than attributes concerning quality, for example. It appears that economic attributes of information assets have seen little progress. However, impact attributes are an increasingly recognised area, and have expanded to encompass strategic and performance-related issues, such as planning and control and managing internal and external operating environments. Similarly, the measurement of the effects of information assets may not be as clear an indication of their value as their impact on overall organisational performance. However, measuring value does have a positive impact on the perceptions of senior managers of information assets.

Value of Information

The literature suggests that the value of information is not objective; indeed, information has no inherent value (Orna, 2004, pp. 131–132). Difficulties with quantifying the value of information, an issue identified in the Reuters (1995, p. 5) report on information as an asset, were also found to be a concern of senior managers. An approach that recognises that information has a unique role as a lubricant, that it enters into all aspects of a business, and that its value increases as it is shared is also relevant. Value comes from people transforming information into knowledge and action. Therefore, only the effects of attributes of information assets help to judge value. The value-added or value-creating role of information can be highlighted using an approach based on future economic benefits. This approach allows information assets to be viewed in much the same way as intangible assets in organisations. The traditional view of assets as static and information and knowledge as dynamic has been overturned by research in the intangible assets field, which highlights the value-creating yet changing nature of intangibles assets.

Organisational Performance

The lack of coverage of organisational effectiveness in the literature has seen recent improvement, most notably the link identified by Marchand et al. (2001b) between the positive IO of an organisation and its business performance. However, the role of information assets in enhancing organisational effectiveness is still unclear. This may not be a negative finding, since there is good recognition that it is the use of information to create business value that improves effectiveness. As it is difficult to separate out the impact of information from other value-creating activities, recognition that information has an underpinning and enabling role in enhancing organisational performance is significant.

The literature on information as an asset (KPMG/IMPACT, 1994; Reuters, 1995; Boisot, 1998) argues that senior UK managers are not aware of the information assets held and used by their organisations and, as a result, are not managing them effectively. The research findings show that senior managers do recognise a range of information assets. However, a distinction appears to exist between the management of those information assets that can be seen to have a direct impact on external business performance (such as customer information) and less tangible information assets (such as communication), which impact on internal effectiveness. While a role for information assets is identified in creating competitive advantage, decision-making and strategy, these do not receive the management attention that more tangible information assets relating to customers and products enjoy.

Finally, the research findings do appear to support a link between enhanced organisational performance and good management of information assets, most notably in the senior managers' concern with competitive advantage. However, it is suggested that this link is somewhat hidden by a concentration on enabling external effectiveness in supporting customers which has the unintended consequence of degrading internal effectiveness which ultimately results in competitive disadvantage.

REFERENCES

Allen, T. J. (1966). *Managing the flow of scientific and technical information.* Cambridge, MA: MIT Press.

Argyris, C., & Schön, D. A. (1996). *Organisational learning II.* Reading: Addison-Wesley.

Arrow, K. (1984). *The economics of information.* London: Blackwell.

Badenoch, D., Reid, C., Burton, P., Gibb, F., & Oppenheim, C. (1994). The value of information. In: M. Feeney & M. Grieves (Eds), *The value and impact of information* (pp. 9–78). West Sussex: Bowker Saur.

Barry, C. A. (1998). Choosing qualitative data analysis software: Atlas/ti and Nudist compared. Sociological Research Online [online], 3 (3). < www.socresonline.org.uk/socresonline/3/ 3/4.html>, [accessed 21.11.02].

Best, D. (1996). Business process and information management. In: D. Best (Ed.), *The fourth resource: Information and its management* (pp. 3–17). Aldershot: Aslib/Gower.

Black, S. H., & Marchand, D. (1982). Assessing the value of information in organisations: A challenge for the 1980s. *The Information Society Journal*, *1*(3), 191–225.

Boisot, M. (1998). *Knowledge assets: Securing competitive advantage in the information economy.* Oxford: Oxford University Press.

Broady-Preston, J., & Williams, T. (2004). Using information to create business value: City of London legal firms, a case study. *Performance Measurement and Metrics*, *5*(1), 5–10.

Burk, C., & Horton, F. (1988). *Infomap: A complete guide to discovering corporate information resources.* Englewood Cliffs, NJ: Prentice-Hall.

Eaton, J. J., & Bawden, D. (1991). What kind of resource is information? *International Journal of Information Management, 11*(2), 156–165.

Fincham, R., & Roslender, R. (2003). *The management of intellectual capital and its implications for business reporting.* Edinburgh: Institute of Chartered Accountants of Scotland.

Glazer, R. (1993). Measuring the value of information: The information-intensive organisation. *IBM Systems Journal, 32*(1), 99–111.

Griffiths, D., & King, J. (1991). Indicators of the use, usefulness and value of scientific and technical information. In: D. Raitt (Ed.), *Online information: Proceedings of the 15th international online meeting, 10–12 December* (pp. 361–377). London: Aslib.

Hawley, R. (1995). Information as an asset: The board agenda. *Information Management and Technology, 28*(6), 237–239.

Horton, F. W. (1993). The strategic role of information management. *Library Science, 30*(1), 1–5.

KPMG/IMPACT. (1994). *Information as an asset: The board agenda.* London: KPMG/IM-PACT.

Marchand, D. A. (Ed.) (2000). *Competing with information: A manager's guide to creating business value with information content.* Chicester: Wiley.

Marchand, D., Kettinger, W. J., & Rollins, J. D. (2001a). *Information orientation: The link to business performance.* New York: Oxford University Press.

Marchand, D., Kettinger, W. J., & Rollins, J. D. (2001b). *Making the invisible visible: How companies win with the right information, people and IT.* Chicester: Wiley.

Marshall, C., & Rossmann, G. B. (1989). *Designing qualitative research.* Newbury Park, CA: Sage.

Orna, E. (1996). Valuing information: Problems and opportunities. In: D. Best (Ed.), *The fourth resource: Information and its management* (pp. 18–40). Aldershot: Aslib/Gower.

Orna, E. (2004). *Information strategy in practice.* Aldershot: Gower.

Owens, I., & Wilson, T. D. (1997). Information and business performance: A study of information systems and services in high performing companies. *Journal of Librarianship and Information Science, 29*(1), 19–28.

Repo, A. J. (1986). The dual approach to the value of information: An appraisal of use and exchange values. *Information Processing and Management, 22*(5), 373–383.

Reuters (1995). *Information as an asset: The invisible goldmine.* London: Reuters.

Richards, T. J., & Richards, L. (1994). Using computers in qualitative research. In: N. K. Denzin & Y. Lincoln (Eds), *Handbook of qualitative research* (pp. 445–462). Thousand Oaks, CA: Sage.

Roberts, D., & Felsted, A. (2002). The secret returns of Brown's PFI gravy train. *Financial Times, Companies and Finance Section*, August 17/18, p.12.

Senge, P. M. (1990). *The fifth discipline: The art and practice of the learning organisation.* London: Century Business.

Strauss, A., & Corbin, J. (1990). *Basics of qualitative research: Grounded theory procedures and techniques.* Newbury Park, CA: Sage.

APPENDIX. CASE STUDY INTERVIEW SCHEDULE

*The Attributes of Information as an Asset, Its Measurement and Role in
Enhancing Organisational Effectiveness*

Explanatory Statement

Information assets comprise "data that is or should be documented
and which has future economic benefit".

An example of an information asset might be as concrete as a customer database or as abstract as employee know-how.

Please note that the term "asset" is used to signify something of
future economic benefit and is not used simply in its conventional
accounting sense.

Theme 1. The organisation and information strategy

Question 1.
Do you agree or disagree with the following statements, for your organ-
isation?
Please explain why you agree or disagree.

(a) Information assets are major assets of the organisation.

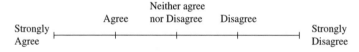

(b) Information assets must be managed as major assets of the organisation.

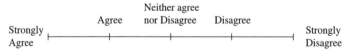

(c) Information investments should be made only in support of the organisations goals and objectives.

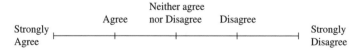

(d) Senior managers and employees throughout the organisation are cus-
todians of the information assets they use.

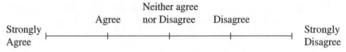

(e) Senior managers and employees have a major responsibility, within
corporate constraints, to use information assets effectively and effi-
ciently and to share them internally and externally.

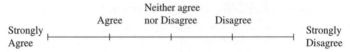

(f) Users are responsible for the planning and control of the information
assets they use.

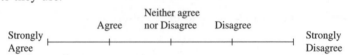

(g) There is a formal management approach to the management of life cycle
phases of information assets, beginning with creation and following
through to retirement or disposal.

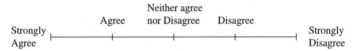

Question 2.

(a) Information assets feature on the management agenda?

Yes ☐

No ☐

(b) In Management meetings, do you discuss the value of information assets?

Yes ☐

No ☐

(c) If the answer to Question 2 (b) was Yes, What issues are raised?
(d) If the answer to Question 2 (b) was No, please describe why you think the value of information assets is not discussed.
(e) Do you put any monetary value on information assets?
(f) Do you rank the value of information assets?

Theme 2. The organisation and effectiveness

Question 3.

(a) Would you describe your organisation as an effective one?

Yes □

No □

(b) What does the term "organisational effectiveness" mean to you and your team?
(c) Is your organisation becoming more or less effective in your view?
(d) What is the role of information assets in enhancing your organisation's effectiveness?

Theme 3. Identifying information assets

Question 4.

(a) Has your organisation identified categories of information you consider significant for the business?

Yes □

No □

(b) If the answer to Question 4 (a) was yes, please describe what the information assets are.
(c) What are the most significant attributes of the information assets you have identified?
(d) What mechanisms are used by your organisation to identify information assets?
(e) What policies are in place to manage and protect them?
(f) Please estimate the cost to your organisation of replacing these information assets and the current level of investment in them.

(g) If the answer to Question 4 (a) was no, is it because identifying information assets is:
  (1) Too difficult   □
  (2) Too expensive   □
  (3) Not important   □
  (4) Not justified   □
  (5) Not useful   □
  (6) Other   (please specify)

Please tick as many as apply.

Theme 4. Using information assets

Question 5.
Please think of a non-routine decision you have made in the previous few months at work. For that decision:

(a) What categories of information did you use?
(b) What categories of information would you have liked to have used?
(c) Was the decision a success in your view? Please justify.
(d) Since you made your decision, has the outcome affected your perception of the value of the information used?

Theme 5. Measuring the effects of information assets

Question 6.

(a) Does your organisation measure the contribution information assets make to the business?

                              Yes □

                              No   □

(b) If the answer to Question 6 (a) was yes, how is this achieved?
(c) If the answer to Question 6 (a) was no, can you suggest any ways in which your organisation might begin to measure in this area?

Finally, do you consider that the identification and management of information assets will become more important, less important or remain unchanged over the next five years?

          More   Less   Unchanged
          Why?

Is there anything else you would like to add?

ABOUT THE AUTHORS

Michael Carpenter is an associate professor in the School of Library and Information Science at Louisiana State University. He holds a Ph.D. in librarianship from the University of California at Berkeley, and an MBA from the University of California at Los Angeles. Prior to pursuing a career in academia, Dr. Carpenter worked at the Library of Congress and was the chief financial officer for an industrial building contractor in Los Angeles.

Linda K. Colding received her MSLS from the Catholic University of America in Washington, DC. After serving as a bibliographer at the Air University Library at Maxwell AFB, Alabama, she arrived at the University of Central Florida, first serving as a reference librarian and then a year later as Library Instruction Coordinator. Dr. Colding received her Doctor of Public Administration from the University of Alabama.

Janine Golden is a library program specialist for the State Library and Archives of Florida with responsibility for leadership development and recruitment for Florida's libraries. Her background includes 33 years in school/public library administration with a research path involving leadership and management positions in public libraries. Dr. Golden holds an M.Ed. from Penn State University, an MLS from Indiana University, and a Ph.D. in Library Science from the University of Pittsburgh. She also teaches at distance for the University of Pittsburgh and Florida State University.

Jeff Luzius earned his BS in Psychology from Troy State University, his MS in Library & Information Studies from Florida State University, and M.Ed. & EdD in Higher Education Administration from Auburn University. Dr. Luzius started his career in librarianship at Troy State University in Troy, AL as an Access Services Librarian and then moved to Auburn University first as the Education Librarian and then as the Head of Document Delivery. In September 2005 he began work as the associate dean for library services at Gadsden State Community College in Gadsden, AL.

Betsy Van der Veer Martens is an assistant professor at the University of Oklahoma School of Library and Information Studies. She was formerly the electronic marketing manager at the Cornell University Press. She received her doctorate in information transfer from the Syracuse University School of Information Studies in 2004.

Jean Mulhern accepted the post of director of the S. Arthur Watson Library at Wilmington College (Ohio) in the fall of 2005. Prior to that she served as the director of the Rembert E. Stokes Library at Wilberforce University where she coordinated that university's regional accreditation processes for several years and served as an instructor in the adult degree completion program. She is completing Ph.D. in Educational Leadership at the University of Dayton.

Joan Stenson has recently completed a part-time Ph.D. in the Department of Information Science, Loughborough University on the attributes of information as an asset. Her research interests include work in knowledge management, intangible assets, e-government and e-democracy, international ICT strategy and e-learning.

James H. Walther became National Director of Research for Greenberg Traurig, LLP in January 2006. Prior to that, he served as director of Staff Development for The New York Public Library where he was named a *2005 Mover and Shaker* by Library Journal. Concurrently, he has teaching appointments at Pratt Institute's School of Information and Library Science and San Jose State University's School of Library and Information Science. His previous positions include manager of library services at Bryan, Cave, LLP, Washington, DC and a faculty appointment at The Catholic University of America, School of Library and Information Science. His degrees are from The George Washington University and the University of Wisconsin-Milwaukee.

Robert C. Ward is an assistant professor in the School of Library and Information Science at Louisiana State University. He holds a Ph.D. in Public Administration and Public Affairs from Virginia Polytechnic Institute and State University. Prior to pursuing a career in academia, Dr. Ward worked for over 30 years as a Public Library Director and Systems Administrator.

Larry Nash White is an assistant professor in the Department of Library Science and Instructional Technology in East Carolina University's College of Education. He earned a doctorate in Library and Information Studies from Florida State University in 2002 with a specialization in administration in information service organizations. White's professional background includes a wide variety of experiences in public and academic libraries, retail management, and management consulting. His research interest includes organizational performance assessment, the use of information by organizational leaders, and intellectual capital assessment.

AUTHOR INDEX

SUBJECT INDEX

SET UP A CONTINUATION ORDER TODAY!

Did you know that you can set up a continuation order on all Elsevier-JAI series and have each new volume sent directly to you upon publication? For details on how to set up a **continuation order**, contact your nearest regional sales office listed below.

To view related series in Sociology, please visit:

www.elsevier.com/sociology

30% Discount for Authors on All Books!

A 30% discount is available to Elsevier book and journal contributors on all books *(except multi-volume reference works)*.

To claim your discount, full payment is required with your order, which must be sent directly to the publisher at the nearest regional sales office above.